AGING MEDICINE

Robert J. Pignolo, MD, PhD; Mary A. Forciea, MD;
Jerry C. Johnson, MD, Series Editors

For further volumes:
http://www.springer.com/series/7622

Amy S. Kelley • Diane E. Meier
Editors

Meeting the Needs of Older Adults with Serious Illness

Challenges and Opportunities
in the Age of Health Care Reform

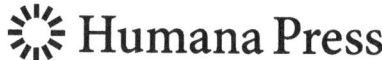

Editors
Amy S. Kelley, M.D., M.S.H.S.
Brookdale Department of Geriatrics
 and Palliative Medicine
Icahn School of Medicine at Mount Sinai
New York, NY, USA

Diane E. Meier, M.D.
Brookdale Department of Geriatrics
 and Palliative Medicine
Icahn School of Medicine at Mount Sinai
New York, NY, USA

ISBN 978-1-4939-0406-8   ISBN 978-1-4939-0407-5 (eBook)
DOI 10.1007/978-1-4939-0407-5
Springer New York Heidelberg Dordrecht London

Library of Congress Control Number: 2014945371

© Springer Science+Business Media New York 2014
This work is subject to copyright. All rights are reserved by the Publisher, whether the whole or part of the material is concerned, specifically the rights of translation, reprinting, reuse of illustrations, recitation, broadcasting, reproduction on microfilms or in any other physical way, and transmission or information storage and retrieval, electronic adaptation, computer software, or by similar or dissimilar methodology now known or hereafter developed. Exempted from this legal reservation are brief excerpts in connection with reviews or scholarly analysis or material supplied specifically for the purpose of being entered and executed on a computer system, for exclusive use by the purchaser of the work. Duplication of this publication or parts thereof is permitted only under the provisions of the Copyright Law of the Publisher's location, in its current version, and permission for use must always be obtained from Springer. Permissions for use may be obtained through RightsLink at the Copyright Clearance Center. Violations are liable to prosecution under the respective Copyright Law.
The use of general descriptive names, registered names, trademarks, service marks, etc. in this publication does not imply, even in the absence of a specific statement, that such names are exempt from the relevant protective laws and regulations and therefore free for general use.
While the advice and information in this book are believed to be true and accurate at the date of publication, neither the authors nor the editors nor the publisher can accept any legal responsibility for any errors or omissions that may be made. The publisher makes no warranty, express or implied, with respect to the material contained herein.

Printed on acid-free paper

Humana Press is a brand of Springer
Springer is part of Springer Science+Business Media (www.springer.com)

Preface

Palliative care is specialized medical care for people with serious illnesses. It focuses on providing patients with relief from the symptoms, pain, and stress of a serious illness—whatever the diagnosis or stage of illness. The goal is to improve quality of life for both the patient and the family. Countless studies have shown that patients with serious and life-threatening illness experience untreated pain and other symptoms; lengthy hospitalizations involving unwanted, often futile, burdensome, and costly medical treatments; and low overall family satisfaction—particularly with the quality of hospital care [1–11].

Encouragingly, a growing body of research supports the evidence for palliative care's positive impact on important clinical outcomes. These include relieved pain and distressing symptoms, improved quality of life for patients and families compared to controls, reduced anxiety and depression, support of ongoing discussion of goals of care and difficult decision-making, spiritual well-being, eased burden on caregivers and improved satisfaction, improvement in patients' ability to complete life-prolonging treatments, improved communication and transition management, and better survival in studies of some cancer and hospice populations. As a consequence of better quality of care—for example, fewer pain and symptom crises leading to 911 calls, emergency department visits, and hospitalizations—palliative care models have been shown in multiple studies to reduce hospital readmissions and costs and to decrease costs in community settings [12–25].

This evidence highlights the ability to enhance healthcare value by improving quality and, by actually meeting patient and family needs, containing costs. For example, a pivotal study by Morrison et al. (2008) found that palliative care programs improve physical and psychological symptoms as well as caregiver outcomes of well-being and family satisfaction [26]. This study also demonstrated net savings of $1,696 in direct hospital costs per admission. A similar study found that patients enrolled in Medicaid who received palliative care incurred $6,900 less in hospital costs than a matched group receiving usual care. The patients receiving palliative care spent less time in the hospital; were less likely to die in intensive care units; and more likely to receive hospice referrals [27]. Likewise, a study of the Advanced Illness and Management (AIM) program launched by Sutter Health in Northern California found that, through integrated home-based and transitional palliative care, patients' needs were met at home, resulting in fewer hospitalizations and lower costs (average savings per patient was approximately $2,000 per month) [28].

The past two decades have witnessed a dramatic period of growth in palliative care services, particularly in hospitals. Over 85 % of large hospitals now offer palliative care services. Yet, fewer than half of public, for-profit, and small community hospitals report presence of a palliative care team. Even in the hospitals where such services exist, only a fraction of those patients and families who could benefit actually receive palliative care. These teams are variably supported by hospital operations dollars, fee for service provider reimbursement, and philanthropy. As a result of inadequate and unreliable resources and the fact that palliative care services are not mandated through regulatory or accreditation processes, most programs are too understaffed to reach all the patients in need. Therefore, public policy is needed to standardize high quality and to assure access for all Americans with serious illness who can benefit from care informed by palliative care principles and practices. Importantly, access to palliative care must be scaled beyond hospitals to community settings where patients and their families live and need help. It is precisely the absence of needed palliative and social supports in the community that forces people to turn to 911 calls, ambulances, and emergency rooms.

The USA is currently facing a crisis in health care marked by unsustainable spending and quality that is poor relative to international benchmarks. A recent report to the Institute of Medicine on the costs of care for the seriously ill revealed that 5 % of the US population account for half of the nation's healthcare spending and only a minority of them, 11 %, are in the last year of life [29]. The ongoing healthcare reform debate centers on how to best care for this seriously ill population, in a manner that supports high quality, person- and family-centered care, so as to improve quality enough to reduce the need for costly crisis care in hospitals. Palliative care must be a key component to those discussions.

Meeting the Needs of Older Adults with Serious Illness: Challenges and Opportunities in the Age of Health care Reform is a platform upon which to build that discussion. In the following chapters, expert researchers and academic leaders have partnered with policy experts and thought leaders to tackle 16 key areas where palliative care could have a substantial role in reform and improvement, and real-world policy options to accomplish these goals. Together these partners highlight the current evidence, outline specific policy recommendations to translate this evidence into practice, and discuss the practical action steps by which these policy changes could be enacted.

The first section of the text, **Current Needs of Older Adults with Serious Illness**, describes the harms of unnecessary testing and treatment, using the *Choosing Wisely* campaign as a case study of an actionable solution [30]; reveals racial, socioeconomic, and regional disparities in access to palliative care services; and delves into the challenges and implications of caregiving among families of the seriously ill. The second segment, **Settings for the Care of the Seriously Ill**, examines the wide arrays of settings for the care of the seriously ill, including community and home-based services, hospice programs and various sites of delivery of hospice services, and long-term care facilities. Next, ***Measuring Quality and Paying for the Care of the Seriously Ill*** begins with a discussion of current efforts to measure the quality of care for the seriously ill, including the limitations of such measures and actionable areas for their improvement. This section also addresses the evidence for palliative care's impact on costs; explores government programs for the seriously ill, including many people dually eligible for Medicare and Medicaid coverage; and examines the perspective of payers providing healthcare insurance coverage to this expensive and vulnerable population. In addition to the policy recommendations and action steps described in the preceding sections, the final segment of the book, ***Platforms for Improvement***, explicitly reviews five areas of active evolution: novel approaches to integrating palliative care into accountable care organizations; healthcare system redesign to facilitate the process of eliciting and incorporating what is most important to patients—their priorities for their life—into clinical practice across the care continuum; advocacy for palliative and person-centered care by disease-specific advocacy groups, including current legislative efforts; research priorities and funding mechanisms to expand the palliative care evidence base; and education and training efforts across the medical, nursing, and other healthcare and allied disciplines.

The recommendations and actionable steps described throughout these chapters are the products of the latest scientific evidence and the collaborative efforts of leading academic, industry, and policy experts in each field. As a whole, ***Meeting the Needs of Older Adults with Serious Illness: Challenges and Opportunities in the Age of Health care Reform*** provides a road map for improving the value of health care for the seriously ill amidst this critical time of transformation.

New York, NY   Amy S. Kelley, M.D., M.S.H.S.
                                                                         Diane E. Meier, M.D.

References

1. Delgado-Guay M, Parsons H, Li Z, Palmer L, Bruera E. Symptom distress, interventions, and outcomes of intensive care unit cancer patients referred to a palliative care consult team. Cancer. 2009;115(2):437–35.
2. Field B, Devich L, Carlson R. Impact of a comprehensive supportive care team on management of hopelessly ill patients with multiple organ failure. Chest. 1989;96(2):353–56.
3. Gade G, Venohr I, Conner D, McGrady K, Beane J, Richardson R, et al. Impact of an inpatient palliative care team: a randomized control trial. J Palliat Med. 2008;11(2):180–90.
4. Gelfman L, Meier D, Morrison R. Does palliative care improve quality? A survey of bereaved family members. J Pain Symptom Manage. 2008;36(1):22–28.
5. Higginson I, Finlay I, Goodwin D. Is there evidence that palliative care teams alter end-of-life. J Pain Symptom Manage. 2003;25(2):150–68.
6. Manfredi P, Morrison R, Goldhirsch S, Carter J, Meier D. Palliative care consultations: how do they impact the care of hospitalized patients? J Pain Symptom Manage. 2000;20(3):166–73.
7. Pierucci R, Kirby R, Leuthner S. End-of-life care for neonates and infants: the experience and effects of a palliative care consultation service. Pediatrics. 2001;108(3):653–60.

8. van Staa A, Visser A, van der Zouwe N. Caring for caregivers: experiences and evaluation of interventions for a palliative care team. Patient Educ Couns. 2000;41(1):93–105.
9. Temel J, Greer J, Muzitkansky A, Gallagher E, Admane S, Jackson V, et al. Early palliative care for patients with metastatic non-small-cell lung cancer. N Engl J Med. 2010;363(8):744–52.
10. Ciemins E, Blum L, Nunley M, Lasher A, Newman J. The economic and clinical impact of an inpatient palliative care consultation service: a multifaceted approach. J Palliat Med. 2007;10:1347–55.
11. Kutner J, Kassner C, Nowels D. Symptom burden at the end of life: hospice providers' perceptions. J Pain Symptom Manage. 2001;21:473–80.
12. Campbell M, Frank R. Experience with end-of-life practice at a university hospital. Crit Care Med. 1997;25(1):197–202.
13. Carr M, Merriman MP. Comparison of death attitudes among hospice workers and health care professionals in other settings. OMEGA—J Death Dying. 1995;32(4):287–301.
14. Du Pen S, Du Pen A, Polissar N, Hansberry J, Miller Kraybill B, Stillman M, et al. Implementing guidelines for cancer pain management: results of a randomized control trial. J Clin Oncol. 1999;17:361.
15. Finn J, Pienta K, Parzuchowski J. Bridging cancer treatment and hospice care. ASCO [abstract]. 2002 ASCO Annual Meeting; 2002.
16. Schneiderman L, Gilmer T, Teetzel H, Dugan D, Blustein J, Cranford R, et al. Effect of ethics consultations on nonbeneficial life-sustaining treatments in the intensive care setting: a randomized control trail. JAMA. 2003;290(9):1166–72.
17. Wright AA, et al. Place of death: correlations with quality of life of patients with cancer and predictors of bereaved caregivers' mental health. J Clin Oncol. 2010;28(29):4457–64.
18. White K, Stover K, Cassel J, Smith T. Nonclinical outcomes of hospital-based palliative care. J Healthc Manag. 2006;51:260–73.
19. Hanson L, Usher B, Spragens L, Bernard S. Clinical and economic impact of palliative care consultation. J Pain Symptom Manage. 2008;35:340–6.
20. Brumley R, Enguidanos S, Cherin D. Effectiveness of a home-based palliative care program for end-of-life. J Palliat Med. 2003;6:715–23.
21. Pantilat S, O'Riordan D, Dibbie S, Landefeld S. Hospital-based palliative medicine consultation: a randomized control trial. Arch Intern Med. 2010;170(22):2038–40
22. Rabow M, Dibble S, Pantilat S, McPhee S. The comprehensive care team: a controlled trial of outpatient palliative medicine consultation. Arch Intern Med. 2004;164(1):83–91.
23. Meyers F, Carducci M, Loscalzo M, Linder J, Greasby T, Beckett L. Effects of a problem-solving intervention (COPE) on quality of life for patients with advanced cancer on clinical trials and their caregivers. simultaneous care educational intervention (SCEI): linking palliation and clinical trials. J Palliat Med. 2011;14(4):465–73.
24. Brumley R, Enguidanos S, Jamison P, Seitz R, Morgenstern N, Saito S, Mcilwane J, Hilary K, Gonzalez J. Increased satisfaction with care and lower costs: results of a randomized trial of in-home palliative care. J Am Geriatr Soc. 2007;55(7):993–1000.
25. Bakitas M, Doyle Lyons K, Hegel M, Balan S, Brokaw F, Seville J, Hull J, Li Z, Tosteson T, Byock I, Ahles T. Effects of a palliative care intervention on clinical outcomes in patients with advanced cancer. JAMA. 2009;302(7):741–9.
26. Morrison RS, Penrod JD, Cassell JB, Causel-Ellenbogen M, Litke A, Spragens L, Meier DE. Cost savings associated with U.S. Hospital Palliative Care Consultation Programs. Arch Intern Med. 2008;168(16):1783–90.
27. Morrison RS, Dietrich J, Ladwig S, Quill T, Sacco J, Tangeman J, et al. Palliative care consultation teams cut hospital costs for Medicaid beneficiaries. Health Aff. 2011;30(3):454–63.
28. Meyer H. Changing the conversation in California about care near the end of life. Health Aff. 2011;30:390–3.
29. Aldridge MD, Kelley AS. Epidemiology of serious illness and high utilization of healthcare; prepared for: Institute of Medicine Committee on Approaching Death: Addressing Key End of Life Issues; 2014.
30. Choosing Wisely. http://www.choosingwisely.org/

Contents

Part I Current Needs of Older Adults with Serious Illness

1 **When More Is Less: Overuse of Medical Services Harms Patients** 3
   Shannon Brownlee, Christine Cassel, and Vikas Saini

2 **Disparities in Access to Palliative Care** 19
   Cardinale B. Smith and Otis W. Brawley

3 **Family Caregiving and Palliative Care: Aligning Theory, Practice, and Policy** 31
   Carol Levine and Carol V. O'Shaughnessy

Part II Settings for the Care of the Seriously Ill

4 **This Is Your Life: Achieving a Comprehensive, Person-Centered Model of Care at the Intersection of Policy, Politics, and Private Sector Innovation** 47
   Brad Stuart and Andrew L. MacPherson

5 **Hospice and Healthcare Reform: What Is the Optimal Path?** 59
   Melissa D. Aldridge and Jean S. Kutner

6 **Palliative Care in the Long-Term Care Setting** 73
   Mary Ersek, Justine S. Sefcik, and David G. Stevenson

Part III Measuring Quality and Paying for the Care of the Seriously Ill

7 **Quality and Outcome Measures** 93
   Laura C. Hanson, Anna P. Schenck, and Helen Burstin

8 Palliative Care's Impact on Utilization and Costs: Implications
for Health Services Research and Policy 109
J. Brian Cassel

9 Long-term Services and Supports: A Necessary
Complement to Palliative Care 127
Judy Feder, Harriet L. Komisar, and Robert A. Berenson

10 The Manifest Destinies of Managed Care and Palliative Care 137
Richard H. Bernstein and Karol K. DiBello

Part IV Platforms for Improvement

11 Models of Care Delivery and Coordination: Palliative Care
Integration Within Accountable Care Organizations 153
Michigan Pioneer ACO & Hospice of Michigan: Dorothy Deremo,
Monique Reese
Partners Health System Pioneer ACO: Susan D. Block, Vicki A. Jackson,
Thomas H. Lee
UnityPoint Health Pioneer ACO: Lori Bishop
Order of Saint Francis Health Care Pioneer ACO: Robert Sawicki

12 Implementing a Care Planning System: How to Fix the Most
Pervasive Errors in Health Care 177
Bernard J. Hammes, Linda A. Briggs, William Silvester,
Kent S. Wilson, Sue Schettle, John R. Maycroft, Julie Sandoval,
Ann E. Orders, and Melissa Stern

13 Igniting Action to Integrate Palliative Care in Our
US Health System: The Role of Disease-Specific
Advocacy Groups—A Cancer Advocacy Case Study 191
Rebecca Kirch and Andy Miller

14 What Do You Mean You Don't Also Offer Palliative Care?
Effective Public Engagement to Harness Demand
to Improve Care for Serious Illness 203
Sharyn M. Sutton and Marian S. Grant

15 Research Priorities in Palliative Care for Older Adults 215
R. Sean Morrison

16 Medical and Nursing Education & Training 225
Charles F. von Gunten and Betty R. Ferrell

Index 237

Contributors

Melissa D. Aldridge, Ph.D., M.B.A. Brookdale Department of Geriatrics and Palliative Medicine, Icahn School of Medicine at Mount Sinai, New York, NY, USA

Robert A. Berenson, M.D. Urban Institute, Washington, DC, USA

Richard H. Bernstein, M.D. Department of Geriatrics and Palliative Medicine, Icahn School of Medicine at Mount Sinai, New York, NY, USA

Lori Bishop, R.N., C.H.P.N. UnityPoint Health/UnityPoint at Home, Urbandale, IA, USA

Susan D. Block, M.D. Department of Psychosocial Oncology and Palliative Care, Dana-Farber Cancer Institute and Brigham and Women's Hospital, Boston, MA, USA

Otis W. Brawley, M.D. American Cancer Society, Inc., Atlanta, GA, USA

Linda A. Briggs, M.A., M.S., R.N. Gundersen Health System, La Crosse, WI, USA

Shannon Brownlee, M.S. Lown Institute, Brookline, MA, USA

Helen Burstin, M.D., M.P.H. National Quality Forum, Washington, DC, USA

Christine Cassel, M.D. National Quality Forum, Washington, DC, USA

J. Brian Cassel, Ph.D. Hematology/Oncology and Palliative Care, Virginia Commonwealth University, Richmond, VA, USA

Karol K. DiBello, D.N.P. Lawrence Medical Associates, New York-Presbyterian/Lawrence Hospital, Bronxville, NY, USA

Dorothy Deremo, R.N., M.S.N., M.H.S.A., F.A.C.H.E. Michigan Pioneer ACO & Hospice of Michigan, Detroit, MI, USA

Mary Ersek, Ph.D., R.N., F.A.A.N. National PROMISE Center, Philadelphia Veterans Affairs Medical Center, Philadelphia, PA, USA

University of Pennsylvania School of Nursing, Philadelphia, PA, USA

Judy Feder, Ph.D. Urban Institute, Washington, DC, USA

Betty R. Ferrell, R.N., Ph.D. Department of Nursing Research and Education, City of Hope, Duarte, CA, USA

Marian S. Grant, D.N.P., M.S.N., B.S.N., B.S. University of Maryland School of Nursing, Baltimore, MD, USA

Bernard J. Hammes, Ph.D. Gundersen Health System, La Crosse, WI, USA

Laura C. Hanson, M.D., M.P.H. Division of Geriatric Medicine and Center for Aging and Health, University of North Carolina School of Medicine, Chapel Hill, NC, USA

Vicki A. Jackson, M.D., M.P.H. Palliative Care Division, Massachusetts General Hospital, Boston, MA, USA

Harvard Medical School, Boston, MA, USA

Rebecca Kirch, J.D. American Cancer Society, Inc., Washington, DC, USA

Harriet L. Komisar, Ph.D. AARP, Washington, DC, USA

Jean S. Kutner, M.D., M.S.P.H. Department of Medicine, University of Colorado School of Medicine, Aurora, CO, USA

Thomas H. Lee, M.D. Chief Medical Officer, Press Ganey, Boston, MA, USA

Carol Levine, M.A. Families and Health Care Project, United Hospital Fund, New York, NY, USA

Andrew L. MacPherson Healthsperien, LLC, Washington, DC, USA

John R. Maycroft, M.P.P. Wisconsin Medical Society, Madison, WI, USA

Andy Miller, M.H.S.E., M.C.H.E.S. MillerStephens & Associates, Austin, TX, USA

R. Sean Morrison, M.D. Brookdale Department of Geriatrics and Palliative Medicine, Icahn School of Medicine at Mount Sinai, New York, NY, USA

Carol V. O'Shaughnessy National Health Policy Forum, George Washington University, Washington, DC, USA

Ann E. Orders, M.H.A. Continuum of Care and Health Care Reform, Kaiser Permanent, Pasadena, CA, USA

Monique Reese, D.N.P., A.R.N.P., F.N.P.-C., A.C.H.P.N. UnityPoint Health, Urbandale, IA, USA

Vikas Saini, M.D. Lown Institute, Brookline, MA, USA

Department of Medicine, Harvard Medical School, Boston, MA, USA

Julie Sandoval, M.D. The Permanente Medical Group, Oakland, CA, USA

Robert Sawicki, M.D. Division of Supportive Care, OSF HealthCare, Peoria, IL, USA

Anna P. Schenck, Ph.D. Public Health Leadership Program, Gillings School of Global Public Health, University of North Carolina, Chapel Hill, NC, USA

Sue Schettle Twin Cities Medical Society, Minneapolis, MN, USA

Justine S. Sefcik, M.S., R.N. Doctoral Student, 2012-2014 National Hartford Centers of Gerontological, Nursing Excellence Patricia G. Archbold Scholar, University of Pennsylvania School of Nursing, Philadelphia, PA, USA

William Silvester, M.D. International Society of Advance Care Planning and End of Life Care, Melbourne, VIC, Australia

Cardinale B. Smith, M.D., M.S.C.R. Division of Hematology Medical Oncology and Brookdale Department of Geriatrics and Palliative Medicine, Icahn School of Medicine at Mount Sinai, New York, NY, USA

Melissa Stern, M.B.A. Life Care Planning, Kaiser Permanente, Pasadena, CA, USA

David G. Stevenson, S.M., Ph.D. Department of Health Policy, Vanderbilt University School of Medicine, Nashville, TN, USA

Brad Stuart, M.D. Advanced Care Innovation Strategies (ACIStrategies), Forestville, CA, USA

Sharyn M. Sutton, Ph.D. Masters of Arts in Communication, The John Hopkins University, Washington, DC, USA

Charles F. von Gunten, M.D., Ph.D. OhioHealth System, Columbus, OH, USA

Kent S. Wilson, M.D. Honoring Choices Minnesota, Minneapolis, MN, USA

Part I
Current Needs of Older Adults with Serious Illness

Chapter 1
When More Is Less: Overuse of Medical Services Harms Patients

Shannon Brownlee, Christine Cassel, and Vikas Saini

A case related in 2012 [6] by Dr. Angelo Volandes, of Harvard Medical School, illustrates how easily one seemingly reasonable clinical decision leads to the next, each contributing to a cascade of harm and overuse. Glenda B. was diagnosed with Alzheimer's while in her late 60s. By the time she was 71, Glenda was no longer able to drive or balance her checkbook; by 80, she was in the advanced stages of her disease: confused, unable to recognize familiar faces, incapable of feeding or dressing herself. She had completed an advance directive while still in the early stages of her disease, indicating that in the event that she lived long enough to develop advanced dementia, she would not want cardiopulmonary resuscitation or to be placed on a ventilator or fed through a tube.

When Glenda fell and broke her hip, she was taken to the emergency department of a Boston teaching hospital, where she was met by her sons. An orthopedic surgeon told them their mother needed surgery to repair her hip, citing the generally recognized and accepted clinical approach; without surgery, he said, their mother would suffer significant pain. When they indicated that their mother's advance directive might not permit her to be intubated for the surgery, they were told the directive could be "temporarily reversed," as this was standard procedure for patients with an advance directive who suffered a femoral fracture. Reluctantly, they agreed to the surgery.

An internist who was called to evaluate Glenda's fitness for the procedure noted an irregular EKG reading and administered a cardiac enzyme test, which was elevated. The internist alerted the attending cardiologist, who informed Glenda's sons that their

---

S. Brownlee, M.S. (✉)
Lown Institute, 21 Longwood Avenue, Brookline, MA 02446, USA
e-mail: brownleesm@gmail.com

C. Cassel, M.D.
National Quality Forum, Washington, DC, USA

V. Saini, M.D.
Lown Institute, 21 Longwood Avenue, Brookline, MA 02446, USA

Department of Medicine, Harvard Medical School, Boston, MA, USA

mother might be suffering a heart attack and needed to be catheterized. (The elevation of cardiac enzymes is a generally accepted marker of heart injury due to coronary disease and is often treated with angioplasty or mechanical revascularization.) They agreed to the procedure, and a coronary stent was placed. During the procedure, and again afterwards, Glenda stopped breathing. Contrary to her advance directive, and presumably arising from the same logic as for the hip surgery, cardiopulmonary resuscitation was performed and she was placed on a ventilator. After a week in the intensive care unit, she was successfully removed from the ventilator. Two days later, she was transferred from the intensive care unit to the operating room, where she was re-intubated for her hip repair. The procedure was uncomplicated, but Glenda could not be removed from the ventilator and was transferred back to the ICU.

At the end of Glenda's second stay in the ICU, her sons were approached for their consent for a tracheostomy (requiring an incision in the throat for placement of a tube to permit long term ventilator dependence) and placement of a feeding tube (requiring an incision through the abdominal wall to place a tube for delivery of artificial nutrition and hydration), another "standard procedure" among patients expected to remain ventilator dependent for a prolonged period. Despite some misgivings about having agreed to allow their mother to be intubated against her expressed wishes, the sons felt she had come too far to give up now. They agreed to the procedures. Glenda was stabilized and transferred back to the long-term care wing of her nursing home. Over the following month, she was transferred back and forth from nursing home to hospital three times for infections and once to re-insert her feeding tube after she pulled it out. This last episode led the nursing home staff to place her in wrist restraints.

During Glenda's last hospitalization, a medical resident helping care for her decided to consult the hospital's palliative care team. The team first approached her sons to discuss their mother's goals of care. Then, over the course of 2 days, the team reviewed her voluminous medical records and queried her various specialists about her prognosis. When they met again with her sons, they told them their mother was unlikely to recover even the limited function and quality of life she had before the original fall. The sons decided that their mother would never have wanted any of the interventions that she had undergone over the last 8 weeks and that hospice—care focusing strictly on her comfort—would be the right choice.

Both the ventilator and the feeding tube were removed. She continued to breathe on her own (as often occurs in such patients) and was able to transfer back to her nursing home's hospice unit, where she died peacefully, surrounded by her sons and grandchildren.

When taken in isolation, each clinical decision—to repair Glenda B.'s broken hip, place a stent during an acute myocardial infarction, perform a tracheostomy after a prolonged period of intubation, and place a feeding tube—undoubtedly seemed reasonable and appropriate to Glenda's clinicians. Indeed, based on standard clinical practice, each decision led to the "right" care, so long as the context of this frail, elderly, demented patient's specific situation was not taken into account. Each step was portrayed to her sons as the most compassionate course. Yet when seen in hindsight and in aggregate, it is possible to view much of the care Glenda received as overuse, even as each decision along the way may also have seemed entirely understandable.

In order for Glenda B.'s clinicians to have made different, more patient-centered decisions, they would have had to resist an array of forces—economic, social, and legal—that so often make overuse the default option in American medicine. Resisting those forces requires ignoring prevailing medical culture, which encourages clinicians to "fix" each isolated condition, and seeing patients as a series of individually failing organ systems and broken parts rather than as whole persons. The orthopedic surgeon encountered a woman in pain from a fractured femur, which could be repaired with a routine surgery. The cardiologist saw a possible heart attack that could be visualized and corrected with catheterization. This practice of focusing on each organ system in isolation, rather than the whole patient, can make it difficult for clinicians to keep in mind the therapeutic cascade that so often occurs in the care of frail and elderly; it makes it almost impossible to perceive an alternative course of care, much less discuss different options with the patient and family.

It is against this backdrop, of a medical culture that often values doing more rather than doing what's best for the individual patient, that palliative care must try to ensure that patients and families understand the potential outcomes of various treatment decisions and that they are protected from unnecessary suffering, both from their illnesses and from iatrogenic harm. While overuse can be particularly pernicious when it comes to the care of frail, elderly patients, regardless of whether they are known to be near the end of life, the suffering it can cause is not confined to this population. Young or old, rich or poor, insured or uninsured, patients are vulnerable to the harms of overuse. This chapter will look at some of the economic and cultural factors that contribute to this problem. It will suggest some broad categories for defining overuse, look at the estimates of its scope and the harm that is caused, and offer several of the remedies that will be needed to shift the medical culture that sustains it.

Definition of Overuse

Overuse is often seen as falling into two main categories, overdiagnosis and overtreatment, but there is considerable overlap between the two, and there are other categories of services that should be, but often are not, considered overuse [1–3]. Overdiagnosis is most likely to occur when tests are used to screen asymptomatic patients for disease. It is also likely when diagnostic tests are used for a patient who has a low pretest likelihood of having the condition; when there is no effective treatment even if the patient does have the condition; or when effective treatment exists but the patient is not an appropriate candidate, so diagnosis will not change the course of therapy. Overtreatment occurs when procedures or tests for which there is no evidence of benefit whatsoever are used; the patient is an inappropriate candidate; the patient is appropriate but his or her preference is ignored; or the totality of the patient's risk, comorbidities, and quality of life are not considered or discussed.

Given the wide variety of clinical situations where overuse is possible, we suggest some broad categories for scrutiny:

- *Ineffective screening tests* that have not been shown to reduce morbidity or mortality, and which are likely to lead to the finding of lesions that will not harm the patient, but must nonetheless be pursued with a diagnostic workup once they are detected (e.g., CA125 test for ovarian cancer [5])
- *Screening tests that commonly lead to* the diagnosis of conditions that likely would not have caused symptoms in the patient's lifetime [7], or who could have been treated equally effectively had they been detected at a later time (e.g., PSA test [8]) or to *overdiagnosis* when the pretest probability of disease is low
- *Ineffective treatments and tests* (e.g., antibiotics for viral infection)
- *Inappropriately used treatments and tests*, or treatments and tests that have been shown to be effective for some patients but are delivered to patients who are unlikely to benefit (e.g., coronary angioplasty for a patient who has no symptoms of ischemic heart disease and CT scan for a pediatric patient with no evidence of intracranial trauma on a neurological exam [9])
- *Non-evidence-based treatments or tests*, which nonetheless become standard of care despite nonexistent, poor, or conflicting evidence for effectiveness or benefit vs. harm (e.g., tissue plasminogen activator (tPA) for stroke [10] and steroids for spinal cord injury [11])
- *Routine but useless tests and procedures*, such as routine anticoagulation for all hospitalized patients [12] or blood and imaging tests whose results will not be read or will not change the course of treatment
- *Futile rescue care*, such as CPR or feeding tube for an elderly patient suffering multiple organ failure or advanced dementia [13]
- *Unwanted elective procedures and tests* that the patient would have chosen to avoid if he or she had been well informed and the clinician had engaged in shared decision-making [14]
- *Unwanted end-of-life care*, or end-of-life care that contravenes wishes stated in an advance directive [15–17]

The delivery of ineffective or inappropriate services is the clearest case of overuse, the easiest to measure, and exceedingly common. For example, two recent studies using records from the American College of Cardiology (ACC) National Cardiovascular Data Registry found that 7 and 11.6 % of patients who underwent elective coronary angioplasty for ischemic heart disease were inappropriate, based on guidelines developed by the ACC [18, 19]. The patients who were deemed inappropriate by the authors either had no symptoms of heart disease or did not have the particular signs and symptoms (e.g., level of coronary artery occlusion) that the guidelines identified as indicating a likelihood of benefit from the procedure. Delivering a treatment to an inappropriate patient is a clear case of overtreatment.

Unfortunately, such tidy definitions for overtreatment are the exception, in part because there have not been definitive studies of many interventions, and those that have valid evidence are often studied only in specific and limited populations. This is especially the case for the frail elderly, for whom large randomized trials of most interventions have not been conducted or published. For example, each specific intervention that Glenda B. endured might have been shown to be effective in isolation, especially in younger, healthier patients, but with the complications of her advanced dementia and frailty, they could not have been expected to offer much chance, if any, of meaningful recovery.

Even in younger people, examples abound of treatments that are used widely in the absence of valid evidence that they work, or without evidence to help clinicians know which patients are most likely to benefit. For example, in the 1990s, at least 41,000 women were subjected to the rigors and risk of high dose chemotherapy for metastatic breast cancer with autologous bone marrow transplant rescue, a treatment that was enthusiastically embraced by oncologists, and particularly hematologists, long before the evidence was in from four randomized controlled trials, which showed it was no better than standard therapy [20]. In other cases, flawed or biased research, or misinterpretation of data, misleads clinicians into using ineffective or sometimes harmful treatments, as was true for rofecoxib (Vioxx) [21, 22]. Patients may also be overtreated when clinicians are reluctant to curb their enthusiasm for an experimental procedure, even after well-conducted clinical trials have thrown the treatment's value into doubt [23, 24].

Perhaps the least recognized form of overuse occurs when patients who are offered elective procedures are not adequately informed about the trade-offs involved in their treatment options [25, 26]. For example, most elective angioplasty patients believe, incorrectly, that the procedure will reduce their risk of heart attack and death [27]. Evidence suggests that patients routinely undergo many types of elective treatments, even surgery, that they would have actively chosen to avoid, had they been better informed of the trade-offs and the level of evidence supporting the procedure and had their clinician done a better job of eliciting their preferences [14]. This situation, dubbed "preference misdiagnosis" in a recent paper by Albert Mulley and colleagues [28], should be considered a form of overuse.

Scope of the Problem

Given the wide variety of medical service overuse, it should come as no surprise that it has been difficult to quantify the total amount of overuse that occurs in the USA in any given year. Data on overuse are scarce, both because it has not been formally recognized as a widespread and serious problem until recently and because many treatments can be appropriate or inappropriate, depending on widely varying clinical circumstances and the patient's preferences. Identifying cases of overuse in large datasets is difficult, and efforts to quantify it have been further hampered by the fact that the USA has no research agenda specifically aimed at defining its scope, causes, or consequences [29, 30].

Despite these difficulties, several credible estimates for the amount of money wasted on overuse have been produced in recent years. Each draws on different types of data, yet all suggest that overuse is a common occurrence in American health care. Using geographic variation in Medicare utilization patterns, John Wennberg and his colleagues estimate that as much as 30 % of Medicare spending, or over $159 billion [31], goes towards overuse [32], and there is some evidence that the patterns of care that lead to overuse in the Medicare population also hold for Americans under age 65 [33]. The Dartmouth researchers attribute much of the difference in care across geographic regions to the overuse of such supply-sensitive (i.e., if the capacity to deliver the service exists, it will be deployed) services as hospital days, time in the ICU, and extra physician visits. Another estimate for overuse comes from the Institute of Medicine, which in 2012 identified a total of $750 billion in unnecessary annual medical spending [34]. Of that $750 billion, the Institute estimated that $210 billion was spent on unnecessary services. Another paper, by Donald Berwick and Andrew Hackbarth, estimated that in addition to overtreatment, another $25–45 billion is spent annually on care that could have been avoided, had care processes been more effective [4]. A PricewaterhouseCoopers paper calls out $210 billion in "defensive medicine," a category that appears to consist almost entirely of overtreatment [35].

While the wide range among these estimates reflects the uncertainty surrounding the true scope of the problem, accumulating evidence suggests that overuse makes up a significant proportion of American health care. And because unnecessary medical services offer no or only marginal benefit, while still posing the risk of harm to patients, the amount of harm being caused by overuse is undoubtedly substantial. The most obvious and worrisome harms are poor patient outcomes—increased pain, serious disability, and death—but there are also significant harms related to "nonclinical" outcomes, such as financial burdens, spending precious remaining time in a hospital instead of at home, and patients' loss of autonomy and diminished ability to participate in daily life. Medical interventions can delay or interfere with physical, spiritual, and emotional comfort and quality of life, especially at the end of life, and deprive both patient and family members of time together that cannot be regained.

What is the extent of harm caused by overuse? Again, there is no systematic collection of such data, and few studies that have looked directly at that question, but the sporadic evidence that does exist suggests the number of patients who suffer harm is likely to be considerable. The most readily available data on harm come from studies of overtreatment, the inappropriate use of a treatment or test. One 2006 systematic review estimated that more than 40 % of antipsychotic, antidepressant, and antianxiety medications in the USA were prescribed inappropriately [36]. The authors did not attempt to quantify the rate of serious side effects, which include akathisia, suicidality, and extrapyramidal symptoms such as Parkinsonism [37]. A recent paper estimated that the four million CT scans performed on children each year are projected to cause 4,870 cancers [38]. As many as one-third of CT imaging tests may be inappropriate [39]; thus approximately 1,600 of those cancers may have been the result of a scan that offered no benefit.

We can also make some reasonable inferences of harm from overuse due to preference misdiagnosis, which occurs when the patient would have chosen a different treatment had he or she been better informed of the options. Several randomized controlled trials have found wide differences in treatment choices among patients who were informed of their options via usual care versus patients who also had access to patient decision aids [14], devices that offer balanced, evidence-based information about elective treatment choices in a manner that most patients can understand. One such study found that patients with access to a decision aid were 20 % less likely to choose elective coronary artery interventions than patients who got usual care [40]. Another recent study found that patients suffering from knee and hip pain due to arthritis, and who had access to patient decision aids, were at least 25 % less likely to opt for joint replacement compared to patients receiving usual care [41]. Overall, studies comparing patients who have access to a patient decision aid show that 20 % fewer patients choose invasive options compared to patients who get usual care [14].

From these sorts of studies we can infer the number of patients who are harmed by a treatment they would not have wanted, had they been better informed of their options. Typical estimates for serious procedural adverse events for coronary artery interventions, including stroke, myocardial infarction, perforation, and death, are around 1 %. That means that of the 80,000 patients who had an elective PCI, but who would not have really wanted one if fully informed, (20 % of the total of 400,000), 800 suffered a serious adverse event. For the 11.6 % of such patients who were inappropriate candidates [19], 464 can be estimated to have suffered a serious side effect.

A similar calculation can be made for knee and hip replacement patients: of the over one million leg joint replacements done each year, around 250,000 would likely have been unwanted. All arthroplasty patients face postoperative pain and a period of rehabilitation. Nearly 4 % [42], or about 10,000 joint replacement patients can be expected to suffer a serious adverse event such as infection, dislocation, myocardial infarction, pulmonary embolism, and death. A little less than 1 % had to undergo a second surgery to repair problems with the first.

For every specific type of overuse that can be imagined, the potential for harm is greatest in the elderly. The old have fewer physiologic reserves than the young, are more likely to live with multiple chronic conditions that interact and influence recovery, are more likely to require hospitalization (with all the attendant risks of nosocomial infection and medical error that each admission entails), and have lower reserve capacity to recover from what might be minor side effects for younger patients. Medicare beneficiaries, particularly those over 75, are at uniquely high risk of suffering harm from overuse. Studies have found, for example, that elderly patients who have multiple comorbidities or limited life expectancy and who undergo screening and treatment for cancer only rarely benefit from treatment; many suffer chart-documented pain and psychological distress [43, 44]. Aggressive treatment, which may be effective in a younger patient, may lead to lower quality of life and an earlier death in an elderly patient [45].

Wasted Resources

In addition to physical harm, overuse is a substantial component of the growing economic burden imposed by healthcare spending, for both the public and private sectors. Rising healthcare spending is a contributor to high unemployment [46] and a cause for concern about high levels of future government debt or tax increases. That fiscal burden poses a threat to the continued provision of health care and other critical public goods such as education, infrastructure, national defense, and poverty reduction. Most importantly, growing healthcare spending (with little or no improvement in population-based outcomes compared with other developed countries [47]) is a principal reason for the slow growth in lower- and middle-class living standards since the 1980s. From 2000 to 2009, nearly a third of a typical worker's compensation growth went to rising healthcare spending [46].

Diminished living standards are not the only form of financial harm. Overtreatment also represents a misallocation of resources, which could be put to better use paying for services that patients want, such as palliative care and home-based care, especially during serious chronic illnesses. Filling hospital beds with patients who do not need to be there and are at risk of harm strains the resources of the medical system [48]; it distracts doctors and nurses from other patients, fills CT scanners and operating rooms at critical moments, and packs emergency departments and clinics with patients who could be more safely and effectively managed elsewhere [49, 50]. The result is longer waits and potentially worse outcomes for those patients with ailments that medicine is actually able to treat or even cure. In areas with high levels of socioeconomic inequality, it seems reasonable to conjecture that overtreatment of the wealthy may contribute to undertreatment of the poor (though there are no data to support this contention).

Collateral Damage: Clinicians and Family

When patients are no longer able to make independent decisions, family members must step in to protect their wishes, but the culture of medicine routinely fails to support them in those efforts. As in Glenda B.'s case, family members often become the focus of medicine's "do everything" culture, even to the point of overturning the patient's already-expressed directives. Overuse can inflict substantial emotional distress and guilt on family members, and stand in the way of their acceptance of the reality of the future course of the illness, especially when patients are nearing the end of life. (In recognizing the harm we do to families, both as decision-makers on behalf of their loved ones and as overburdened family caregivers, we must also recognize that the system is failing to provide needed supports for them, too.)

Overuse can also hurt clinicians, diminishing their satisfaction in their work and damaging their sense of pride in their professionalism [51]. Overuse is connected to clinician burnout and moral distress, a well-documented phenomenon, particularly among nurses, that is the result of internal conflict—knowing the right thing to do for the patient and being unable to do it because of institutional or other constraints [52].

Causes of Overuse

Various observers offer different reasons for the prevalence of overuse. Health policy analysts often blame fee-for-service payment, which rewards clinicians and the entire healthcare industry for the volume rather than value of services [53]. Clinicians often point to defensive medicine, their constant worry that a patient may sue for a missed diagnosis or failure to treat [54]. Medical training, particularly the "hidden curriculum" (the transfer by example of idiosyncratic patterns of practice from instructors to trainees), has a powerful effect on clinician behavior, including their tendency to overtreat [55]. Anecdotal reports suggest that trainees, particularly during residency, are more likely to suffer rebuke for failing to perform tests than for overtreatment. On the other side of the stethoscope, patients themselves may demand unnecessary care; certainly clinicians believe that much overuse can be laid at their feet [56].

Many have commented on the role of fragmentation in the dysfunctions of our healthcare system. In our view another major factor in the growth of overuse has been the fragmentation of clinical thinking itself. The reductionist approach which accompanied the arrival of scientific medicine after the Flexner report ushered in an era of intensive search for ultimate causes. With growing technologic power, such causes were sought in smaller and smaller units of analysis, right up to current science on the nanoscale. When evidence has been generated for individual drugs, devices, or procedures, trials have tended to ignore the effects of multiple factors on health and well-being and have actually excluded research subjects who are elderly or have multiple chronic conditions—the very population most likely to receive these treatments. This increasingly reductionist approach often results in inappropriate interpretations of the generalizability and applicability of specific treatments to individual patients, and unexpected harms.

All of these factors contribute to overuse, because they are a manifestations of a larger problem, a medical culture emphasizes what can be *done* to the patient—the physical, medical, technological fixes for each of patients' clinical problems. Patients' needs for communication, plain English information and decision supports, understanding, empathy, and comfort may be lost in the storm of diagnoses, tests, and treatments. The desire to help a patient, or to demonstrate caring, combined with a medical culture of doing, means that clinicians have come to view the mother of a child with belly pain who leaves the emergency room without a CT scan as a lawsuit waiting to happen, and the frail and elderly patient who dies of natural causes without rescue care as a medical failure.

This focus on doing can impair clinicians' ability to perceive the true reason the patient is seeking care and prevent them from appropriately addressing the patient's goals. The adult children of a frail and demented older person who are demanding treatment for a cancer diagnosis do not realize the potential dangers that chemotherapy and radiation pose in such patients. All they know is that they want to do the best for their mother, and they assume that the treatment recommendations have taken into account the patient's frailty and other chronic conditions, and are likely to restore her to health. The clinician fears that the children who are expecting

-the-art cancer treatment might sue if he or she explains that leaving the untreated is actually safer than subjecting her to risks and toxicities she is unlikely to tolerate. And so the physician complies with the adult children's demands, knowing it is the wrong thing to do. Tort reform, the most commonly proposed solution to defensive medicine, cannot address this communication gap between the frightened patient and family and the lawsuit-averse clinician [57, 58], though better communication does lead to lower risk of a lawsuit [59, 60].

Our reliance on medical solutions to illness, disability, and even the inevitability of death has also fed our overconfidence in them, to the point where clinicians may have trouble acknowledging evidence that a treatment does not work. Treatments remain in common use years or decades after negative results from well-conducted clinical trials should have led clinicians to restrain their enthusiasm. For example, vertebroplasty was hailed early on as a relatively safe treatment for back pain caused by osteoporotic vertebral fracture, with a "90 % rate of effectiveness" [61]. In 2009, the *New England Journal of Medicine* published two randomized controlled clinical trials of the procedure [23, 62]. The trials, both of which compared the procedure to sham surgery, found no difference in pain relief or functional status. Yet back surgeons and other interventionalists continue to champion the procedure, pointing to less powerful studies, including case-controlled studies, studies with short follow-up, and case series, all of which have less power to demonstrate benefit [63]. Other common practices are never even tested, so strong is our faith in their power to heal.

* * *

While we believe the culture of medicine is the driving force behind a huge amount of overuse, there are other factors that should be acknowledged. One of the most important findings from the Dartmouth Atlas research is the powerful influence the supply of resources has on the volume of services delivered to patient, particularly the chronically ill. Dartmouth researchers point to "supply-sensitive care," medical services whose rate of utilization is driven by the local supply of medical resources [32]. This care is largely the result of discretionary decisions made when patients are hospitalized—and many of these decisions have little if any valid evidence to guide them. For example, clinicians (often emergency room physicians) routinely decide whether or not a patient with influenza-like illness needs to be admitted to the hospital. A search of PubMed turned up only one study examining criteria clinicians may use, and no published guidelines. Under such conditions, the availability of beds becomes a factor in the decision [64]. Similarly, the availability of other clinicians (particularly specialists) can influence referral decisions. For example, compared to a region where fewer gastroenterologists are available, in a region where more such specialists are available primary care physicians may be more likely to refer a patient with typical gastroesophageal reflux than they would in an area with fewer specialists [65, 66]. The SUPPORT study found that the primary predictor of place of death among 9,000 seriously ill persons was the number of hospital beds per capita in the study community [67]. Thus variation in hospital bed availability, not patient or family or physician preference, drove the "decision" for where the patient would die and how he or she would be treated during this vulnerable period of life. When it comes to supply-sensitive care, including hospitalization, ordering of imaging studies, ICU stays, and referrals to other physicians, equally sick patients in high-supply areas will receive substantially more treatment than patients in low-supply areas, yet there is little evidence to show that regions where patients receive more care have better outcomes [68–70]. The lack of benefit, the substantial cost of supply-sensitive services [71], and the disruption of patients' lives are all reasons to think at least some supply-sensitive care represents overuse.

Solutions

Eliminating overuse will require many technical remedies to guide clinicians towards more appropriate treatment. We need more and better evidence for the effectiveness and generalizability of many treatments currently in use, and a clearer understanding of the risk of harm, especially for high-risk vulnerable patient populations. The Patient-Centered Outcomes Research Institute (PCORI) should help supply some of the needed data. We will also need more effective means of disseminating valid, evidence-based guidelines and getting clinicians to follow them. Choosing Wisely, the campaign launched by the American Board of Internal Medicine Foundation in 2012, has successfully persuaded more than three dozen specialty societies to identify procedures and tests that are ineffective or often used inappropriately [72], including treatments and tests routinely and inappropriately administered to frail elders and patients in need of palliative care [73]. Each specialty society has produced a list of at least five such overused treatments and several have launched campaigns to encourage their members to stop doing them—or in some cases to stop doing them on the wrong patients.

Choosing Wisely represents an essential start down the road towards reducing overuse, and its effects will be amplified if other methods are employed at the same time. For example, the ABIM Foundation supports teaching tools to help physicians gain needed communications skills. Shared decision-making, a formal process for informing patients of their treatment options and eliciting their preferences, should be encouraged through training at all levels and through incentives such as quality guidelines and payment. We need better systems for ensuring that advance directives and person-determined goals for care are first sought and then respected. One possible means to accomplish that goal: making rates of completion of and compliance with advance directives a reportable quality measure. Another reportable measure: the percentage of elective surgery patients who have access to shared decision-making and high-quality patient decision aids. The rate at which palliative care is employed should be measured, not just for the dying but for any patient who is diagnosed with a serious, life-threatening, or painful disease. And as many health policy experts have already pointed out, payment models that value effective care directed at patient goals over simply performing more procedures will make room in the system for better care. Patients and families can begin to help themselves avoid suffering unnecessary medical services by asking some simple questions (see Fig. 1.1).

1. **Don't recommend percutaneous feeding tubes in patients with advanced dementia; instead, offer oral assisted feeding.**
In advanced dementia, studies have found feeding tubes do not result in improved survival, prevention of aspiration pneumonia, or improved healing of pressure ulcers. Feeding tube use in such patients has actually been associated with pressure ulcer development, use of physical and pharmacological restraints, and patient distress about the tube itself. Assistance with oral feeding is an evidence-based approach to provide nutrition for patients with advanced dementia and feeding problems; in the final phase of this disease, assisted feeding may focus on comfort and human interaction more than nutritional goals.

2. **Don't delay palliative care for a patient with serious illness who has physical, psychological, social or spiritual distress because they are pursuing disease-directed treatment.**
Numerous studies—including randomized trials—provide evidence that palliative care improves pain and symptom control, improves family satisfaction with care and reduces costs. Palliative care does not accelerate death, and may prolong life in selected populations.

3. **Don't leave an implantable cardioverter-defibrillator (ICD) activated when it is inconsistent with the patient/family goals of care.**
In about a quarter of patients with ICDs, the defibrillator fires within weeks preceding death. For patients with advanced irreversible diseases, defibrillator shocks rarely prevent death, may be painful to patients and are distressing to caregivers/family members. Currently there are no formal practice protocols to address deactivation; fewer than 10% of hospices have official policies. Advance care planning discussions should include the option of deactivating the ICD when it no longer supports the patient's goals.

4. **Don't recommend more than a single fraction of palliative radiation for an uncomplicated painful bone metastasis.**
As stated in the American Society for Radiation Oncology (ASTRO) 2011 guideline, single-fraction radiation to a previously un-irradiated peripheral bone or vertebral metastasis provides comparable pain relief and morbidity compared to multiple-fraction regimens while optimizing patient and caregiver convenience. Although it results in a higher incidence of later need for retreatment (20% vs. 8% for multi-fraction regimens), the decreased patient burden usually outweighs any considerations of long-term effectiveness for those with a limited life expectancy.

5. **Don't use topical lorazepam (Ativan), diphenhydramine (Benadryl), haloperidol (Haldol) ("ABH") gel for nausea.**
Topical drugs can be safe and effective, such as topical non-steroidal anti-inflammatory drugs for local arthritis symptoms. However, while topical gels are commonly prescribed in hospice practice, anti-nausea gels have not been proven effective in any large, well-designed or placebo-controlled trials. The active ingredients in ABH are not absorbed to systemic levels that could be effective. Only diphenhydramine (Benadryl) is absorbed via the skin, and then only after several hours and erratically at subtherapeutic levels. It is therefore not appropriate for "as needed" use. The use of agents given via inappropriate routes may delay or prevent the use of more effective interventions.

Fig. 1.1 Choosing Wisely: Five things physicians and patients should question, American Geriatrics Society

All of these fixes can help cut overuse and the harm that it causes, and many will be necessary in the coming years. However, we believe these fixes will not be sufficient to tackle the outsized problem of overuse without a dramatic shift in medical culture, towards "doing more *for* the patient, and less *to* the patient," in the words of cardiologist and humanitarian Bernard Lown. Palliative care has a central role to play in that shift. Its practitioners recognize, whether explicitly or not, that patients and families must be helped towards having concrete and achievable goals for care, and they need to understand both the potential benefits and the harms of alternative paths, and the limits to what medicine can do to improve the quality of life and lengthen it. Patients and their families must be helped to understand there are trade-offs involved in virtually every medical choice. Palliative care recognizes the wide gulf that exists between what patients want, how they express it, and what clinicians may subsequently feel compelled to deliver, and between patient-centered care and tests and treatments applied by harried and risk-averse clinicians, who work in hospitals, nursing homes, or other sites of care that are not organized around the needs of patients. This is especially true for the frail elderly, where personalized home care can improve quality of life, even length of life, while dramatically reducing hospitalizations and the use of expensive but potentially harmful and futile technology [74].

If we want to break the cycle of overuse, certainly we must give clinicians the evidence and other tools they need to know what the right care is, and a legal system that ensures they won't be sued if that's what they deliver. And we must train them to be better communicators and appraisers of evidence. We need a research agenda for the problem of overuse, and ways of measuring compliance with guidelines for best practices. But more than all of these, we need to change the culture of medicine and the implicit belief on the part of both clinicians and patients that more is better. The fact is that less is very often more.

References

1. Abramson J. Overdosed America: the broken promise of American medicine. New York: Harper Perrenial; 2004. p. 384.
2. Brownlee S. Overtreated : why too much medicine is making us sicker and poorer. 1st ed. New York: Bloomsbury; 2007. p. 343.
3. Welch HG, Schwartz L, Woloshin S. Overdiagnosed: making people sick in the pursuit of health, vol. xvii. Boston: Beacon Press; 2011. 228 p.
4. Berwick DM, Hackbarth AD. Eliminating waste in US health care. JAMA. 2012;307(14): 1513–6.
5. Moyer VA. Screening for ovarian cancer: U.S. Preventive Services Task Force reaffirmation recommendation statement. Ann Intern Med. 2012;157(12):900–4.
6. Lenzer J. Unnecessary care: are doctors in denial and is profit driven healthcare to blame? BMJ. 2012;345:e6230.
7. Welch HG, Black WC. Overdiagnosis in cancer. J Natl Cancer Inst. 2010;102(9):605–13.
8. Lin K, et al. Benefits and harms of prostate-specific antigen screening for prostate cancer: an evidence update for the U.S. Preventive Services Task Force. Ann Intern Med. 2008;149(3): 192–9.

9. Schachar JL, et al. External validation of the New Orleans Criteria (NOC), the Canadian CT Head Rule (CCHR) and the National Emergency X-Radiography Utilization Study II (NEXUS II) for CT scanning in pediatric patients with minor head injury in a non-trauma center. Pediatr Radiol. 2011;41(8):971–9.
10. Brown SG, Macdonald SP, Hankey GJ. Do risks outweigh benefits in thrombolysis for stroke? BMJ. 2013;347:f5215.
11. Bydon M et al. The role of steroids in acute spinal cord injury. World Neurosurg. 2013. http://www.worldneurosurgery.org/article/S1878-8750(13)00348-3/abstract.
12. Lederle FA, et al. Venous thromboembolism prophylaxis in hospitalized medical patients and those with stroke: a background review for an American College of Physicians Clinical Practice Guideline. Ann Intern Med. 2011;155(9):602–15.
13. Teno JM, et al. Does feeding tube insertion and its timing improve survival? J Am Geriatr Soc. 2012;60(10):1918–21.
14. Stacey D, et al. Decision aids for people facing health treatment or screening decisions. Cochrane Database Syst Rev. 2011;10, CD001431.
15. Volandes AE, et al. Randomized controlled trial of a video decision support tool for cardiopulmonary resuscitation decision making in advanced cancer. J Clin Oncol. 2013;31(3):380–6.
16. Volandes AE, et al. A randomized controlled trial of a goals-of-care video for elderly patients admitted to skilled nursing facilities. J Palliat Med. 2012;15(7):805–11.
17. Downey L, et al. Life-sustaining treatment preferences: matches and mismatches between patients' preferences and clinicians' perceptions. J Pain Symptom Manage. 2013;46(1):9–19.
18. Anderson HV, et al. Relationship between procedure indications and outcomes of percutaneous coronary interventions by American College of Cardiology/American Heart Association Task Force Guidelines. Circulation. 2005;112(18):2786–91.
19. Chan PS, et al. Appropriateness of percutaneous coronary intervention. JAMA. 2011;306(1):53–61.
20. Mello MM, Brennan TA. The controversy over high-dose chemotherapy with autologous bone marrow transplant for breast cancer. Health Aff. 2001;20(5):101–17.
21. Curfman GD, Morrissey S, Drazen JM. Expression of concern: Bombardier et al., "Comparison of upper gastrointestinal toxicity of rofecoxib and naproxen in patients with rheumatoid arthritis," N Engl J Med 2000;343:1520-8. N Engl J Med. 2005;353(26):2813–4.
22. Curfman GD, Morrissey S, Drazen JM. Expression of concern reaffirmed. N Engl J Med. 2006;354(11):1193.
23. Kallmes DF, et al. A randomized trial of vertebroplasty for osteoporotic spinal fractures. N Engl J Med. 2009;361(6):569–79.
24. Buchbinder R, et al. A randomized trial of vertebroplasty for painful osteoporotic vertebral fractures. N Engl J Med. 2009;361(6):557–68.
25. Sepucha KR, et al. How does feeling informed relate to being informed? The DECISIONS survey. Med Decis Making. 2010;30(5 Suppl):77S–84S.
26. Zikmund-Fisher BJ, et al. The DECISIONS study: a nationwide survey of United States adults regarding 9 common medical decisions. Med Decis Making. 2010;30(5 Suppl):20S–34S.
27. Rothberg MB, et al. Patients' and cardiologists' perceptions of the benefits of percutaneous coronary intervention for stable coronary disease. Ann Intern Med. 2010;153(5):307–13.
28. Mulley AG, Trimble C, Elwyn G. Stop the silent misdiagnosis: patients' preferences matter. BMJ. 2012;345:e6572.
29. Korenstein D, et al. Overuse of health care services in the United States: an understudied problem. Arch Intern Med. 2012;172(2):171–8.
30. Keyhani S, Siu AL. The underuse of overuse research. Health Serv Res. 2008;43(6):1923–30.
31. The Henry J. Kaiser Family Foundation. Medicare spending and financing fact sheet. [2012 11/14/12 6/11/2013]. http://kff.org/medicare/fact-sheet/medicare-spending-and-financing-fact-sheet/
32. Wennberg JE, Fisher ES, Skinner JS. Geography and the debate over Medicare reform. Health Aff (Millwood), 2002. Suppl Web Exclusives. W96–114.
33. Wennberg JE, Cooper MM, editors. The Dartmouth atlas of health care in Michigan. Detroit: Blue Cross/Blue Shield of Michigan; 2000.

34. Smith MD, Institute of Medicine (US), Committee on the Learning Health Care System in America. Best care at lower cost: the path to continuously learning health care in America. Washington, DC: National Academies Press; 2012.
35. PricewaterhouseCoopers. The price of excess: identifying waste in healthcare spending. Alabama: PricewaterhouseCoopers Health Research Institute; 2008.
36. Jureidini J, Tonkin A. Overuse of antidepressant drugs for the treatment of depression. CNS Drugs. 2006;20(8):623–32.
37. Govoni S, et al. Extrapyramidal symptoms and antidepressant drugs: neuropharmacological aspects of a frequent interaction in the elderly. Mol Psychiatry. 2001;6(2):134–42.
38. Miglioretti DL, et al. The use of computed tomography in pediatrics and the associated radiation exposure and estimated cancer risk. JAMA Pediatr. 2013;167(8):700–7.
39. Melnick ER, et al. CT overuse for mild traumatic brain injury. Jt Comm J Qual Patient Saf. 2012;38(11):483–9.
40. Morgan MW, et al. Randomized, controlled trial of an interactive videodisc decision aid for patients with ischemic heart disease. J Gen Intern Med. 2000;15(10):685–93.
41. Arterburn D, et al. Introducing decision aids at Group Health was linked to sharply lower hip and knee surgery rates and costs. Health Aff. 2012;31(9):2094–104.
42. Soohoo NF, et al. Factors that predict short-term complication rates after total hip arthroplasty. Clin Orthop Relat Res. 2010;468(9):2363–71.
43. Walter LC, Covinsky KE. Cancer screening in elderly patients: a framework for individualized decision making. JAMA. 2001;285(21):2750–6.
44. Walter LC, Eng C, Covinsky KE. Screening mammography for frail older women: what are the burdens? J Gen Intern Med. 2001;16(11):779–84.
45. Temel JS, et al. Early palliative care for patients with metastatic non-small-cell lung cancer. N Engl J Med. 2010;363(8):733–42.
46. Nyce SA, Schieber SJ. How rising health costs slow wage growth. Washington, DC: Progressive Policy Institute; 2012.
47. Woolf SH, Aron LY. The US health disadvantage relative to other high-income countries: findings from a National Research Council/Institute of Medicine report. JAMA. 2013;309(8):771–2.
48. Savino JS, et al. Practice pattern variability for myocardial revascularization: impact on resource use across 24 centers. J Cardiothorac Vasc Anesth. 2002;16(2):149–56.
49. Xu KT, et al. Over-prescribing of antibiotics and imaging in the management of uncomplicated URIs in emergency departments. BMC Emerg Med. 2013;13:7.
50. Siddiqui S, Ogbeide DO. Utilization of emergency services in a community hospital. Saudi Med J. 2002;23(1):69–72.
51. Meier DE, Back AL, Morrison RS. The inner life of physicians and care of the seriously ill. JAMA. 2001;286(23):3007–14.
52. Pauly BM, Varcoe C, Storch J. Framing the issues: moral distress in health care. HEC Forum. 2012;24(1):1–11.
53. Porter ME. A strategy for health care reform—toward a value-based system. N Engl J Med. 2009;361(2):109–12.
54. Bishop TF, Federman AD, Keyhani S. Physicians' views on defensive medicine: a national survey. Arch Intern Med. 2010;170(12):1081–3.
55. Lucas FL, et al. Variation in cardiologists' propensity to test and treat: is it associated with regional variation in utilization? Circ Cardiovasc Qual Outcomes. 2010;3(3):253–60.
56. Campbell EG, et al. Professionalism in medicine: results of a national survey of physicians. Ann Intern Med. 2007;147(11):795–802.
57. Sloan FA, Shadle JH. Is there empirical evidence for "defensive medicine"? A reassessment. J Health Econ. 2009;28(2):481–91.
58. Carrier ER, et al. Physicians' fears of malpractice lawsuits are not assuaged by tort reforms. Health Aff. 2010;29(9):1585–92.
59. Levinson W, et al. Physician-patient communication. The relationship with malpractice claims among primary care physicians and surgeons. JAMA. 1997;277(7):553–9.

60. Kachalia A, et al. Liability claims and costs before and after implementation of a medical error disclosure program. Ann Intern Med. 2010;153(4):213–21.
61. Hacein-Bey L, et al. Treating osteoporotic and neoplastic vertebral compression fractures with vertebroplasty and kyphoplasty. J Palliat Med. 2005;8(5):931–8.
62. Buchbinder R, Osborne RH, Kallmes D. Vertebroplasty appears no better than placebo for painful osteoporotic spinal fractures, and has potential to cause harm. Med J Aust. 2009;191(9):476–7.
63. Papanastassiou ID, et al. Comparing effects of kyphoplasty, vertebroplasty, and non-surgical management in a systematic review of randomized and non-randomized controlled studies. Eur Spine J. 2012;21(9):1826–43.
64. Wennberg J. Tracking medicine: a researcher's quest to understand health care. New York: Oxford University Press; 2010.
65. Fisher ES, Bynum JP, Skinner JS. Slowing the growth of health care costs—lessons from regional variation. N Engl J Med. 2009;360(9):849–52.
66. Sirovich B, et al. Discretionary decision making by primary care physicians and the cost of U.S. Health Care. Health Aff. 2008;27(3):813–23.
67. Pritchard RS, et al. Influence of patient preferences and local health system characteristics on the place of death. SUPPORT Investigators Study to Understand Prognoses and Preferences for Risks and Outcomes of Treatment. J Am Geriatr Soc. 1998;46(10):1242–50.
68. Ong MK, et al. Looking forward, looking back: assessing variations in hospital resource use and outcomes for elderly patients with heart failure. Circ Cardiovasc Qual Outcomes. 2009;2(6):548–57.
69. Fisher ES, et al. The implications of regional variations in Medicare spending. Part 1: the content, quality, and accessibility of care. Ann Intern Med. 2003;138(4):273–87.
70. Fisher ES, et al. The implications of regional variations in Medicare spending. Part 2: health outcomes and satisfaction with care. Ann Intern Med. 2003;138(4):288–98.
71. Wennberg JE. Understanding geographic variations in health care delivery. N Engl J Med. 1999;340(1):52–3.
72. Cassel CK, Guest JA. Choosing wisely: helping physicians and patients make smart decisions about their care. JAMA. 2012;307(17):1801–2.
73. AGS Choosing Wisely. Workgroup American Geriatrics Society identifies five things that healthcare providers and patients should question. J Am Geriatr Soc. 2013;61(4):622–31.
74. Klein E. If this was a pill, you'd do anything to get it, in Wonkblog. Washington, DC: Washington Post; 2013.

Chapter 2
Disparities in Access to Palliative Care

Cardinale B. Smith and Otis W. Brawley

The Institute of Medicine (IOM) defines disparities in health care as racial or ethnic differences in the quality of health care that are not due to clinical needs, preferences, and appropriateness of intervention [1]. Disparities in health care have been well documented in the USA and are consistent across a range of illnesses. A higher proportion of racial and ethnic minority patients have inferior disease outcomes as a result of more advanced stages of disease at diagnosis and lower likelihood of receiving high quality treatment [2–4]. These differences often persist after controlling for access-related factors such as insurance. Palliative care is an element of high quality treatment that is often lacking, hence the importance of study of disparities in access and use of palliative care.

The IOM describes a model in which healthcare disparities arise from a complex interplay of economic, social, and cultural factors. Socioeconomic status (SES) influences disease risk through factors such as safe neighborhoods and housing, adequacy of social supports, tobacco use, poor nutrition, physical inactivity, and obesity. Income, education, and health insurance coverage are elements of SES. SES influences access to appropriate preventive services, early detection, diagnosis, treatment, and palliative care. Social inequities, such as the legacy of racial discrimination in the USA, can still influence the interactions between patients and physicians [1]. Some patients have mistrust of medical professionals; cultural factors and religiosity also play a role in health behaviors and attitudes toward illness and belief in

---

C.B. Smith, M.D., M.S.C.R. (✉)
Division of Hematology Medical Oncology and Brookdale Department of Geriatrics
and Palliative Medicine, Icahn School of Medicine at Mount Sinai, 1 Gustave L. Levy Place,
PO Box 1079, New York, NY 10029, USA
e-mail: cardinale.smith@mssm.edu

O.W. Brawley, M.D.
American Cancer Society, Inc., 250 Williams St., Atlanta, GA 30303, USA

modern medicine versus alternative forms of healing. Additionally, some racial and ethnic minorities display health beliefs that are overly fatalistic. For most diseases, socioeconomic factors that disproportionately plague minorities such as poverty, inadequate education, and lack of health insurance appear to play a more important role in disparate outcomes as opposed to inherent biological differences [5].

The goal of palliative care is to relieve suffering and provide the best possible quality of life for people facing pain, symptoms, and stresses from serious illness. Palliative care is appropriate for patients at any age or illness stage and can be provided along with curative or life-prolonging therapies. Unlike hospice, which is directed at patients who are dying and who have opted to forego life-prolonging treatments, palliative care ideally should be provided at the time of diagnosis of a serious illness and in conjunction with all other appropriate disease-directed treatments.

Palliative care is associated with improved symptom control [6], clearer understanding of diagnosis and prognosis [6], more efficient utilization of healthcare resources [7], and greater patient and family satisfaction [6–9]. Recent data show that early integration of palliative care with standard oncologic care for patients with advanced lung cancer is associated with improvements in quality of life, mood, and survival [10].

There is literature demonstrating that a significant proportion of racial and ethnic minorities experience poor quality palliative care. Racial and ethnic minorities are more likely to receive inadequate pain assessment and management. They are less likely to complete advance directives and utilize hospice, are more likely to undergo aggressive life-sustaining treatments, and have a higher utilization of healthcare resources at the end of life (EOL) [11–13].

There is also an incomplete literature concerning public beliefs and attitudes about the use of palliative care. Similarly, not much is known about the impact of specialty palliative care on the perceptions of care among minority patients and the full extent to which this care improves the outcomes of minority patients. While there are data regarding the racial and ethnic disparities in the utilization of certain components of palliative care (specifically hospice care at the EOL), there is an overall paucity of literature about the utilization of specialist palliative care services and organized palliative care teams. Racial/ethnic disparities in the use of palliative care services are likely to persist as palliative care services become more available in the hospital and community setting throughout the USA.

The following discussion will focus on what is known about the disparities that exist regarding specific areas of palliative care, describe future work needed to elicit the beliefs of minority patients about specialty palliative care consultation, and discuss relevant policy measures to help improve the palliative care outcomes of minority patients with serious illness. In describing the available literature we will follow the conceptual framework used in the National Healthcare Disparities Report that describes three major attributes of care: access to care (entry, structural, and cultural barriers), receipt of care (including use and cost of services), and quality of care (as measured by effectiveness, safety, timeliness, patient centeredness, and efficiency) [14].

Access to Care

The availability of palliative care has increased tremendously over the last decade. Among all hospitals, 63 % report having the presence of a palliative care team, and among large hospitals (≥300 beds), 85 % report a palliative care team [15]. Unfortunately, only 54 % of public safety net hospitals have a palliative care team [15]. This almost certainly contributes to underutilization of palliative care among minority patients.

The literature consistently shows that minority patients do not have equal access to pain care in the USA. This spans across all healthcare settings, including emergency rooms, inpatient services, outpatient clinics, and nursing homes [16]. This observed disparity is often attributed to system-related factors such as reduced access to specialty care and lack of adequate health insurance [17, 18]. As a result, racial/ethnic minority patients are less likely to report finding pain specialists available to them compared to non-Hispanic white patients [12].

Even when SES is held constant, minority patients remain at risk for disparities in pain care [19]. Availability of analgesic medications is a potential barrier to pain management. Pharmacies located in minority neighborhoods are more likely to have inadequate opioid stocks [20, 21]. A study of pharmacies in New York City revealed that 72 % of pharmacies in predominantly white neighborhoods stocked opioids sufficient to treat severe pain, but only 25 % of pharmacies in predominantly nonwhite neighborhoods had similar pain medications available [20]. The reasons cited for this included the additional paperwork required, regulatory oversights and monitoring, and the fear of penalties imposed by state and federal drug-enforcement agencies.

In an effort to curtail the rising rates of controlled substance abuse and diversion, increasing restrictions on prescribing practices of physicians are being developed at both the state and federal level. State Medicaid programs cover high numbers of minority populations. Many programs have created strict criteria for authorization and coverage of opioids. These regulations lead to decreased prescribing practices [22, 23], which in turn may widen the observed disparity in access of appropriate pain management among minorities.

Cultural beliefs can also prevent adequate pain treatment [24–26]. Some Hispanic and African-American patients are not prescribed analgesics because they do not mention pain to their healthcare provider. They are often stoic and believe that pain is inevitable [24, 26]. African-American patients in particular fear that they will become addicted to the analgesics used to treat pain. Some minority patients also fear developing tolerance to the drugs, or having intolerable side effects [26]. Studies of Hispanic and African-American patients have found that a significant proportion rely on alternative and complementary pain treatments and prefer to take analgesics only when pain is very severe [26, 27].

In addition to healthcare system and patient barriers, physician barriers contribute to the underutilization of palliative care by minorities. In surveys, a high proportion of minority patients report that physicians seem not to believe they have pain or do not understand their pain. It has been shown that physicians tend to underestimate the pain of patients of different cultures [28]. In a study of barriers to referral to inpatient palliative care the providers' culture, religion, and ethnicity played an active role in their decision to explain palliative care to patients and to participate in decision-making about palliative care. When providers and patients differed in culture, religion, and ethnicity, the providers were less likely to explain palliative care. Furthermore, physicians are often the primary source of education and referrals for their patients, but they too often lack knowledge of the range of services provided by palliative care. Referral of patients with serious illness for palliative care is often infrequent and delayed until after discontinuation of disease-directed treatment [29, 30]. Many lung cancer physicians refer less than 25 % of their lung cancer patients for palliative care consultation [31] despite evidence that early use of palliative care improves the quality of life, mood, and survival of patients with lung cancer [10].

Receipt of Care

There are racial/ethnic differences in the receipt of and preferences for advance care planning, aggressive disease-directed treatments, and life-sustaining technologies in the context of end-stage disease. Several studies have reported racial/ethnic differences in knowledge of, attitudes toward, and initiation of advance care planning. African-Americans and Hispanics are less likely than whites to have completed advance directives and do-not-resuscitate (DNR) orders or be interested in doing so [32, 33]. Similarly, minority patients more often want more intensive intervention and life-prolonging treatment in the face of serious illness [34, 35]. In a survey conducted to assess patients' wishes for advance care planning by Blackhall et al., non-Hispanic whites were least likely to accept or want life support, Hispanics were positive about life support and would want life support (they believed life support would not be suggested if a case was truly hopeless), and African-Americans were more likely to feel it was acceptable to withhold or withdraw life support, but would personally want it for themselves [36]. In fact, minority patients report a higher willingness to exhaust personal financial resources on medical care in an attempt to extend life [37].

Factors often cited as explanations for higher proportion of African-American patients preferring more aggressive disease-specific therapies and lower rate of advance directive completion include barriers to access of high-quality health care, reliance on spiritual support and other cultural norms to cope with illness, decreased health literacy, and mistrust of the US health care system [38, 39]. Among Hispanics, immigration status, decreased health literacy, reluctance to openly discuss terminal illness, and religious and cultural beliefs that interfere with identification and treatment of disease contribute to preferences for aggressive disease-modifying therapies and lower rate of advance directive completion [40, 41].

Disparities also exist in receipt of appropriate patient–physician communication. In several studies physicians appear to deliver less information and communicate less support to African-American and Hispanic patients compared to white patients, even in the same care settings [42, 43]. Similarly, a higher proportion of minority patients surveyed feel they have had inadequate conversations related to prognosis and treatment. They also feel that family members often are not included [44]. Even when minority patients with serious illness report desires to discuss care preferences with a physician, they often do so at a rate much less than whites. The Study to Understand Prognoses and Preferences for Outcomes and Risks of Treatments (SUPPORT) found that African-Americans wished to discuss resuscitation preferences with their physicians more often than whites, but they were less likely to have this type of discussion [45].

Minority patients often do not receive treatment consistent with their wishes even when their wishes are known. It is known that a higher proportion of racial/ethnic minorities prefer more life-prolonging technology at EOL. Despite the disproportionate preference for intensive EOL care among African-American patients, it has been demonstrated that white patients who prefer intensive EOL care were nearly three times more likely to receive it than African-American patients with the same preferences [46]. Of particular relevance to EOL care are study results that show that African-American patients receive less resource-intensive care than do other hospitalized patients, despite their preferences for more life-prolonging measures [45]. Conversely, poor patient–physician communication may lead to aggressive care in many racial/ethnic minorities who do not want it [45].

Quality of Care

The IOM defines superior quality care as care that is effective, safe, timely, patient centered, efficient, and equitable [47]. There are few studies examining the impact of specialty palliative care consultation quality on outcomes of minority patients. The literature suggests that minority patients with access to hospital-based palliative care services benefit in the same ways as nonminorities [9, 48]. One study specifically examining the impact of palliative care consultation on pain outcomes demonstrated similar and significant reductions in pain among racial/ethnic minorities [49]. The minority population included in this study was predominantly Asian and Pacific Islander. In another study, the effectiveness of inpatient palliative care consultations on completion of advance directives and DNR orders by racial and ethnic minorities was assessed. African-American and Hispanic patients had higher rates of advance directives and DNR orders when a palliative care consultation occurred [50].

The timing of referral of patients with advanced cancer to outpatient specialty palliative care and the outcome on symptom burden were evaluated by race and ethnicity in a single center study [51]. Although the timing of referral was similar, there was less improvement in the symptom burden (pain, depression, and fatigue) for minority compared to nonminority patients [51]. Decreased adherence to treatment among minorities and the likelihood that minority patients are less likely to receive targeted treatment for symptoms have been hypothesized as a contributor to the observed disparity [28]; however, the exact reasons for the limited symptom improvement among minority patients in this study are unknown.

The National Healthcare Quality Report (NHQR) and the National Healthcare Disparities Report (NHDR) are published annually by the Agency for Healthcare Research and Quality. These reports track five measures of palliative care delivered by home health agencies, nursing homes, and hospices: dyspnea among home healthcare patients, pressure sores in nursing home residents, help with emotional and spiritual needs provided to hospice patients, effective communication about what to expect among hospice family caregivers, and provision of care consistent with patients' wishes among those enrolled in hospice [52]. These reports have identified racial and ethnic disparities across all measures with minority patients consistently receiving poorer quality care. With the exception of the measures focusing on the care of hospice patients, the influence of specialty palliative care physicians and other important metrics in palliative care is not currently measured.

Policy Changes

There is a plethora of literature describing the racial and ethnic disparities in access to appropriate medical care. Several things must occur to improve and ensure that minorities have access to quality specialty palliative care.

First, more research is needed to recognize how care providers can better determine and understand the needs and care priorities of minority patients facing serious illness. More research should focus on the common beliefs and attitudes of minority patients and their caregivers that may affect the utilization of specialty palliative care.

Understanding the components of care that are most important to minorities will assist with developing palliative care programs that are culturally appropriate. Currently, only 0.2 % of all grants from the National Institutes of Health (NIH) are related to palliative care [53]. More resources devoted to palliative care research are needed. Similarly, career development awards should also be designated to ensure that junior researchers (medical, nursing, and social work) have the ability to enter the field.

The Patient Centered Quality Care for Life Act (HR 1666, introduced April 23, 2013) aims to expand the palliative care research base, improve training, and broaden access to palliative care. The proposed legislation would engage health professionals, patients, public and private payers, and state and federal health officials in the development of solutions and models of best practices for providing palliative care to those in need.

Second, the public's awareness of palliative care in minority and majority populations must increase. The vast majority of patients are unaware of the existence of palliative care and the value of the care provided by this specialty [55]. Studies show that most patients believe palliative care is important and beneficial when it is explained to them. Most believe that palliative care should be made available for patients with serious illness and would consider it for a loved one if they had a serious illness [55].

A significant barrier to receipt of care among minorities is mistrust and a belief that they will be deprived of beneficial life-prolonging medical care. Palliative care is perceived as an inappropriate substitute for costly healthcare technology. This can be overcome by integrating simultaneous palliative care into the current healthcare delivery infrastructure. Multidisciplinary programs combining disease-directed treatment and palliative care should be developed. Major accreditation and certification organizations should require access to palliative care as a condition of accreditation and certification. Similarly, financial incentives to healthcare systems that provide access to palliative care and penalties for failure in providing these services should also be created. A simultaneous effort is needed to engage community-based organizations to promote public awareness campaigns using individuals from the community as educators, spokespersons, outreach workers, and liaisons to stimulate the development of these integrated programs.

Third, in order to ensure that minorities have access to providers with expertise in palliative care, there needs to be an increase in the professional workforce capacity. To accomplish this, postgraduate training opportunities for all disciplines involved in providing palliative care, such as graduate medical education slots, should be increased. There is an inadequate medical and nursing workforce with expertise in palliative care. Acknowledging that education is an important strategy for overcoming barriers to palliative care, there is a critical need to develop interdisciplinary learning opportunities for healthcare professionals, clergy, and social workers who will provide services to minority patients facing serious illness and their families.

Specific loan forgiveness programs for physicians and advance-practice nurses should also be established to encourage and support entry into this field. The Palliative Care and Hospice Education and Training Act is legislation that addresses a major barrier facing the expansion of palliative care by training medical school faculty and creating new incentives for the training and development of interdisciplinary health professionals in palliative care [54].

A renewed focus on teaching basic primary palliative care skills to practitioners in each medical specialty is paramount to ensuring that minority patients receive the core aspects of palliative care. Core palliative care competencies should be mandated in undergraduate and postgraduate education as a condition of accreditation. This teaching must include content on cultural traditions, values, beliefs, and attitudes of a number of commonly encountered races and ethnicity so that service providers will better understand, acknowledge, and act to overcome the effects of racism, discrimination, and bias on patient participation in and response to beneficial interventions.

Lastly, it is critical that public policy reflects the specific needs and challenges faced by members of minority populations with serious illness. To that end, national initiatives must be funded to evaluate novel models of care delivery to promote efforts to improve access to palliative care among members of minority populations. This is especially important as the number of older minorities in community settings, such as nursing homes, is continuing to rise [56]. Providing longitudinal, community-based palliative care to patients living with serious illness who are well enough to be in home-like settings yet, who experience the very real burdens of advanced and progressive illness, is critically important. These models can serve as a system for coordination of care and can assist with streamlining the transition from palliative to end-of-life care when disease-focused treatments are no longer effective or their burden clearly outweighs their benefit. Funding of these demonstration projects and integration of the models that are most effective in providing culturally competent palliative care will be essential in improving the access to palliative care among minorities.

Conclusion

With the rapidly aging minority population and commensurate increases in chronic, serious illnesses, the need for access to high-quality palliative care for minorities is imperative. The barriers to access to palliative care services by minority groups are common and complex and often further complicated by a lack of suitable models of culturally appropriate care to meet patient and family needs. Overcoming these barriers will require that an evidence base exists to ensure high quality care that is aligned with minority patients' preferences; that minority populations understand what palliative care is and have resources available to access it; that healthcare providers be trained to deliver this kind of care; that healthcare organizations expand their ability to deliver palliative care; and that new models of care delivery are developed and implemented where they are most needed. Achieving these goals will ensure that palliative care is reliably available for minority patients with serious illness and their families throughout the trajectory of serious illness.

References

1. Institute of Medicine. Unequal treatment. Confronting racial and ethnic disparities in healthcare. Washington, DC: The National Academies Press; 2003.
2. Epstein AM, Ayanian JZ. Racial disparities in medical care. N Engl J Med. 2001;344(19): 1471–3.
3. Clegg LX, Li FP, Hankey BF, Chu K, Edwards BK. Cancer survival among US whites and minorities: a SEER (Surveillance, Epidemiology, and End Results) Program population-based study. Arch Intern Med. 2002;162(17):1985–93.
4. Heisler M, Smith DM, Hayward RA, Krein SL, Kerr EA. Racial disparities in diabetes care processes, outcomes, and treatment intensity. Med Care. 2003;41(11):1221–32.
5. Ward E, Jemal A, Cokkinides V, et al. Cancer disparities by race/ethnicity and socioeconomic status. CA Cancer J Clin. 2004;54(2):78–93.
6. Ellershaw JE, Peat SJ, Boys LC. Assessing the effectiveness of a hospital palliative care team. Palliat Med. 1995;9(2):145–52.
7. Morrison RS, Penrod JD, Cassel JB, et al. Cost savings associated with US hospital palliative care consultation programs. Arch Intern Med. 2008;168(16):1783–90.
8. Ringdal GI, Jordhoy MS, Kaasa S. Family satisfaction with end-of-life care for cancer patients in a cluster randomized trial. J Pain Symptom Manage. 2002;24(1):53–63.

9. Manfredi PL, Morrison RS, Morris J, Goldhirsch SL, Carter JM, Meier DE. Palliative care consultations: how do they impact the care of hospitalized patients? J Pain Symptom Manage. 2000;20(3):166–73.
10. Temel JS, Greer JA, Muzikansky A, et al. Early palliative care for patients with metastatic non-small-cell lung cancer. N Engl J Med. 2010;363(8):733–42.
11. Hanchate A, Kronman AC, Young-Xu Y, Ash AS, Emanuel E. Racial and ethnic differences in end-of-life costs: why do minorities cost more than whites? Arch Intern Med. 2009;169(5):493–501.
12. Cintron A, Morrison RS. Pain and ethnicity in the United States: a systematic review. J Palliat Med. 2006;9(6):1454–73.
13. Fishman J, O'Dwyer P, Lu HL, Henderson H, Asch DA, Casarett DJ. Race, treatment preferences, and hospice enrollment: eligibility criteria may exclude patients with the greatest needs for care. Cancer. 2009;115(3):689–97.
14. Agency for Healthcare Research and Quality. Conceptual framework: national healthcare disparities report. Rockville: AHRQ; 2002.
15. Morrison RS, Augustin R, Souvanna P, Meier DE. America's care of serious illness: a state-by-state report card on access to palliative care in our nation's hospitals. J Palliat Med. 2011;14(10):1094–6.
16. Bonham VL. Race, ethnicity, and pain treatment: striving to understand the causes and solutions to the disparities in pain treatment. J Law Med Ethics. Spring 2001;29(1):52-68.
17. Green CR, Anderson KO, Baker TA, et al. The unequal burden of pain: confronting racial and ethnic disparities in pain. Pain Med. 2003;4(3):277–94.
18. Green CR. The healthcare bubble through the lens of pain research, practice, and policy: advice for the new president and congress. J Pain. 2008;9(12):1071–3.
19. Fuentes M, Hart-Johnson T, Green CR. The association among neighborhood socioeconomic status, race and chronic pain in black and white older adults. J Natl Med Assoc. 2007;99(10):1160–9.
20. Morrison RS, Wallenstein S, Natale DK, Senzel RS, Huang L-L. "We don't carry that"—failure of pharmacies in predominantly nonwhite neighborhoods to stock opioid analgesics. N Engl J Med. 2000;342(14):1023–6.
21. Green CR, Ndao-Brumblay SK, West B, Washington T. Differences in prescription opioid analgesic availability: comparing minority and white pharmacies across Michigan. J Pain. 2005;6(10):689–99.
22. Ross-Degnan D, Simoni-Wastila L, Brown JS, et al. A controlled study of the effects of state surveillance on indicators of problematic and non-problematic benzodiazepine use in a Medicaid population. Int J Psychiatry Med. 2004;34(2):103–23.
23. Brushwood DB. Maximizing the value of electronic prescription monitoring programs. J Law Med Ethics. Spring 2003;31(1):41-54.
24. Meghani SH, Keane A. Preference for analgesic treatment for cancer pain among African Americans. J Pain Symptom Manage. 2007;34(2):136–47.
25. Ward SE, Goldberg N, Miller-McCauley V, et al. Patient-related barriers to management of cancer pain. Pain. 1993;52(3):319–24.
26. Anderson KO, Green CR, Payne R. Racial and ethnic disparities in pain: causes and consequences of unequal care. J Pain. 2009;10(12):1187–204.
27. Juarez G, Ferrell B, Borneman T. Influence of culture on cancer pain management in Hispanic patients. Cancer Pract. 1998;6(5):262–9.
28. Anderson KO, Mendoza TR, Valero V, et al. Minority cancer patients and their providers: pain management attitudes and practice. Cancer. 2000;88(8):1929–38.
29. Osta BE, Palmer JL, Paraskevopoulos T, et al. Interval between first palliative care consult and death in patients diagnosed with advanced cancer at a comprehensive cancer center. J Palliat Med. 2008;11(1):51–7.
30. Reville B, Miller MN, Toner RW, Reifsnyder J. End-of-life care for hospitalized patients with lung cancer: utilization of a palliative care service. J Palliat Med. 2010;13(10):1261–6.

31. Smith CB, Nelson JE, Berman AR, et al. Lung cancer physicians' referral practices for palliative care consultation. Ann Oncol. 2012;23(2):382–7.
32. Hopp FP. Preferences for surrogate decision makers, informal communication, and advance directives among community-dwelling elders: results from a national study. Gerontologist. 2000;40(4):449–57.
33. Phipps E, True G, Harris D, et al. Approaching the end of life: attitudes, preferences, and behaviors of African-American and white patients and their family caregivers. J Clin Oncol. 2003;21(3):549–54.
34. Wright AA, Zhang B, Ray A, et al. Associations between end-of-life discussions, patient mental health, medical care near death, and caregiver bereavement adjustment. JAMA. 2008;300(14):1665–73.
35. Earle CC, Landrum MB, Souza JM, Neville BA, Weeks JC, Ayanian JZ. Aggressiveness of cancer care near the end of life: is it a quality-of-care issue? J Clin Oncol. 2008;26(23):3860–6.
36. Blackhall LJ, Frank G, Murphy ST, Michel V, Palmer JM, Azen SP. Ethnicity and attitudes towards life sustaining technology. Soc Sci Med. 1999;48(12):1779–89.
37. Martin MY, Pisu M, Oster RA, et al. Racial variation in willingness to trade financial resources for life-prolonging cancer treatment. Cancer. 2011;117(15):3476–84.
38. Goldsmith B, Dietrich J, Du Q, Morrison RS. Variability in access to hospital palliative care in the United States. J Palliat Med. 2008;11(8):1094–102.
39. Krakauer EL, Crenner C, Fox K. Barriers to optimum end-of-life care for minority patients. J Am Geriatr Soc. 2002;50(1):182–90.
40. Smith AK, Sudore RL, Perez-Stable EJ. Palliative care for Latino patients and their families: whenever we prayed, she wept. JAMA. 2009;301(10):1047-1057, E1041.
41. Ortega AN, Fang H, Perez VH, et al. Health care access, use of services, and experiences among undocumented Mexicans and other Latinos. Arch Intern Med. 2007;167(21):2354–60.
42. Ross CE, Mirowsky J, Duff RS. Physician status characteristics and client satisfaction in two types of medical practice. J Health Soc Behav. 1982;23(4):317–29.
43. Hooper EM, Comstock LM, Goodwin JM, Goodwin JS. Patient characteristics that influence physician behavior. Med Care. 1982;20(6):630–8.
44. Royak-Schaler R, Passmore SR, Gadalla S, et al. Exploring patient-physician communication in breast cancer care for African American women following primary treatment. Oncol Nurs Forum. 2008;35(5):836–43.
45. Borum ML, Lynn J, Zhong Z. The effects of patient race on outcomes in seriously ill patients in SUPPORT: an overview of economic impact, medical intervention, and end-of-life decisions. Study to Understand Prognoses and Preferences for Outcomes and Risks of Treatments. J Am Geriatr Soc. 2000;48(5 Suppl):S194–8.
46. Mack JW, Paulk ME, Viswanath K, Prigerson HG. Racial disparities in the outcomes of communication on medical care received near death. Arch Intern Med. 2010;170(17):1533–40.
47. Institute of Medicine. Crossing the quality chasm: a new health system for the 21st century. Washington, DC: National Academy Press; 2001.
48. Braiteh F, El Osta B, Palmer JL, Reddy SK, Bruera E. Characteristics, findings, and outcomes of palliative care inpatient consultations at a comprehensive cancer center. J Palliat Med. 2007;10(4):948–55.
49. Bell CL, Kuriya M, Fischberg D. Pain outcomes of inpatient pain and palliative care consultations: differences by race and diagnosis. J Palliat Med. 2011;14(10):1142–8.
50. Sacco J, Carr DRD, Viola D. The effects of the palliative medicine consultation on the DNR status of African Americans in a safety-net hospital. Am J Hosp Palliat Care. 2013;30(4):363–9.
51. Reyes-Gibby CC, Anderson KO, Shete S, Bruera E, Yennurajalingam S. Early referral to supportive care specialists for symptom burden in lung cancer patients: a comparison of non-Hispanic Whites Hispanics, and non-Hispanic Blacks. Cancer. 2012;118(3):856–63.
52. Report NHQ. Effectiveness of care (Chapter 2). Rockville: Agency for Healthcare Research and Quality; 2012.

53. Gelfman LP, Du Q, Morrison RS. An update: NIH research funding for palliative medicine 2006 to 2010. J Palliat Med. 2013;16(2):125–9.
54. American Cancer Society Cancer Action Network. Quality of life: American Cancer Society Cancer Action Network Legislative Initiatives. http://acscan.org/content/wp-content/uploads/2013/02/2013-ACS-CAN-Quality-of-Life-legislation.pdf. Accessed September 17, 2013.
55. Center to Advance Palliative Care. Public opinion research on palliative care 2011. New York: Center to Advance Palliative Care; 2011.
56. Feng Z, Fennell ML, Tyler DA, Clark M, Mor V. The care span: growth of racial and ethnic minorities in US nursing homes driven by demographics and possible disparities in options. Health Aff (Millwood). 2011;30(7):1358–65.

Chapter 3
Family Caregiving and Palliative Care: Aligning Theory, Practice, and Policy

Carol Levine and Carol V. O'Shaughnessy

Family members are understandably distraught when they see a relative in severe pain, having difficulty breathing, or wracked by nausea. If a nurse or doctor says, "Let me see what we can do to make your mother more comfortable," the response is almost always, "Thank you. It's so hard to see her suffer." And yet, if the professional says, "It would be a good idea to call in a palliative care team at this point," the response, if not an outright "no," may be more guarded. "What do you mean? Are you giving up on her?"

For every person like Amy Berman [1], who decided, with her mother's support, to choose palliative care over aggressive treatment when she was diagnosed with a particularly virulent form of breast cancer, there are many more patients and family members who say, after long and difficult courses of treatment, "Why didn't someone tell me about palliative care earlier?" And at the other end of the spectrum, there are some family members who say, like the daughter of a gravely ill 92-year-old man, "He doesn't have quit in him." In this case, as recounted by Dr. Ira Byock, even after the man's inevitable death, his daughter complained that Dr. Byock was "heavy-handed in pressuring him to die against his will" [2].

Carol Levine Directs the Families and Health Care Project at the United Hospital Fund
Carol O'Shaughnessy is a Principal Policy Analyst at the National Health Policy Forum. The views expressed in this chapter do not necessarily represent those of the National Health Policy Forum.

C. Levine, M.A. (✉)
Families and Health Care Project, United Hospital Fund,
1411 Broadway, 12th Floor, New York, NY 10018, USA
e-mail: clevine@uhfnyc.org

C.V. O'Shaughnessy
National Health Policy Forum, George Washington University, Washington, DC, USA

Opening a discussion of palliative care—and its equally misunderstood counterpart, hospice—brings up fears of professional abandonment, suspicions about financial reasons to reduce expensive curative treatments, concerns that death is imminent, guilt, anger, and other emotions. Thinking about the policy implications of addressing family caregivers' needs in palliative care has to start with the reality that most patients and family caregivers do not know very much about palliative care. In a public opinion poll conducted by the Center to Advance Palliative Care, only 3 % said that they were "knowledgeable" about palliative care [3]. People are often introduced to palliative care during a crisis when it is difficult to accept and integrate new knowledge. If they do know something, it may be incomplete or inaccurate. And even when they do get appropriate information, they may choose to ignore it.

With the aging of American society and advances in healthcare technology, more people with serious illnesses are living longer, increasing the extent and intensity of care and support needed. Although a large analytic base documents the key role that family caregivers play in providing essential care to persons with chronic or life-threatening illnesses, and some practice protocols and guidelines call for expanded caregiver support, assessment, and training, the value of caregiver labor has largely been absent from policy discussions.

The issues inherent in providing adequate, appropriate, and sustained assistance to all caregivers are even more pronounced in palliative care, which requires skills, monitoring, and attention to emotional and spiritual factors as well as complex clinical care. Although research on family caregiving and palliative care has documented caregiver needs, most policy discussions have focused on professional, clinical, regulatory, and financial aspects of palliative care. This chapter addresses some of the gaps while recognizing the diversity of families and the complexity of the situations in which palliative care is an option.

Background on Family Caregivers

Most discussions of family caregivers today use a broad definition, one that includes partners, neighbors, and friends, as well as spouses, children, and other relatives. The defining characteristic is the role the person plays in providing or managing the person's care, not the legal relationship or lack of it.

How many family caregivers are there? The estimates range widely, depending on the definition of caregiving, the population surveyed, and the methodology, for example, whether caregivers were identified by people with disabilities or by people who identified themselves as caregivers [4]. According to the AARP Public Policy Institute, there were about 42.1 million adult family caregivers in 2009. Their unpaid care is currently valued at $450 billion a year, a significant increase from the $196 billion estimated in 1999 in the first use of this methodology [5].

The surveys agree that the majority (two-thirds) of family caregivers are women in their middle years taking care of older women. In the 2009 National Alliance on Caregiving/AARP Public Policy Institute survey, the average age of caregivers taking care of people over the age of 50 was 50 and the average care recipient was 77 [6].

But the composite should not conceal the picture's diverse elements. Caregivers are men as well as women, spouses and partners, adult children, minor children, friends and neighbors, people of all religious, economic, and ethnic backgrounds.

On average, family caregivers spend about 20 h a week assisting their family member. Like the composite description, this average is made up of caregivers who spend 8–10 h a week as well as those who have to be available all day, every day (and what is even harder, all night, every night). The big picture also includes caregivers whose responsibilities are fairly routine, such as shopping and making meals and just checking in, as well as those who do complex medication management and operation of medical equipment like feeding tubes, ventilators, and IV infusions, and keeping a person with advanced dementia safe and comfortable.

A recent report from the AARP Public Policy Institute and the United Hospital Fund, based on a nationally representative survey of family caregivers, found that 46 % performed one or more "skilled" medical/nursing tasks [7]. Medication management and wound care were among the most difficult tasks, according to respondents. Even though many of the people they were caring for had been hospitalized overnight or had gone to emergency rooms in the previous year, the caregivers reported that they had little or no training in performing these challenging tasks. Many of these tasks are the kind that would be expected of family caregivers in a home-based palliative care service.

Impact of Caregiving on Mental, Physical, and Financial Health

Emotional Impact

Substantial research has documented that the stresses of caregiving take a toll emotionally, physically, and financially. Some of the stress results from seeing the family member decline as well as the specific stresses of caregiving over time. Between 40 and 70 % of family caregivers have clinically significant symptoms of depression. Placing the family member in a nursing home does not necessarily lessen anxiety and depression because of guilt, loss of control, and worries about the quality of care. Caregivers who provide 36 or more hours a week of care have the highest level of depression. The Evercare® study of "Caregivers in Decline" found that "when caregivers talk about their worsened health, stress seems to be the most pervasive health problem in their lives" [8]. Caregivers feel angry, drained, guilty, helpless, and isolated.

Stress from Dealing with the Healthcare "System"

Most studies focus on stress related to the demands of caregiving, balancing different roles and responsibilities, or the dynamics of the relationship with the care recipient or other family members. Unfortunately, few studies ask whether the difficulty of dealing with healthcare or social service professionals or the bureaucracies in which they work is a significant source of stress. One of the few studies to ask about this aspect of caregiving is the 2008 study of employed current and former caregivers conducted by the Work and Family Institute [9]. When asked about their top wishes for the way in which doctors, nurses, and others in the healthcare system could support family caregivers, they reported: "more frequent and better quality two-way communication; less overworked, more compassionate staff at medical and nursing facilities with the skills to listen and learn from the caregivers and the elders; and a more user-friendly easier-to-navigate and less costly health care system."

Physical Impact

Caregivers' physical health also suffers as well as their mental health. They are generally in worse health than their non-caregiving peers. They are at increased risk of heart disease, stroke, and dementia. Immune system deficiencies have been well documented; if a caregiver actually finds time to get a flu shot (as frequently advised), its protection is not as strong because of the lowered immune response. Joint and muscle problems are common, often exacerbated by the lifting, moving, and pushing needed to take care of someone who has mobility problems or is in a wheelchair. Sleep deprivation is very common. Increased mortality is the ultimate caregiver sacrifice. In one study older caregivers who reported strain were 63 % more likely to die than their non-caregiving peers [10].

Financial Impact

Most caregivers do not like to dwell on the financial sacrifices they make or even to tally them. Only 15 % of the respondents to the 2009 National Alliance for Caregiving reported serious financial hardship, with the highest percentage (22 %) among the lowest income group. But the financial impact of caregiving does take a toll. Out-of-pocket expenses can be a constant drain, especially travel for long-distance caregivers. Expenditures for all the things not covered by Medicare and commercial insurance—copays, disposable items, extra help, assistive devices, home modifications, or a customized wheelchair—add up. If caregivers do not think a lot about the short-term drain on their finances, they are largely oblivious to the long-term impact on their own retirement and long-term care needs.

Half of all caregivers are employed full- or part-time. In the 2009 National Alliance on Caregiving/AARP study, 70 % of workers reported that caregiving had an impact on employment. Two-thirds went to their jobs late, left early, or took time off. Twenty percent took a leave of absence. Some caregivers turn down promotions or opportunities for enhancing their skills. Some large employers have established flexible policies for family caregivers, but most have not. Some businesses are totally supportive or generally tolerant. Others do not make any adjustments for caregivers. For their part caregiving employees are reluctant to acknowledge their dual responsibilities in their workplaces lest this be seen as shirking their workload and perhaps jeopardizing their job.

Vulnerability in Caregiver Experience

Despite this litany of problems, it is important to remember that not all caregivers are equally vulnerable. Older caregivers are particularly at risk, as are poor caregivers and those with chronic health problems. Caregivers with language or health literacy difficulties have a hard time navigating the various systems. Caregivers taking care of more than one person are obviously doubly challenged. But all caregivers may be at risk in different ways, such as financially and emotionally.

For many caregivers, there are rewards as well as stresses and strains. Many caregivers learn new skills. They may enjoy the extended time spent with their family member and gain a new perspective on that person's life. Some feel satisfaction, a sense of a duty fulfilled, even if they do not have a particularly loving relationship with their family member. Many caregivers report spiritual growth.

Interestingly, the Families and Work Institute study found that only 14 % of current caregivers reported that caregiving has improved their relationship with the person they care for [9]. That percentage rose dramatically—to 60 %—when caregivers whose relative had died were interviewed. The authors suggest that "Quite possibly, caregivers do not have enough time or mental resources to reflect on the caregiving experience and the relationship with the care recipient until after [it] is over" (underline in original). Hospice or palliative care bereavement services should allow for individuals to search for their own meaning, a healing process that cannot be rushed.

Palliative Care and Family Caregivers: The Practice Arena

In principle person- and family-centered care recognizes and supports the role of family caregivers, addresses the needs of both the recipient of care and his or her caregiver, promotes communication and shared decision-making as well as coordination and collaboration by healthcare delivery teams with family caregivers. While these concepts have been recognized and supported by advocates, researchers, and clinicians, they are generally more an ideal than a reality [11].

> **Box 3.1**
>
> The National Consensus Project (NCP) on Palliative Care Excerpts include guidelines recognize the centrality of family caregivers in clinical practice.
>
> **Guideline 1.1. A comprehensive and timely interdisciplinary assessment of the patient and family forms the basis of the plan of care.**
>
> **Criteria:**
>
> - The IDT [interdisciplinary team] documents assessments of the patient and family perception and understanding of the serious of life limiting illness, including patient and family expectations of treatment, goals for care, quality of life, and preferences for the type and site of care.
>
> **Guideline 1.2. The care plan is based on the identified and expressed preferences, values, goals, and needs of the patient and family and is developed with professional guidance and support for patient–family decision making.** *Family* **is defined by the patient…**
>
> **Criteria:**
>
> - The IDT supports patient–family decision-making and then develops, implements, and coordinates the care plan in collaboration with the patient and family. The team promotes patient and family education and assures communication of the care plan to all involved health professionals. Particular attention is necessary when a patient transfers to a different care setting, with the imperative to communicate with the receiving provider.
>
> Clinical Practice Guidelines for Quality Palliative Care, Third Edition, 2013. pp. 14–15. See full text at http://www.nationalconsensusproject.org/NCP_Clinical_Practice_Guidelines_3rd_Edition.pdf

In February 2012, the National Quality Forum (NQF) endorsed principles of patient- and family- centered care recommending a set of voluntary clinical practice guidelines to guide the growth and expansion of palliative care [12]. These principles were based on work of the National Consensus Project (NCP) on Palliative Care that first developed guidelines in 2004 and updated in 2013 (see Box 3.1). The measures apply to palliative care across healthcare settings, including hospitals, care at home and outpatient facilities. The principles include explicit family-centered care and support to caregivers across a number of domains, including comprehensive interdisciplinary assessment, identified and expressed needs, informed choice, education, physical environment, and specifically for families, grief, and bereavement services. The NQF endorsement should help advance patient- and family-centered approaches to palliative care but implementation will take time.

Building on the work of the NQF and the NCP, in 2011 the Joint Commission launched an advanced certification program for hospital-based palliative care.

The certification program recognizes hospital inpatient programs that demonstrate exceptional patient- and family-centered care and optimize the quality of life for patients with serious illness. Among the criteria for certification is special focus on family engagement in the process of palliative care [13].

Hospital palliative care teams, like hospice teams, see the family as the unit of care. In this view both the patient and the family should be treated as the unit of services. Some experts say that a structured approach to include families as an integral part of the palliative care process does not exist [14].

A comprehensive review of palliative care research and caregiving has pointed to an absence of a strong empirical base for how to respond to the needs of caregivers, indicating that "empirical inquiry regarding effective ways to provide support to family caregivers is still in its infancy." Further, "[s]upport for family caregivers is often lacking and is in need of a codified framework based on best evidence and empirical research" [15].

More is known about palliative care in hospitals than in nursing homes or in patient's homes. A home care agency or hospice may be involved in patient care, but family caregivers are still the main providers of care. While there is no specific Medicare benefit for home-based palliative care as there is for hospice care, the same attention to family caregiver needs that is stressed by hospital teams should carry over to other care settings. Where this is being done, the results are positive [16].

What Should Palliative Care Teams Do to Support Family Caregivers?

Family caregivers often have substantial unmet needs during the last stages of patient illness. These include lack of training about symptom management, poor physician communication about medical decision-making, lack of emotional support, and caregiver belief that the patient was not treated with respect. Teno et al. found that family members were concerned about quality of care that their family member received at the end of life care regardless of whether care was provided in the hospital or a nursing home. Only when care was provided in the home were there fewer unmet needs [17].

Interdisciplinary palliative care teams can assess family caregivers' needs for information, training, and ongoing support. Building this information into the care plan not only eases patients' and family caregivers' worries but also helps ensure that the interventions are carried out correctly at home, where a team is less likely to be available. The most important factors in caregiver support are likely to be teamwork, sharing information, and valuing the patient as a person and the family as a unit.

It is important to develop protocol-supported practices to overcome barriers to adequate caregiver support in palliative care protocols [18]. Barriers include both challenges implicit in family dynamics and funding constraints on the delivery of palliative care by healthcare services. Among barriers cited are:

- Incongruent patient and caregiver perceptions about the level and type of care to be requested [18].
- Incongruent goals of care among healthcare professionals and patient/caregiver units.
- While physicians tend to focus on clinical aspects of care, patients and caregivers tend to view the illness within a spiritual or psychosocial context [19].
- Inadequate communication about what palliative care is and ambivalent caregiver receptivity to supportive services [18].
- Poor or nonexistent communication by physicians to caregivers about what to expect in terms of patient life expectancy or the seriousness of the course of illness [20].
- Caregiver rejection of support offered [18].
- Tendency by healthcare professionals to view the patient as the only person appropriate for their attention. If the family caregiver is considered at all, it is as the mirror image of the patient—the "patient/caregiver" without an understanding the family caregiver's limitations and other responsibilities. Some healthcare professionals are openly hostile to family involvement, seeing it as intrusive, disruptive, and counter to what they perceive as the patient's best interests, or their own professional control [21].

Palliative Care and Family Caregivers: The Policy Arena

Family caregiving is a latecomer to the healthcare policy arena for a number of reasons. One reason is policymakers' fear that family caregivers will reduce their efforts if public or private insurers pay for care. As Bruce Vladeck puts it, with characteristic bluntness, "Policy makers have perceived the problem as one of trying to avoid paying for something that they have been accustomed to getting for free" [22].

Reasons for Lack of Policy Support for Family Caregivers

This stance has been largely unchallenged partly because the terms used to define and measure family caregiving present it as a relatively simple and straightforward set of domestic chores. These measures—activities of daily living (ADLs) and instrumental activities of daily living (IADLs)—were never intended to be applied to family caregivers but were developed in the 1960s to monitor older patients' recovery from hip fractures [23]. They were introduced into the policy world in the 1980s and have become entrenched there as well as in practice, even though they are inadequate measures of family caregiving today.

A second, related reason may be the lack of standards and requirements for team-based care and a failure to appreciate its value in nonhospital settings. Interdisciplinary teams that include social workers are more likely to respond to the psychosocial needs of both patients and family caregivers and to be attuned to environmental and socioeconomic issues that affect caregiving. Although over the last two decades interdisciplinary team-based approaches focusing on care coordination have been tested by Centers for Medicare & Medicaid Services (CMS)-sponsored research, outside of integrated healthcare plans use of interdisciplinary team-based care is relatively rare. Some innovative models of care such as Geriatric Resources for Assessment and Care of Elders (GRACE) [24] and Guided Care [25] offer examples of how interdisciplinary teams can be used to more effectively address patient and family needs.

A third reason that family caregivers are absent from policy discussions is that they are absent from insurance benefits and therefore payment schedules. Only the Medicare hospice benefit deems caregivers eligible for services. In palliative care, as in all medical practice, only the beneficiary is entitled to services, even though support for the family is acknowledged to be an essential aspect of care.

In contrast to the relative absence of recognition to family caregivers by the mainstream healthcare sector, policy and practice in the long-term services and supports (LTSS) sector have had a longer and somewhat better, although still uneven, track record. Most state Medicaid programs provide a wide range of LTSS to the Medicaid-eligible population, primarily through home- and community-based waiver programs. These services are generally recognized to benefit not only consumers with disabilities but also, indirectly, their caregivers.

Despite the lack of caregiver support benefits, the key role of family caregiving has been documented in the federal research agenda for LTSS over the past several decades. For example, special surveys of caregivers of the Medicare population were conducted as part of the National Long-Term Care Survey (NLTCS), a nationally representative survey fielded in various years from 1982 to 2004. (The National Health and Aging Trends Study, its successor, released its first data in 2012.) In part the NLTCS research led to the creation of the National Family Caregiver Support Program under the Older Americans Act in 2000. Although the legislation recognized the importance of providing federal assistance to states to develop caregiver support programs, most programs are small and poorly funded. Access to support services varies geographically. Importantly, these programs do not generally address the needs of caregivers whose family members need palliative care for serious or multiple chronic conditions.

Nonetheless policymakers anxious to control healthcare costs are beginning to recognize the value that caregivers play in care transitions from hospital to home. Eric A. Coleman, a geriatrician, has pointed out that "... in the majority of care transitions, the patient and caregiver are the only common thread between sites of care and by default have been given the added responsibility of facilitating their care transitions, often without the necessary skills or confidence to do so" [26]. The Patient Protection and Affordable Care Act (PPACA) requirement that penalizes hospitals for "excess readmissions" for certain Medicare patients is prompting hospitals to improve their discharge planning procedures. CMS has encouraged hospitals to adopt models that improve care transitions and initiate improved coordination [27]. Few of these specifically require attention to family caregiver needs, however [28].

Despite the recent intense interest in reducing hospital readmissions as a result of the PPACA provision, very few studies look at the role of family caregivers in medication reconciliation and management, follow-up appointments, and other points at which vulnerable and sick patients need assistance. In the United Hospital Fund's Transitions in Care Quality Improvement Collaborative (TC-QuIC), none of the 44 participating hospitals, home care agencies, hospices, or nursing home rehab programs had at the outset a systematic way of even identifying the family caregiver, much less assessing his or her needs. Those institutions that had electronic health records were at a disadvantage because none had a field for entering the family caregiver's name and contact information. Yet when changes were introduced, hospital readmissions decreased as did emergency room visits from a nursing home [29].

Other federal programs such as the Family and Medical Leave Act, the Medicaid home and community-based waiver program, the Social Services Block Grant program, and the Lifespan Respite Care Program offer important assistance to some families, but their scope is quite limited. Moreover, their services are generally not targeted to help caregivers whose family members have serious and advanced or complex illness. In its analysis of healthcare personnel in an aging society, the Institute of Medicine (IOM) stated that federal caregiver programs "…are generally small, poorly funded, and fragmented across the federal, state and local levels" [30].

Possible Future Actions

A number of actions should be considered by payers, providers, caregiver organizations, and the research community to improve support for family caregivers providing palliative care (Table 3.1). Some analysts and practitioners are calling for explicit adherence to principles of person- and family-centered care in implementation of federal healthcare programs—Medicare, Medicaid, and public health services, and social services programs such as the Older Americans Act. Programs designed to improve care coordination such as Accountable Care Organizations and Patient-Centered Medical Homes, as well as Community Care Transition Programs, could add explicit attention to family caregivers in their protocols.

As healthcare, social services, or LTSS programs are created or implemented and research and demonstration efforts are undertaken, the role of family caregivers should be evaluated for its potential impact on quality of care, patient healthcare outcomes, and costs, and include protocols for caregiver support. Short of having Medicare adopt a palliative care benefit, Medicare guidelines and conditions of participation for hospitals, skilled nursing facilities, and home healthcare agencies should explicitly recognize the crucial role that family caregivers play in care of persons with serious and multiple chronic conditions and bring them into the process of care at early stages. Beyond these recommendations, some policymakers are also calling for greater attention to caregiver assessment and training. For example, legislation was introduced in the 112th Congress to amend the National Family Caregiver Support Program to provide grants to states to develop standardized

Table 3.1 Recommended actions for improving support to family caregivers providing palliative care

Stakeholder category	Actions
Providers	
Hospitals, primary care physicians, home health agencies, hospice providers, integrated care systems, community-based service providers, and other health care agencies and organizations	Assure that all palliative care providers adhere to the National Quality Forum's (NQF) National Consensus Project Guidelines for Quality Palliative Care related to the role of family caregivers Assure that all entities that provide or administer services for people with advanced and serious illnesses implement patient- and family-centered protocols Develop education and training tools to identify caregiver needs and interventions for use by staff who provide services to patients with advanced and serious illnesses and their families
Payers	
Centers for Medicare & Medicaid Services, Administration on Community Living, Agency for Healthcare Research and Quality (AHRQ), state Medicaid agencies, private insurers	Assure that all entities that provide or administer services for people with advanced and serious illnesses include patient- and family-centered assessment and support protocols as a condition of receiving federal, state, and/or private funds Sponsor and encourage demonstrations and models that support implementation of palliative care and family caregiver protocols across settings and payers Explore the feasibility of payment for assessment and training for family caregivers providing palliative care Develop options for reimbursement for coordination of family-provided services for patients who are receiving palliative care Target existing federal family caregiver programs authorized by the Older Americans Act and the Lifespan Respite Act on the needs of caregivers who provide palliative care
Caregiver support organizations	
Many national organizations provide support to caregivers, including the Family Caregiver Alliance, Alzheimer's Association, National Alliance for Caregiving, and Caregiver Action Network. Also, many state and local organizations support caregivers, including area agencies on aging, developmental disability councils, centers for independent living, and departments of human or social services	Improve family caregiver knowledge about palliative care through development of various information modalities, including fact sheets, webinars, links to palliative care organizations, and outreach to employers that sponsor workplace caregiver programs Working with state and local organizations and payers, disseminate tools such as getpalliativecare.org that help family caregivers identify hospital- and community-based palliative care programs and services and assist families to access these programs and services Initiate state and community programs and meetings to improve family caregiver awareness about palliative care In collaboration with health care providers, develop programs that provide support to family caregivers who provide home-based medical care Develop/implement family caregiver assessment and training tools that focus on palliative care and management of patient transition across care settings (e.g., recognition and management of pain, nausea, constipation)

(continued)

Table 3.1 (continued)

Stakeholder category	Actions
Health research agencies and organizations	
Centers for Medicare & Medicaid, Agency for Healthcare Research and Quality, Patient-Centered Outcomes Research Institute, National Institutes of Health; Institute of Medicine, National Institute on Nursing Research	Develop research agendas that focus on gaps in knowledge about successful interventions to help caregivers assume palliative care roles including: • Specific interventions to reduce unmet caregiver needs, provide appropriate and just in time training, and to increase caregiver receptivity to palliative care services • Focus on specific underserved populations, including young caregivers and those from racial or ethnic minorities and living in rural areas Develop research on ways to improve physician–patient–caregiver communication about palliative care, including ways to ameliorate incongruent goals about levels and types of care to be delivered Conduct research on the role of family caregivers who provide home-based palliative care, including their role in medication management and home-based medical care Design and implement a national study (similar to an Institute of Medicine study panel) on the needs of family caregivers as part of the healthcare and long-term services and supports workforce including palliative care

assessments of caregiver needs and appropriate caregiver support services. IOM has recommended that public, private, and community organizations provide funding for caregiver training opportunities.

In addition, given the relatively limited amount of funding for caregiver support programs, policymakers may want to consider how to better target services available under the National Family Caregiver Support Program to meet the needs of family caregivers of the highest risk and highest cost groups—those with serious and multiple chronic conditions. Another step that may be needed is a research agenda to fill gaps in knowledge of how palliative care protocols can best meet caregiver needs. Gaps that have been identified include development of specific interventions to assist caregivers, lack of research on certain family caregiver populations, such as young caregivers and ethnic minorities, and ways to assess unmet needs [31].

Public policy needs to keep pace with addressing the realities of high cost and poor quality health care for the sickest and most vulnerable. The principles and practice of palliative care demonstrably improve quality of care and, as an epiphenomenon of this improved quality, reduce need for emergency department and hospital care. The mediator of this impact is the support provided by palliative care teams to the family caregivers, who, when well supported, can honor their loved ones wishes by caring for them at home. The opportunities are there and the time is right for increased attention, funding, and support.

References

1. Berman A. Living life in my own way—and dying that way as well. Health Aff. 2012;31(4):871–4.
2. Byock I. The best care possible: a physician's quest to transform care through the end of life. New York: Avery Books; 2012. p. 91–3.
3. Center to Advance Palliative Care. 2011 Public opinion research on palliative care. http://www.capc.org/tools-for-palliative-care-programs/marketing/public-opinion-research/2011-public-opinion-research-on-palliative-care.pdf
4. Giovanetti ER, Wolff JL. Cross-survey differences in national estimates of numbers of caregivers of disabled older adults. Milbank Q. 2011;88(3) (2010): 310-349. http://assets.aarp.org/rgcenter/ppi/ltc/i51-caregiving.pdf
5. Arno P, Levine C, Memmott MM. The economic value of informal caregiving. Health Aff. 1999;18(2):182–8.
6. National Alliance for Caregiving and AARP. Caregiving in the U.S. 2009. http://www.caregiving.org/pdf/research/Caregiving_in_the_US_2009_full_report.pdf
7. Reinhard SC, Levine C, Samis S. Home alone: family caregivers providing complex chronic care. 2012. Available at: http://www.uhfnyc.org/publications/880853
8. National Alliance for Caregiving. Evercare® Study of caregivers in decline: a close-up look at the health risks of caring for a loved one. 2006. http://www.caregiving.org/pdf/research/Caregivers%20in%20Decline%20Study-FINAL-lowres.pdf
9. Aumann K, Galinsky E, Sakai K, et al. The elder care study: everyday realities and wishes for change. New York: Families and Work Institute; 2010. http://familiesandwork.org/site/research/reports/elder_care.pdf.
10. Schulz R, Beach SR. Caregiving as a risk factor for mortality: the caregiver health effects study. JAMA. 1999;282(23):2215–9.
11. Feinberg L. Moving toward person- and family-centered care. AARP public policy institute, insight on the issues, March 2012. www.aarp.org/content/dam/aarp/research/public_policy_institute/ltc/2012/moving-towardperson-and-family-centered-care-insight-AARP-ppi-ltc.pdf
12. National Quality Forum's Framework for Hospice and Palliative Care. National Consensus Project. http://www.nationalconsensusproject.org/DisplayPage.aspx?Title=Downloads; NQF, Endorsement summary: palliative care and end-of-life care measures. http://www.qualityforum.org/News_And_Resources/Endorsement_Summaries/Endorsement_Summaries.aspx
13. The Joint Commission. Advanced Certification for Palliative Care Programs. http://www.jointcommission.org/certification/palliative_care.aspx
14. Tse Man Wah D. Care for the family in palliative care, Palliative Medicine Doctors' Meeting, HKSPM Newsletter April and August 2007.
15. Hudson PL et al. Family caregivers and palliative care: current status and agenda for the future. J Palliat Med. 2011;14(7):864–9.
16. Brumley RD, Enguidanos S, Cherin DA. Effectiveness of a home-based palliative care program for end-of-life. J Palliat Med. 2003;6(5):715–24.
17. Teno JM et al. Family perspectives on end-of-life care at the last place of care. In: Meier DE, Isaacs SL, Hughes RG, editors. Palliative care: transforming the care of serious illness. Princeton: Robert Wood Johnson Foundation; 2009.
18. Hudson PL et al. Meeting the supportive needs of family caregivers in palliative care: challenges for health professionals. J Palliat Med. 2004;7(1):19–25.
19. Steinhauser, KE et al. Factors considered important at the end of life by patients, family, physicians, and other care providers. In: Diane E. Meier, Stephen L. Isaacs, Robert G. Hughes (eds) Palliative care: transforming the care of serious illness. Robert Wood Johnson Foundation: 2009.
20. Cherlin E et al. Communication between physicians and family caregivers about care at the end of life: when do discussions occur and what is said? J Palliat Med. 2005;8(6):1176–85.
21. Levine C, Zuckerman C. The trouble with families: toward an ethic of accommodation. Ann Intern Med. 1999;130(2):148–52.

22. Vladeck B. You can't get there from here: dimensions of caregiving and dementias of policy-making. In: Levine C, editor. Family caregivers on the job: moving beyond ADLs and IADLs. New York: United Hospital Fund; 2004. p. 124.
23. Reinhard SC. The work of caregiving: What do ADLs and IADLs tell us? In: Levine C, editor. Family caregivers on the job: moving beyond ADLs and IADLs. New York: United Hospital Fund; 2004. p. 37–66.
24. Counsell SR et al. Geriatric Resources for Assessment and Care of Elders (GRACE): a new model of primary care for low-income seniors. J Am Geriatr Soc. 2006;54(7):1136–41.
25. Wolff JL, Rand-Giovanetti E, Palmer S, et al. Caregiving and chronic care: the guided care program for families and friends. J Gerontol A Biol Sci Med Sci. 2009;64(7):785–91.
26. Coleman EA. Falling through the cracks: challenges and opportunities for improving transitional care for persons with continuous complex care needs. J Am Geriatr Soc. 2003;5(4):549–55.
27. Centers for Medicare & Medicaid Services (CMS). Medicare Program: hospital inpatient prospective payment systems for acute care hospitals and the long-term care hospital prospective payment system and fy2012 rates; hospitals' FTE resident caps for graduate medical education payment. Federal Register, vol. 76, no. 160, August 18, 2011. Final Rule. Hospital Readmission Reduction Program rule begins on page 51660. http://www.gpo.gov/fdsys/pkg/FR-2011-08-18/pdf/2011-19719.pdf
28. Gibson JH, Kelley KA, Kaplan AK. Family caregiving and transitional care: a critical review. 2012. Family caregiver alliance. http://caregiver.org/caregiver/jsp/content/pdfs/FamilyCGing_andTransCare_CR_FINAL10.29.2012.pdf
29. Levine C, Halper DE, Rutberg JL, Gould DA. Engaging families as partners in transitions. New York: United Hospital Fund, 2013. http://www.uhfnyc.org/publication/880905
30. Institute of Medicine (IOM). Patients and informal caregivers (Chapter 6). In: Retooling for an aging America, building the health care workforce; 2008. Washington, DC: The National Academies Press. www.nap.edu/openbook.php?record_id=12089&page=241
31. Hudson PL et al. Research priorities associated with family caregivers in palliative care: international perspectives. J Palliat Med. 2011;14(4):397–401.

Part II
Settings for the Care of the Seriously Ill

Chapter 4
This Is Your Life: Achieving a Comprehensive, Person-Centered Model of Care at the Intersection of Policy, Politics, and Private Sector Innovation

Brad Stuart and Andrew L. MacPherson

Case Narrative

Mary woke to the familiar blare of sirens. It was her third 911 call this month. Once again, heart failure had filled her lungs with fluid. Strapped to the cold steel gurney as the ambulance jolted toward the hospital, she felt the nylon cutting into the skin of her forearms. She tried to speak, but no sound came out. Instead her teeth clenched on a hard plastic tube that jutted down her windpipe. A ventilator hissed, pumping cold air into her lungs. That was a good thing; she was too tired to breathe. Only 5 days ago as she left the hospital in a wheelchair, the cardiologist had teased her, "See you soon." What did he know about how she starved for air, so exhausted that she could not walk to the bathroom?

Mary spent 3 long days in the intensive care unit before they got her off the ventilator, out of the ICU, and out to the medical ward. Soon she could go back home. But how long, she wondered, before the nightmare started all over again?

Then Dr. Bryce, a palliative care specialist, stopped by her room. Mary talked about her family, how frazzled her husband and adult children had become, how their savings were running out. Dr. Bryce recommended medication for Mary's pain and breathing trouble. Then she recommended hospice. No one had brought this up before. Mary said no. She needed time to think about her situation—and her life.

B. Stuart, M.D. (✉)
Advanced Care Innovation Strategies (ACIStrategies),
5912 Anderson Road, Forestville, CA 95436, USA
e-mail: brad@acistrategies.com

A.L. MacPherson
Healthsperien, LLC, Washington, DC, USA

As Dr. Bryce left the hospital room, she said, "Tomorrow morning I'm bringing someone from our Advanced Illness Management team. We call it AIM. They'll start seeing you here in the hospital, and then visit you after you get back home."

Lynn, an AIM nurse, showed up the next morning with Dr. Bryce, who announced, "Lynn and I are on the same team. Actually, so are you."

Instead of making her come to the hospital for care, they told Mary how they would bring care to her home. "We need to learn what you want in your own life, not just in your medical treatment," said Lynn. "Then we'll design your care to help you live the life you choose."

"Great," said Mary. "But I live half my life in the hospital. I don't choose that—it chooses me."

"Maybe we can break that cycle," Lynn replied.

Two days later, Mary went home with the usual stack of prescriptions and discharge instructions. The next day a nurse and social worker from AIM rang her doorbell. They sorted out her medications and doctor's appointments. They taught her what symptoms to watch for so she could prevent the 911 calls. Then they helped her figure out what she wanted in her own life: to be as independent as she could, see her grandkids every week, and get a ride to church each Sunday. Suddenly, instead of trying to "do what the doctor says," she felt the support of a team she trusted.

Over the next few weeks, they discussed what might happen as her life neared its end. These conversations took place at Mary's own pace without any pressure or arm twisting. She learned to articulate her needs and preferences so her family knew exactly what she wanted: to stay safe and comfortable at home. By her own choice, she never went back to the hospital.

After several weeks in the AIM program, Mary decided to enroll in hospice. When the end of her life finally came, she was at home in peace, comfort, and dignity, surrounded by the people she loved.

Changing the Status Quo by Promoting Personal Engagement

"Usual care" for people with advanced illness in the United States is often episodic, crisis-driven, and hospital-based. The Institute of Medicine (IOM) recently reported that Americans want to know all their healthcare options, wish their care to be coordinated, and seek to be actively engaged with their clinicians. However, there is a wide gap between what Americans want and what they get from the nation's fragmented healthcare system [1].

Engaging people with serious illness in their own care produces better clinical outcomes and more satisfaction with care decisions [2]. Personal engagement helps them avoid treatment they do not want, which in turn benefits society by preventing unwanted utilization of healthcare services and associated costs [3].

This chapter proposes concepts of person-centered care that have bipartisan appeal, and examines new care models that operationalize them. However, successful innovation today does not guarantee future sustainability. These new models will die on the vine without the support of federal policy initiatives that remove obstacles to more coordinated, person-centered care. Therefore we explore bipartisan principles that can stimulate policy change, promote robust political strategy, and foster constructive messaging. We outline a combined clinical and policy plan that can result in meaningful and lasting health system change. This strategy can support the quality, effectiveness, and sustainability of federal entitlement programs, and beyond that, American economic viability.

Private Sector Solutions: A Clinical Model of Person-Centered Advanced Illness Care

Innovative programs like Advanced Illness Management (AIM®) at Sutter Health and Aetna's Compassionate Care® help people with advanced illness navigate the complex US health system so that they get only the care they want and need. AIM reports that over the 30-day period following enrollment, compared to the 30 days before, hospitalizations were reduced by 68 %. Sutter System internal financial analysis showed that, accounting for all inpatient direct care cost savings and revenue foregone by preventing admissions, as well as net costs and savings to physicians, home health, and hospice, the system basically broke even. However, from the payor standpoint, and after accounting for program costs, Medicare realized savings of over $2,000 per enrollee per month extending past 90 days post enrollment [4]. Days in intensive care were reduced by over 70 % and physician office visits were cut in half. Patient and physician satisfaction scores were excellent.

The services of programs like AIM and Compassionate Care are accepted enthusiastically by patients, families, and physicians. They enhance quality of life and quality of care and in so doing reduce cost by moving the focus of care for advanced chronic illness out of the hospital and into home and community. Most importantly, they reduce hospitalization not by rationing, but by following the preferences and meeting the needs of *persons* with advanced illness, so that they do not have to become *patients* in ambulances, ERs, ICUs, and hospitals unless they need or choose to do so.

Unifying principles and practices distilled from palliative care, the Wagner chronic illness schema [5], the Naylor [6] and Coleman [7] transition models, and disease management, these services coordinate care across space (settings including hospital, physician office, home, and community) and time (tracking evolving personal care preferences from diagnosis of serious illness through the end of life). AIM and similar programs transcend the artificial distinction between "treatable" and "terminal" illness and, as a fortunate side benefit, reduce utilization and cost, primarily by meeting needs at home and thus preventing crises that lead to hospitalization.

For example, the AIM model provides:

- A customized mix of curative and comfort care
- Seamless care transitions from hospital to home
- Extension of palliative care from inpatient to ambulatory settings

- Education, counseling, and support for people with advanced illness, their loved ones, and their caregivers
- Advance care planning in real time, at the ill person's own pace, in the comfort and safety of home
- An expanded range of home services to provide practical support to family and paid caregivers
- Crisis prevention through real-time communication and self-management
- Free choice of care options in all settings and at all times

The population eligible for Sutter Health's AIM Program consists of people with multiple chronic illnesses, including but not limited to metastatic cancer, heart failure, chronic lung disease, diabetes with end-organ dysfunction, neurological illness, or geriatric frailty syndrome; over half will have two or more diagnoses. In addition, advanced chronic illness is characterized by one or more of the following factors [8, 9]:

- Evidence of progressive clinical decline, e.g., multiple diagnosis-related subspecialty and ED visits and hospitalizations
- Questionable response to disease-modifying treatment, e.g., inadequate response to cancer chemotherapy
- Progressively reduced functional and or cognitive status, e.g., recent onset of dependence for activities of daily living (ADLs)
- Progressively reduced nutritional status, e.g., significant non-intentional weight loss

Many, but not all, candidates for programs like AIM would be eligible for hospice, but instead they choose to continue potentially life-prolonging treatment, or they (and/or their family or physicians) are unwilling to consider hospice enrollment. However, unlike hospice, palliative care and advanced care do not use life expectancy but rely on need as the criterion for enrollment. Clinicians are unable, and often unwilling, to predict prognosis as is required for hospice eligibility [10]. Although people with advanced illness must eventually come to terms with the fact that life expectancy may be limited, in the AIM program this is not discussed until the ill person wants to talk about it.

Trained interdisciplinary teams of nurses, social workers and others, under the direction of a physician, form the backbone of the AIM model [11]. Team members, who communicate in real time via electronic health record (EHR) or conventional methods, are stationed in major care settings:

- Hospital: AIM care managers interface with hospitalists, specialists, emergency staff, case managers, discharge planners, inpatient and ambulatory palliative care teams, and others. They assess and enroll patients, initiating transition processes that will continue when the ill person returns to their residence in the community
- Physician office: AIM care managers are embedded in large medical groups to consult directly with physicians and office/clinic staff, and to provide telemanagement support
- Call centers: AIM care telemanagers with access to the EHR provide 24/7 coverage
- Home: AIM teams provide high-touch home visits as needed

Core duties and responsibilities of the AIM team include transition management; goal setting and advance care planning; ensuring follow-up appointments; medication reconciliation and management; critical symptom recognition, self-management, and reporting; and crisis planning and prevention. Close relationships with attending physicians, particularly primary care doctors, are critical. Many physicians report that the AIM staff is "their" team.

Continuous performance improvement and program sustainability are supported by data gathering, aggregation, analysis and reporting systems. Valid and accurate measurement of utilization and costs in all settings is critical. Calculation of net savings to both providers and payers from program enrollment, accounting for all revenue and costs including reimbursement lost to the hospital through avoided hospitalizations, is particularly important.

Person-Centered Advanced Illness Care and Provider Integration

Implementing the advanced care model connects providers in all clinical settings, promoting clinical integration to facilitate accountable care [12]. Because of AIM team support, hospitals, physician groups, home-based care, and community services automatically integrate their activities and communications, which

- Develops systems out of disparate provider groups
- Promotes care management interventions for the larger chronically ill population
- Incentivizes adoption of beneficial technology, e.g., EHRs
- Builds the foundation for shared risk/shared savings arrangements that will eventually supersede fee-for-service reimbursement

In this scenario, advanced care implementation can help providers form "virtual ACOs" that can help them move from fragmented fee-for-service billing toward shared risk/shared savings reimbursement. Early-adopter organizations can lead by designing, implementing, and testing innovative advanced care models. Data from these efforts can then be used to drive policy change. Through an action network, leading organizations could bootstrap the process of clinical integration and accelerate the pace of healthcare reform significantly. Collaboration among health systems, health services research, CMS/HHS, and Congress would support this movement.

Personal Choice and Responsibility: A Bipartisan Foundation for Reform

Modern medicine offers a growing array of treatment options to individuals with advanced chronic illness. But this care comes at a high cost, both financially and personally, without any assurance that life will be extended in ways that are personally meaningful to people who undergo these treatments [13]. A *patient* may receive "appropriate care," but it may not feel this way to the *person* living inside the patient identity.

"Patient-centered care" has become a mantra for health system reformers. However, the *patient* may undergo treatment that adheres to the highest standards of clinical practice, while the *person* suffers at the hands of clinicians who never think to inquire whether the person actually wants this kind of "care." This "preference misdiagnosis" is a powerful but unacknowledged cause of overtreatment and rising costs [14].

Personal choice should become a more fundamental reform concept than "patient choice." "Patient-centered care" is actually a provider-centric construct. It focuses on things like clinician behavior and hospital utilization, but ignores the fact that *persons* might not choose to be *patients* at all if they could avoid it. Thus "patient-centered" thinking misses opportunities to promote choice, improve quality, and reduce costs.

Advancing illness does not necessarily require repeated hospitalization. New care models can help even the sickest people remain safe and comfortable at home. Decades of hospice, and more recent experience with palliative care, clearly demonstrate the ability of these models to improve quality, satisfaction and survival, and as a result, to reduce occurrence of crisis hospitalization. What we need now is universal access to a new kind of care for people who, because they want to continue treatment or because they are not ready to self-identify as the "dying," and therefore do not fit into the narrow confines of hospice eligibility.

Personal choice is a complex, iterative, and evolving process that includes eliciting critical aspects of the person's inner world, contemplating and discussing them, and finally making healthcare decisions solidly based on what matters most to each individual. Healthcare choices are driven by values, feelings, cultural influences, perceptions of family desires, and other factors that the person may not consciously recognize. Standard "one-shot" discussions in hospital or office may not yield a viable plan that stands up to the passage of time, the challenges of illness progression, and changing personal circumstances. Decision making that proceeds at the person's own pace, over time as illness advances, in a setting where that person feels safe and secure, can provide better results.

A natural complement to personal choice in advanced illness is *personal responsibility*. People with chronic conditions are now taught to self-manage certain aspects of their care. Beyond this, however, they should make explicit choices about their future care while their mental and emotional clarity and competence remain intact. When providers ignore the foreseeable or continue with disease treatment on autopilot, the crises that inevitably result can force difficult choices on loved ones. The resulting emotional trauma and burden can be heavy and long-lasting. Moreover, some families push for intensive treatment that the ill person would not have chosen while competent. After advancing illness renders these people powerless to resist, physicians may succumb to family pressure to initiate treatment. In situations where no one helps people to articulate what matters most to them, the system defaults to aggressive and costly hospital treatment, independent of the likelihood of benefit or what matters most to the person and their family.

Advance care planning over time can prevent these mishaps. Personal responsibility on the part of persons who are ill and their providers therefore benefits loved ones, the community, and society.

Political and Policy Challenges to Achieving High-Quality, Comprehensive Advanced Illness Care

Political Challenges

Until the passage of the *Affordable Care Act* (ACA) in March 2010, the promise of healthcare reform had remained unfulfilled. The reason is simple: Health care is a deeply personal issue. In politics, healthcare reform becomes a crucible for conflicting feelings about self and physical being, family, community, responsibility, and the impact of government on all these. In today's partisan environment, a functional healthcare debate can turn quickly into an exchange of highly emotional political rhetoric. When personal mortality is added to this highly charged mix, rational discussion can degenerate into a race to the rhetorical bottom, where political toxicity stymies progress.

Policymakers exercise a complex calculus of risk and reward to determine their priorities. They evaluate many factors, including personal values, issue objectives, constituent (especially likely voter) needs and desires, state or district economic interests, and of course the potential for both personal and issue success. When an issue carries potential risk without any counterbalancing reward, policymakers may have no choice but to back away. Any momentum toward positive change then stalls or evaporates completely.

Just such a seismic shift occurred in December 2010 following the enactment of the ACA. The law granted the Secretary of Health and Human Services (HHS) authority to support innovative delivery reforms to achieve the "triple aim" of improving care and population health while constraining cost growth. Expansion of access to doctor-patient conversation about advanced care planning and care management clearly had the potential to contribute to this goal.

However, novel suggestions for care of advanced illness were suppressed by blowback from the rancorous debate over the ACA. Opponents of the law sought to marry the concepts of advanced care planning with fears of rationing and big government [15]. When the Obama administration allowed regulations that permitted voluntary advanced care planning consults to occur as part of the annual Medicare exam [16], press reports asserted that the Administration was trying by stealth to reinsert the same language that had originally promoted "death panel" rhetoric [17]. With no visible stakeholder support and no bipartisan champions to provide cover, the Administration was forced to make a risk/reward decision. The policy was abandoned a few days later.

Ironically, when Americans are asked whether they would support federal policy interventions to ensure access to services provided in a person-centered, comprehensive advanced or palliative care model, they unequivocally embrace this, just as they support components of the law itself despite confusion about it as a whole [18–20].

Policy Challenges

Despite significant local, state, regional, and even federal innovations in advanced illness care delivery, Federal policy barriers inhibit dissemination of innovations developed within leading health systems, health plans, and academic centers. Examples include lack of federal coverage for care management services that would ameliorate health system fragmentation (and conversely, current law that promotes and incentivizes fragmented care); regulations that inhibit innovation by limiting scope of practice and preventing full collaboration across provider settings; payment incentives in fee-for-service Medicare that encourage volume of services with no relationship to quality or outcomes; and failure to update a delivery system that is designed to treat acute, rather than chronic, conditions.

The current Federal debate over debt and deficit reduction presents unique challenges to advocates working to improve person-centered and person-determined care during serious illness. While Medicare expenditures are currently growing at a historically low rate (less than GDP per capita [21]), higher growth rates are projected outside the 10-year Congressional Budget Office (CBO) window [22]. Even so, in the short term, the dollar amount and percentage of federal Medicare investment will increase from $550 billion and 15.4 % respectively in 2013 to over $1 trillion and 19.3 % by 2022 [23]. Congress will continue to be in the hunt for policy "savers," or legislative interventions that will constrain the growth of federal healthcare outlays over a 10-year period.

Innovative, person-centered advanced or palliative care models should help achieve savings, not just to the federal government but to all payers, including insurers, provider groups, hospitals, state and local governments, and, as importantly consumers. However, this creates a rhetorical paradox for advocates of such interventions. Targeting the costs accrued by people with advanced illness, a cohort that represents high potential for savings, is easily mislabeled by opponents of reform as rationing of care by big government.

Legislative and Regulatory Proposals to Improve Advanced Illness Care

Federal legislative and regulatory action on improving advanced illness care has been limited over the past several congresses, with a few notable exceptions. The *Medicare Modernization Act of 2003*, which created the Medicare Part D prescription drug benefit, also provided for a "welcome to Medicare" assessment for all new beneficiaries, including a voluntary advanced care planning consultation by a physician

[24]. In 2009, several bills were introduced to expand access to AIM and palliative and hospice services. Senator Jay Rockefeller (D-W.Va.) and Congressman Earl Blumenauer (D-Ore.) introduced legislation that would expand physician services to include Medicare and Medicaid coverage of advanced care planning, advanced directive discussions, and expansion of palliative and hospice benefits [25]. In 2013, Congressman Blumenauer reintroduced this legislation with bipartisan support [26]. In the 111th and 112th Congresses, Senator Mark Warner (D-Va.) introduced the *Senior Navigation and Planning Act*, which provides for the reimbursement of advanced care management and coordination services in Medicare, and more recently the similar *Care Planning Act*, along with Senator Johnny Isakson (R-Ga.), that not only establishes reimbursement for "Advanced Illness Planning and Coordination," but also require the Center for Medicare and Medicaid Innovation to an begin a 5-year "Advanced Illness Coordination Services (AICS) Project" demonstration to assess and test this model[1] [27, 28].

The early legislative proposals faced stiff political headwinds. However, the momentum may be shifting as healthcare stakeholders and innovators in the private sector recognize the importance of addressing the needs of this population, joined by bipartisan members of both houses of Congress, creating a foundation for new federal policy.

The Path Forward: Political Consensus and Policy Initiatives to Scale Up Private Sector Innovation

Three important dimensions must be addressed to bolster federal support for system change: (1) Policy; (2) Process; and (3) Partnerships.

Potentially viable *policy* proposals include coverage of advanced care planning services in Medicare and Medicaid, expanded hospice service options including removal of concurrent care exclusions and extension of the hospice 6-month survival requirement, expansion of federal coverage of palliative care services, quality improvement and measurement incenting delivery of quality palliative care, and redesign of post-acute care benefits. New policy must be targeted to a defined population, scorable by independent analysts and the CBO, and supported by key opinion leaders. Policy initiatives must be well constructed and thoughtfully designed to withstand scrutiny from public and private stakeholders that will validate them.

Second, attention to *process* is critical. Policy is a multidimensional strategic product of many pathways, each strewn with its own set of navigational obstacles. Both legislative and regulatory processes must contend with power mechanisms, gatekeepers, champions, committees, leadership, vehicles, and individual personalities.

Legislative champions must decide strategically to make improvement of advanced care their personal political and policy priority. These members will lobby

---

[1] These are just two of the most visible recent legislative proposals intended to improve advanced illness care. Many more such bills have been introduced, but an analysis of their design and impact is beyond the scope of this chapter

colleagues, committee members, and chairpersons, collaborate with key stakeholder groups, and take necessary steps to move the initiative forward, usually attaching their bill to a larger moving vehicle related to health care rather than introducing "stand-alone" legislation.[2] Support must be enlisted from the chairman of the Senate Finance Committee, which has jurisdiction over Titles 18 and 19 of the Social Security Act governing Medicare and Medicaid respectively, as well as Congressional leadership.

Finally, crafting of successful public policy relies on strategic *partnerships* that can accommodate opposition from other policymakers and outside interest groups. This is especially important for advanced and palliative care, given its political sensitivity. Bipartisanship is essential and must be built upon, as are broad-based coalition partnerships that include all interested stakeholder groups, e.g., providers, plans, advocacy organizations, consumers, employers, and faith-based organizations. These groups contribute analytical and messaging support to provide policymakers the political validation they need to publicly address the advanced care issue.[3]

Potential Winning Message: Comprehensive, Person-Centered Advanced Illness Care

Political and policy initiatives are either fueled by supportive public opinion or abandoned for lack of it. A robust and persuasive public message is critical to the success of advanced care.

The core message must be that personal priorities drive the care plan. The advanced care model rests on the core principle of palliative care, placing the person at the center of the decision making process, neutralizing claims of rationing or government control. Hospitalizations are avoided because they are unwanted and unnecessary as proactive measures avert crises that would otherwise have led to a call to 911. Unwanted and unnecessary admissions constitute medical waste, which most reasonable people agree should be eliminated.

Free choice, however, is not enough. Responsibility is also important on individual and societal levels. Persons who are ill and their providers are responsible for timely decisions about care priorities so that loved ones are spared from having to make hard choices without clear guidance from their loved one, and so that clinicians do not feel compelled to "do everything" because they cannot know what a seriously ill but unresponsive or non-communicative patient might have wanted.

---

[2] With some exceptions, Congress typically moves major legislative vehicles by issue area—tax, appropriations, health care, etc. Policy pertaining to advanced care would likely "ride" on one of these major moving vehicles.

[3] An example is the Coalition to Transform Advanced Care (C-TAC). Formed in 2011, C-TAC represents a broad cross-section of health care stakeholders, including payers, providers, business, consumers, faith-based groups, and many others. C-TAC and groups like it play an important role in providing stakeholder "cover" to advance policymaking on this issue.

Responsibility in turn is linked with accountability, a guiding principle of healthcare reform. Providers must become accountable for both the quality of care they provide and its costs. In serious and advanced illness, quality is inextricably linked with personal priorities and responsibility for decision making. Cost savings benefit society by strengthening Medicare's sustainability and ensuring that care goes to those who really benefit according to valid and reliable evidence. This reinforces healthcare reform's intention to provide real value.

The advanced care model of palliative care delivery, and policy that supports its broad-based implementation, provide for more, not fewer, services that individuals want and need to honor their values and preferences, with a greater emphasis on access to care in the home setting and expanded coordination of social and medical services. Access to traditional care will not be reduced, and beneficial services will not be denied at the whim of payers or the government. Large-scale implementation of a truly person-centered care model requires that Medicare coverage continues for all currently guaranteed services.

Conclusion

In the opening vignette, Mary found that her treatment, and indeed the quality of her day-to-day life, changed dramatically when her providers aligned her care plan with her own priorities and wishes. Healthcare reform should include new care models that focus explicitly on this process. Meaningful delivery reform and relatively non-controversial cost containment can be achieved by providing new services that maximize support for each person's responsibility to expressing their own priorities and preferences and then organizing the delivery system to honor and implement them. Private sector innovations supported by accurate and clear messaging, thoughtful policy development, public engagement in the political process, and robust strategic partnerships can all be combined to change the standards of practice for this vulnerable population, and to create lasting system change.

References

1. Novelli WD, Halvorsen GC, Santa J. Recognizing an opinion: findings from the IOM Evidence Communication Innovation Collaborative. JAMA. 2012;308:1531–2.
2. O'Connor AM, Wennberg JE, Legare F, et al. Toward the "tipping point:" decision aids and informed patient choice. Health Aff (Millwood). 2007;26:716–25.
3. Milstein A, Shortell S. Innovations in care delivery to slow the growth of US health care spending. JAMA. 2012;308:1439–40.
4. Labson MC, Sacco MM, Weissman D, Gornet B, Stuart B. Innovative models of home-based palliative care. Cleveland Clin J Med. 2013;80(eSuppl 1):eS30–5.
5. Wagner EH, Austin BT, Davis C, et al. Improving chronic illness care: translating evidence into action. Health Aff. 2001;20:64–78.

6. Naylor MD, Brooten DA, Campbell RL, et al. Transitional care of older adults hospitalized with heart failure: a randomized controlled trial. J Am Geriatr Soc. 2004;52:675–84.
7. Coleman EA, Parry C, Chalmers S, Min SJ. The care transitions intervention: results of a randomized controlled trial. Arch Intern Med. 2006;166:1822–8.
8. Salpeter SR, Malter DS, Luo EJ, Lin AY, Stuart B. Systematic review of cancer presentations with a median survival of six months or less. J Palliat Med. 2012;15:175–85.
9. Salpeter SR, Luo EJ, Malter DS, Stuart B. Systematic review of non-cancer presentations with a median survival of 6 months or less. Am J Med. 2011;125(5):512.e1–6. Epub 2011 Oct 24.
10. Lamont EB, Christakis NA. Complexities in prognostication in advanced cancer: "to help them live the lives the way they want to". JAMA. 2003;290:98–104.
11. Wynia MK, Von Kohorn I, Mitchell PH. Challenges at the intersection of team-based and patient-centered health care: insights from an IOM working group. JAMA. 2012;308: 1327–8.
12. Crosson FJ. 21st-century health care: the case for integrated delivery systems. N Engl J Med. 2009;361:1324–5.
13. Calfo S, Smith J, Zezza M. Last year of life study. Centers for Medicare & Medicaid Services; 2008. Available at http://www.cms.gov/Research-Statistics-Data-and-Systems/Research/ActuarialStudies/Last_Year_of_Life.html. Accessed 26 Nov 2012.
14. Mulley AG, Trimble C, Elwyn G. Stop the silent misdiagnosis: patient preferences matter. BMJ. 2012;345:e6572.
15. Kaiser Family Foundation. Kaiser health tracking poll, March 2010. Key findings. p. 6–8. http://www.kff.org/kaiserpolls/upload/8285-F.pdf
16. Medicare Program; Amendment to Payment Policies Under the Physician Fee Schedule and Other Revisions to Part B for CY 2011. Federal Register. 2011;76(6). 42 CFR Part 410.
17. Pear R. Obama returns to end-of-life plan that caused stir. New York Times; 25 Dec 2010. Accessed 2 Jan 2013. http://www.nytimes.com/2010/12/26/us/politics/26death.html?pagewanted=all
18. Kaiser Family Foundation. Kaiser Health tracking poll. Key findings; Nov 2011.
19. National Journal and The Regence Foundation. Living well at the end of life poll; Feb 2011. http://syndication.nationaljournal.com/communications/NationalJournalRegenceToplines.pdf
20. Center to Advance Palliative Care Public Opinion Poll. Accessed 20 July 2013. http://www.capc.org/tools-for-palliative-care-programs/marketing/public-opinion-research/2011-public-opinion-research-on-palliative-care.pdf
21. The Urban Institute. Medicare, medicaid and the deficit debate. p. 6; April 2012. http://www.urban.org/UploadedPDF/412544-Medicare-Medicaid-and-the-Deficit-Debate.pdf
22. Manchester J. CBO's long-term projections for medicare and medicaid spending in the United States. Congressional Budget Office; Nov 2012. http://www.cbo.gov/sites/default/files/cbofiles/attachments/11-30-2012-OECD_Presentation.pdf
23. Congressional Budget Office (CBO). The 2012 long-term budget outlook; June 2012. http://www.cbo.gov/sites/default/files/cbofiles/attachments/06-05-Long-Term_Budget_Outlook_2.pdf
24. 42 USC. §1395x(ww)(3) and 42 CFR 410.16(a).
25. H.R. 3962 as passed by the House of Representatives, section 1223; 2009.
26. Blumenauer Introduces Bill to Modernize Medicare Advance-Care Planning. Accessed 25 July 2013. http://blumenauer.house.gov/index.php?option=com_content&view=article&id=2187
27. Senator Mark Warner. Senior navigation and planning act. http://thomas.loc.gov/cgi-bin/bdquery/D?d112:16:./temp/~bdNB38::
28. Sens. Warner and Isakson Introduce Bipartisan Care Planning Act of 2013. Access 2 Aug 2013. http://www.isakson.senate.gov/public/index.cfm/news-releases?ID=010950ec-7cbd-414f-87e5-19c309524b4b

Chapter 5
Hospice and Healthcare Reform: What Is the Optimal Path?

Melissa D. Aldridge and Jean S. Kutner

Hospice is a model consistent with the country's stated healthcare reform goals: hospice is person centered, improves clinical outcomes such as pain and satisfaction, uses a multidisciplinary care team, is coordinated across settings, reduces unnecessary hospitalizations, and saves healthcare dollars [1–7]. Studies have consistently demonstrated that hospice improves quality for patients and families by reducing symptom distress, improving caregiver outcomes, and, if used continuously, reducing hospitalizations near the end of life, including emergency department visits and intensive care unit stays and hospital death [3, 6, 8–10]. Hospice care in the United States is growing, and there is much to celebrate in terms of the increase in the number of hospice agencies, the number of patient and family beneficiaries of hospice care, and the diversity of conditions and diagnoses being served by hospice [11]. In 2011, there were more than 3,500 hospice providers—an increase of 53 % from 2000—caring for 1.2 million Medicare beneficiaries at a cost of $13.8 billion [12]. Ninety-eight percent of the US population lives close enough to a hospice to receive care (Fig. 5.1) [13].

Although an estimated 40 % of all deaths in the US are under the care of a hospice program [14], hospice length of stay is often short with 36 % of hospice users receiving less than 1 week of hospice care prior to death [11]. A recent analysis of Medicare beneficiaries found that more people are dying at home with hospice services at the same time as hospital and intensive care unit stays in the last month of life just prior to hospice referral have increased, and multiple transitions across healthcare settings near the end of life are occurring [15].

M.D. Aldridge, Ph.D., M.B.A. (✉)
Brookdale Department of Geriatrics and Palliative Medicine, Icahn School of Medicine at Mount Sinai, One Gustave L. Levy Place, New York, NY 10029, USA
e-mail: melissa.aldridge@mssm.edu

J.S. Kutner, M.D., M.S.P.H.
Department of Medicine, University of Colorado School of Medicine,
Aurora, CO, USA

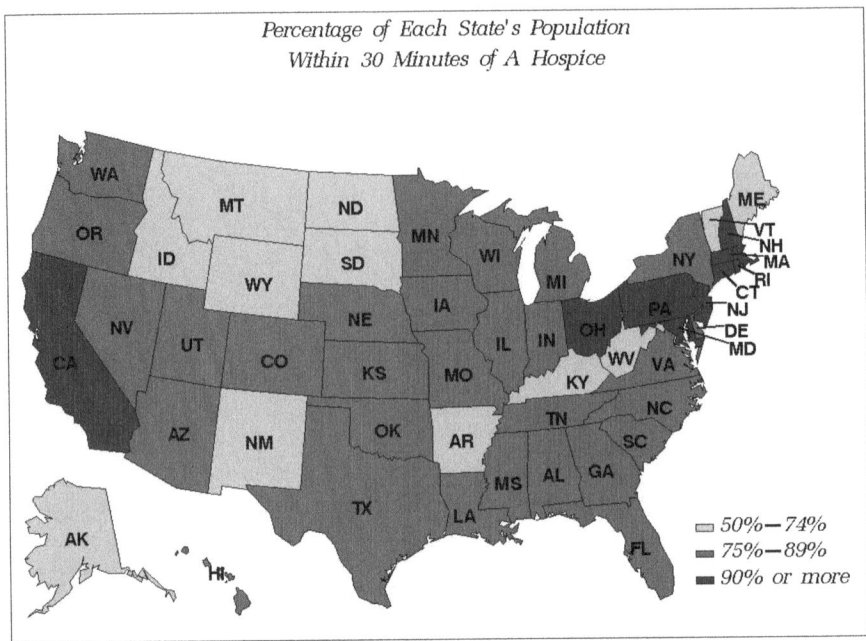

Fig. 5.1 Percentage of each state's population residing within 30 min of a Medicare certified hospice in 2008

The statutory eligibility restrictions of the Medicare Hospice Benefit (MHB) are viewed as a barrier to the use of hospice, leading to calls for eliminating the requirement to give up disease-modifying therapies or the 6-month prognostic criterion [16–19]. The goal is to improve access to hospice care by both increasing the rate of referral and increasing hospice length of stay through earlier referral.

The purpose of this chapter is to delineate the implications of various policy options for improving access to high quality care near the end of life.

The Origins of Hospice

Hospice care in the United States began in the 1970s as a social movement that focused on an alternative to the hospital setting, where dying patients often suffered from significant pain and discomfort, and patients and families did not receive the emotional and spiritual support necessary to cope during the dying process [20]. Hospice was originally provided by "charitable" [20] and "charismatic" [21] leaders working individually or through nonprofit community-based agencies, caring for patients in their own homes and relying on charitable donations as the sole revenue source. Despite growing support in the early 1970s for hospice, the concept (comfort rather than curative care), setting (home rather than hospital care), and focus (person and family centeredness rather than a medical model) of hospice care were still considered experimental in nature.

The passing of the Tax Equity and Fiscal Responsibility Act (TEFRA) in 1982 marked a critical turning point for hospice, enabling Medicare reimbursement for hospice services. The number of Medicare certified hospices rapidly increased from 45 in 1983 to 814 in 1989. A 20 % increase in reimbursement rates as part of the Omnibus Reconciliation Act of 1989 [22] resulted in more than 2,500 [12] new Medicare certified hospice agencies including for-profit hospice agencies, which increased from only 5 % of all hospices in 1990 [23, 24] to an estimated 60 % of agencies by 2011 [11]. During this time, Medicare spending for hospice increased from $445 million (in 1991) to $13.8 billion (in 2011) [12], and the number of Medicare beneficiaries using hospice increased more than sixfold.

Policy Issue: Improving Access to Hospice Care

Despite growth in the number of hospice agencies and beneficiaries, the MHB remains one of Medicare's smallest programs in terms of annual spending and is used by fewer than half of Medicare beneficiaries prior to death [14]. The extent to which this percentage reflects underuse of hospice is unknown as it likely reflects a combination of regulatory barriers, patient and family preferences, and sudden or unpredictable death where there is no time to engage hospice. Potential barriers to hospice care include lack of knowledge, variable availability, and ineligibility, either because of prognostic uncertainty or need for continued disease treatment.

Some studies [25–28] suggest that lack of public awareness is a barrier to receipt and timeliness of hospice. Although hospice is available nationwide [13], there is significant geographic state-by-state variation [4, 29]. Figure 5.1 depicts the percentage of each state's population residing within 30 min of a Medicare certified hospice in 2008. Eleven states had <10 % of their population in communities >30 min from a hospice while [13] eight states had >30 % of their population >30 min from a hospice [13]. Rural areas have lower hospice availability [30] and use [31, 32] compared with urban areas.

Studies have also evaluated how the MHB eligibility criteria pose a barrier to hospice. Patients are eligible to receive hospice care under the MHB if their physician certifies that they have a life expectancy of 6 months or less if their disease follows its expected course. A number of studies suggest that prognostic uncertainty limits use of hospice [16, 19, 27, 28, 33–41]. Further, MHB enrollment requires that an individual forgoes Medicare reimbursement for ongoing disease-modifying treatment related to the terminal diagnosis, another factor limiting use of hospice [16, 19, 28, 42, 43]. As a result, policy options for increasing access to hospice focus on revising MHB eligibility criteria.

Policy Challenge: Who Is the Target Population for Hospice Care?

The central issue facing policy makers and the hospice industry is the appropriate target population for hospice care. Specifically, should hospice: (1) serve a defined population of patients with a predictably limited life expectancy who agree to forego disease-modifying treatments (current MHB); or (2) expand "upstream" to include patients with serious chronic diseases, unpredictable prognosis, and palliative care needs (symptom distress, family caregiver burden, and/or inadequate coordination and communication across the care continuum) who desire palliative and supportive services in concert with disease-modifying treatments regardless of life expectancy.

The restricted prognosis [44] and waiver of Medicare reimbursement for the "curative" treatment of the terminal condition [45] were intended to maintain control over the cost of the MHB by narrowly defining the target hospice population. The advantage of the current MHB eligibility criteria is that it retains a comprehensive benefit customized to the needs of those dying soon, including interdisciplinary care provided primarily in the home, for a targeted population within a few weeks or months of death consistent with the core mission of hospice's early founders. The disadvantages of retaining the current eligibility criteria are restricted access to hospice for the 78 % of Medicare beneficiaries with chronic non-cancer illnesses, highly uncertain and unpredictable prognoses, and continued benefit from disease-modifying treatments in terms of both quality and length of life (e.g., management of congestive heart failure is both palliative—improves quality of life—and life prolonging). In support of this concern, despite significant growth in the range of diagnoses of individuals receiving hospice care [11], prognostic difficulty (i.e., difficulty in certifying that a patient has 6 months or less to live as required by the MHB) remains a barrier to hospice referral [36, 39–41], particularly for individuals with non-cancer diagnoses. Similarly, the distinction between life prolonging and palliative treatment is increasingly meaningless as many effective life-prolonging treatments simultaneously provide symptom relief. Given the need of such patients for both expert disease management and the home- and community-based palliative support that hospice provides, restrictions on their access fail to address the needs of a growing population of Medicare beneficiaries. Further, given early indications that both palliative care and hospice may be associated with better survival [5, 46, 47], systematic exclusion of frail, multimorbid, and functionally and cognitively impaired persons with indeterminate prognoses from hospice represents a denial of evidence-based quality care.

An alternative involves shifting eligibility from a prognosis-based to a needs-based criterion with no restriction on the ability to receive Medicare reimbursement for life-prolonging treatments while receiving hospice. A needs-based criterion could be focused on patients who have some combination of serious illnesses, functional limitations, frailty, and cognitive impairment. Screening to assess need for hospice services could come at any point in the patient's disease trajectory as well as at points of care transitions, such as admission to the hospital or nursing home.

In doing so, hospice care could be integrated earlier in the course of the treatment of individuals with serious disease, and hospice services could be provided *in conjunction* with life-prolonging treatments. With a needs-based eligibility criterion, more individuals would be covered by the MHB, life-prolonging treatments and palliative care could be delivered simultaneously, and the balance of life prolonging and palliative care could occur in response to progression of disease and shifting benefit–burden ratios of medical interventions and patients' clinical needs. Hospice care would no longer be focused on the care of individuals in the last few weeks of incurable illness but would be more broadly focused on the care of individuals with serious illnesses needing multidisciplinary services. This could begin to reduce the death stigma associated with hospice enrollment, leading to earlier referral, better quality of care, quality of life, survival, and the potential for either budget neutrality or cost savings depending on the degree of resulting reduction in acute care services.

Implications of Expanding Medicare Hospice Benefit Eligibility

Expanding MHB eligibility poses substantial challenges. First, in terms of implementation, how would a "needs-based" criterion be defined? When in the course of disease would "need" be assessed? Precisely defining the target population under an expanded vision of hospice care is a nontrivial, critical first step in estimating the size, cost, and practicality of this alternative.

Second, expanding MHB eligibility has cost implications for the overall Medicare program. The number of individuals who would enroll in the MHB would likely substantially increase, increasing overall program costs. However, hospital palliative care programs have led to cost savings due to care coordination, clarified treatment goals, and the avoidance of expensive, non-beneficial treatments covered by Medicare Part A [48–50]. The extent to which expanded hospice programs would achieve similar cost savings is unknown. Expanded MHB eligibility may result in policies to reduce the comprehensiveness (and cost) of the current benefit in order to match services more precisely to needs (higher at outset and end of service, lower during periods of stability), and potentially maintain "budget neutrality." Substantial alteration of the existing MHB could cover more people in need for a longer period of time if care was taken to maintain the resource intense model needed during the last few weeks and months of life.

Third, hospices would need to retrain personnel to care for patients earlier in the course of their disease, as these patients have different medical, nursing, social, and spiritual needs that require different expertise, skills, and scope of services. This integration may be challenging for hospice clinicians to the extent that it appears to dilute hospice's focused commitment to the needs of the predictably dying. As hospice originated in a counter-cultural effort to establish an alternative to mainstream medical care, integration into mainstream medical care may require a major adjustment in hospice culture, as well as training.

Restrictive state licensure requirements would need to be adjusted. Hospice programs would need to integrate into all areas of mainstream medicine to better coordinate palliative and life-prolonging care and would need to enlarge and expand their scope of services to serve a broader population of patients.

Expanding MHB eligibility also has implications for the evolving structure of palliative care delivery in the United States. There has been dramatic recent growth in the number of non-hospice palliative care programs, the dominant model being hospital-based palliative care programs [51, 52]. The number of hospitals with palliative care teams has increased from 24.5 % in 2000 to 67 % in 2011 [51]. At present these programs primarily serve patients on an inpatient or consult basis during their stay in the hospital and focus on defining the patient's goals of care and managing pain and symptoms. Expansion of palliative care services to clinic, home, and nursing home settings has begun in many communities. Although physicians and advanced practice nurses may bill for services, there is no Medicare reimbursement for the interdisciplinary palliative care *team*, which includes social workers, chaplains, counselors, and other professionals. Hospital palliative care programs have grown rapidly to serve the needs of hospitalized seriously ill persons. Also contributing to the rise of palliative care programs are the overwhelming caregiving burdens faced by patients' families [51].

Hospitals with palliative care programs are almost twice as likely to own a hospice program as hospitals without palliative care programs [53]. Expanding eligibility for hospice services may serve to strengthen the pathway between hospital palliative care and hospice care by increasing the incentive for hospitals to purchase or develop their own hospice programs thus enabling a more efficient allocation between the two services. Another component of expanding MHB eligibility criteria is whether the conditions of participation (COP) in hospice might allow more and different provider types to become certified providers.

The Emergence of New Models for Providing Hospice Services

In advance of major policy changes and in anticipation of changes arising from the implementation of healthcare reform, hospices themselves are developing new models of care to meet the needs of patients with serious illness not dying soon, often in partnership with the commercial or private sector, and risk bearing entities such as Accountable Care Organizations (ACOs).

1. Hospice open access

    The gap between patient need for palliative care services and hospice eligibility has led to development of open-access hospice policies, providing palliative and social support while retaining access to disease-modifying treatments. Recent evidence [54] finds that more than one-quarter of hospices report such policies, which may also lead to increased hospice enrollment and length of stay. Although a longer length of hospice stay is financially beneficial, because open access programs must absorb the cost of caring for a patient prior to the patient's eligibility and enrollment in the MHB, declining hospice margins jeopardize the continuation of these programs [55].

Nonprofit hospices are more than twice as likely as for-profit hospices to have open-access policies [54], limiting spread given the substantial growth in the for-profit hospice sector during the past decade [56]. Between 2000 and 2009, four out of five hospice providers that entered the US market were for-profit [56] and by 2011 more than 60 % of hospices were for-profit owned [11]. Changes in hospice eligibility or reimbursement are necessary if open-access policies are to be economically sustainable for hospices, especially as the market share of nonprofit hospices continues to erode.

2. Hospice of Michigan @HOMe Support Program

Another innovative model for operating outside the silo of the MHB is exemplified by the @HOMe Support program of the Hospice of Michigan. The @HOMe Support program is a wholly owned nonprofit subsidiary of the Hospice of Michigan that addresses the needs of patients with a serious illness while ineligible for hospice care. The model is funded through partnership with regional ACOs and Blue Cross Blue Shield of Michigan. Approximately 80 % of patients ultimately transition to hospice. Preliminary outcomes include a 9 % decrease in emergency department utilization, a 33 % decrease in hospital admissions, a 57 % decrease in hospital readmissions, and high patient/family satisfaction scores [57].

Replicating this model requires significant organizational leadership, vision, and cooperation. Challenges include creating awareness among providers, real-time data sharing among differing electronic systems, and developing network relationships within the hospital systems, emergency departments, community providers, nursing facilities, and palliative care initiatives. The @HOMe team is marketing tools and technical assistance to help other communities replicate their proprietary model. This palliative care delivery model exemplifies the opportunities for incorporation of home- and community-based services into ACOs to include post-acute care, complex care management, social supports, palliative care, as well as hospice end of life care (see Chap. 11 for further discussion of @HOMe and the integration of palliative care into ACOs).

3. Mandate for hospice in patient-centered medical homes (PCMHs) and ACOs

The PCMH is a team-based model that provides comprehensive and continuous care, increasing satisfaction, and improved health. An essential component is care coordination across settings for patients with serious illness.

Appropriately coordinated care depends on the individual patient and the complexity of their needs. These complexities include the existence of multiple chronic conditions, functional dependencies, family caregiver burden, cognitive vulnerability, preferences and goals of care, ability to communicate, ability to organize their own care, and the social environment of the patient. Such complexity typically requires a care team that can explicitly provide and assume responsibility for care coordination for patients identified as highest risk.

Because hospice and palliative care models reliably reduce acute care utilization, and PCMHs and ACOs involve assumption of financial risk, attention to service integration is warranted. The Centers for Medicare and Medicaid Services (CMS) needs to consider a mechanism for ensuring that palliative and hospice care are a robust part of the care networks associated with risk-bearing models [55]. This could be achieved by a requirement to provide access to palliative care and hospice services as a condition of receiving designation as a Medicare Advantage plan, an ACO, or a PCMH. Such a requirement would be an important first step in improving access to these services and catalyzing integration of community-based care models into the ACO/PCMH model and payment mechanisms [55].

Actionable Policy Steps to Increase Use of Hospice

1. Adjusting the hospice per diem rate for high-cost patients

   Recent evidence suggests that acknowledging the financial risk of caring for hospice patients with high-cost needs may be an important factor for access to hospice care [54]. A reimbursement policy related to the intensity of services and thus one that varies with patient need may be an important step in improving access to care.

   The MHB's per diem reimbursement creates incentives to restrict enrollment of high-cost patients. This is important because the MHB accounts for 84 % of hospice revenue [11]. Once enrolled in the MHB, all care related to the terminal illness must be paid for by hospice. Since average hospice per diem payment is $153 per day [12], many treatments are prohibitively expensive for hospices [35]. For example, chemotherapy or radiation serve many palliative purposes, as do transfusions for low blood cell counts, and can cost more than $10,000 per month [58]. Tube feeding, total parenteral nutrition, an intrathecal catheter, as well as personal support for those who lack a caregiver in the home, may also be too expensive.

   Recent evidence [54] finds that patients who are receiving high-cost palliative treatments might not have access to hospice services. In a nationally representative survey, 61 % of hospices reported that they would not enroll patients receiving palliative chemotherapy, 55 % would not enroll patients receiving total parenteral nutrition, and 30 % would not enroll patients receiving palliative radiation [54]. If the hospice per diem reimbursement was increased for high-cost needs, such patients would not be as financially risky for hospices, and enrollment policies might become less restrictive.

   MedPAC recently recommended an increase in the per diem rate for the first and last days of every patient's enrollment with hospice [35, 59–61]. The rationale is that hospice costs follow a U-shaped cost curve, and compensation should match actual costs. Under existing hospice per diem reimbursement, the high-cost first and last days of care are averaged with the lower-cost days in the middle of the stay, creating an incentive for longer hospice length of stay with a greater proportion of low-cost but fully reimbursed days.

   The U-shaped adjustment to the per diem rate may create an incentive for shorter hospice lengths of stay, which might not be in patients' best interest. Furthermore, the proposed adjustment does not address the issue of high-cost patients with intensive needs throughout their stay, not merely on their first and last days of hospice care. Risk adjusted compensation for patients with high-cost needs would reduce financial risk, while preserving current incentives for earlier referral to hospice care [54].

2. Adjusting the hospice per diem rate for increased regulatory burden

Providers have called for either increasing in the hospice per diem rate to account for the increasing costs of hospice regulations or decreasing the number of costly regulations that have not been directly linked to improving quality of care [62]. One example of these costly regulations is the requirement for face-to-face recertification of hospice patients [62]. Similarly, the requirement for detailed documentation of medications and the content and frequency of staff visits have also increased costs, particularly for those hospices without electronic medical records [62]. There is also significant concern regarding the financial risk that hospices face from Medicare audits, further limiting willingness to accept patients with uncertain prognosis or costly treatment needs [62]. Hospices found to have enrolled patients who were not eligible for the MHB, perhaps because they lived too long, or lacked "proof" of being terminal, have been required to repay Medicare for reimbursement related to those patients.

Although the intent of CMS in requesting these data is not clear, there is concern that CMS is focusing on regulations that are easy to document as opposed to ones that have been proven to improve quality for patients and families [62].

3. Standardizing eligibility criteria regarding concurrent life-prolonging and palliative care

There is wide variation in the interpretation of the MHB eligibility criteria related to the provision of care that serves both life-prolonging and palliative purposes. CMS regulations state that to elect the MHB, an individual "waives all rights to Medicare payments … related to the treatment of the terminal condition for which hospice care was elected" [63]. Many treatments—such as management of congestive heart failure, emphysema, or infection—are both life-prolonging and palliative. As a result, what constitutes hospice-appropriate care may be interpreted differently by hospices and referring physicians, as well as by patients and families.

Enrolling patients who require costly services even when their primary purpose is palliative (such as radiation therapy for bone metastases) is thus risky for small hospices, which are less likely than larger hospices to be able to absorb the cost. Small hospices have significantly more restrictive enrollment policies compared with larger hospices suggesting that these regulations are adversely impacting access to hospice care [54].

Provision of concurrent hospice and life-prolonging services is the subject of a pilot project called for by section 3131 of the Affordable Care Act, although funds have not yet been appropriated.

4. Hospice disenrollment rate as a reportable quality measure

Approximately 10–15 % of hospice beneficiaries disenroll from hospice prior to death [64–66]. Disenrollment is associated with greater likelihood of hospitalization, emergency department and intensive care unit admission, and hospital death [66]. Patients who disenroll from hospice are almost five times more expensive to the Medicare program, on average, than those who remain with hospice until death [66]. In addition, hospice disenrollment may be a marker for poor quality care and may limit access to interdisciplinary palliative care services at the end of life.

Hospice disenrollment may be initiated either by the patient or the hospice. Patients may revoke hospice due to dissatisfaction with care, a change in preferences, or the desire to pursue treatments not covered under the MHB (e.g., radiation or chemotherapy). A hospice may discharge a patient if it determines the patient is no longer eligible (i.e., not predictably dying soon); the patient moves from the service area; or the patient is admitted to a hospital that does not have a hospice contract. Previous studies, focused exclusively on patient-level factors, have identified younger age [65, 67], non-White race [67], male gender [65], and non-cancer diagnosis [65, 67] as associated with hospice disenrollment.

A large national study [68] of more than 1,300 hospices in the United States demonstrated highly variable disenrollment rates suggesting that disenrollment may be a marker for poor quality care. Some hospices had no patients disenroll during the study period, and other hospices had disenrollment rates as high as 38 %. Hospice disenrollment varied by provider characteristics, including type of hospice, the fiscal intermediary, and the market in which the hospice operated. Newer (within 5 years of initial Medicare certification) and smaller (with 13 or fewer full-time equivalent employees) hospices had higher disenrollment rates than larger, more established hospices. Over the past several decades, the population served by hospice has become increasingly complex [11] with multiple medical, nursing, and caregiver needs. The fact that newer and smaller hospices had higher disenrollment rates suggests that these programs may not be able to meet the needs of their patients or may lack the ability to appropriately select patients who meet Medicare hospice eligibility criteria. Further, patients served by newer hospices were more likely to disenroll and be immediately hospitalized indicating that newer hospices have difficulty managing clinical crises at home.

Recent evidence also finds higher disenrollment rates at for-profit compared with nonprofit hospices and may be related to exceeding the Medicare aggregate cap [69]. The aggregate annual cap was established by Medicare as a regulatory measure to control length of hospice stay and is the only fiscal constraint on the growth of Medicare hospice expenditures. Under the cap, if a hospice's total annual reimbursement from Medicare exceeds its total number of Medicare beneficiaries served multiplied by the cap amount ($25,337 in 2012), it must repay the excess [12]. Given Medicare's per diem hospice reimbursement, exceeding the cap indicates a length of stay profile that is too long [69]. For-profit hospices that report exceeding the cap have higher disenrollment rates than for-profit hospices that do not report exceeding the cap while there is no comparable difference for nonprofit hospices [69].

Another important source of variation in disenrollment is the hospice's fiscal intermediary [68]. Fiscal intermediaries administer the MHB program for CMS by processing claims, reimbursing hospices for Medicare-covered services, tracking beneficiary eligibility, and auditing hospice enrollment and services. Although guidelines exist to aid hospices in determining prognosis (MHB eligibility requirements), some hospice-eligible patients may stabilize or progress slowly or even improve while on hospice and may live longer than 6 months. Such patients are often scrutinized and may be discharged from hospice for "failure to die in a timely fashion." Fiscal intermediaries face competition for CMS contracts and thus have incentives to demonstrate that they are reducing hospice expenditures and rigorously overseeing hospice utilization. Some fiscal intermediaries interpret the Medicare prognostic guidelines more narrowly than others, and exert pressure on hospices to disenroll long-stay patients, contributing to the observed variation in hospice disenrollment.

Policy interventions to reduce disenrollment variation could target both the hospice and the fiscal intermediary by requiring reporting of disenrollment rates and reasons. CMS could also standardize interpretation of hospice eligibility criteria across fiscal intermediaries. A recent MedPAC report on hospice [70] found inadequate guidance on identification of eligible patients across diagnoses and disease categories. Consistent application of eligibility could reduce the disenrollment of individuals believed no longer eligible who die within weeks of hospice disenrollment. Further, public reporting of disenrollment rates creates disincentives for targeting long-stay patients and was recently proposed as a reportable hospice quality measure by a technical expert panel of hospice clinicians and researchers [12].

Conclusion

Although there is widespread support for improving access to hospice, there is uncertainty regarding if and how to change the MHB to achieve this goal. A decision to substantially alter eligibility for the MHB will fundamentally restructure palliative care delivery. The advantages and challenges of such a decision, and its effect on patients and families, must be carefully considered and compared with the consequences of retaining the existing benefit. Given the substantial variation across hospice agencies in clinical sophistication, quality, and service scope [71], demonstration projects may be required to evaluate policy options. Research is needed to quantify the change in demand for hospice services if eligibility was broadened; the potential cost of initiating some version of hospice earlier in the disease; the structure of various models of concurrent hospice and non-hospice palliative care programs; and the implications of an expanded or modified MHB on patient and family experiences and outcomes.

There are, however, a number of options that could be implemented to improve access without changing the MHB, including adjustment of the hospice per diem rate to incorporate variation in patient complexity and treatment requirements; increases in reimbursement to reflect additional regulatory requirements; and public reporting of disenrollment rates as a quality metric. Further, incentives or requirements for integration of palliative care and hospice into Medicare Advantage and new delivery and payment models, such as ACOs and PCMHs, have the potential to improve access for patients without the challenges of modifying the existing MHB.

References

1. Meier DE. Increased access to palliative care and hospice services: opportunities to improve value in health care. Milbank Q. 2011;89:343–80.
2. Taylor Jr DH, Ostermann J, Van Houtven CH, Tulsky JA, Steinhauser K. What length of hospice use maximizes reduction in medical expenditures near death in the US Medicare program? Soc Sci Med. 2007;65:1466–78.
3. Carlson MDA, Herrin J, Du Q, et al. Impact of hospice disenrollment on health care use and medicare expenditures for patients with cancer. J Clin Oncol. 2010;28:4371–5.
4. Wennberg JE, Fisher ES, Stukel TA, Skinner JS, Sharp SM, Bronner KK. Use of hospitals, physician visits, and hospice care during last six months of life among cohorts loyal to highly respected hospitals in the United States. BMJ. 2004;328:607.
5. Pyenson B, Connor S, Fitch K, Kinzbrunner B. Medicare cost in matched hospice and non-hospice cohorts. J Pain Symptom Manage. 2004;28:200–10.
6. Teno JM, Clarridge BR, Casey V, et al. Family perspectives on end-of-life care at the last place of care. JAMA. 2004;291:88–93.
7. Kelley AS, Deb P, Du Q, Aldridge Carlson MD, Morrison RS. Hospice enrollment saves money for Medicare and improves care quality across a number of different lengths-of-stay. Health Aff (Millwood). 2013;32:552–61.
8. Wright AA, Keating NL, Balboni TA, Matulonis UA, Block SD, Prigerson HG. Place of death: correlations with quality of life of patients with cancer and predictors of bereaved caregivers' mental health. J Clin Oncol. 2010;28:4457–64.
9. Bradley EH, Prigerson H, Carlson MDA, Cherlin E, Johnson-Hurzeler R, Kasl SV. Depression among surviving caregivers: does length of hospice enrollment matter? Am J Psychiatry. 2004;161:2257–62.
10. Teno JM, Shu JE, Casarett D, Spence C, Rhodes R, Connor S. Timing of referral to hospice and quality of care: length of stay and bereaved family members' perceptions of the timing of hospice referral. J Pain Symptom Manage. 2007;34:120–5.
11. NHPCO facts and figures: hospice care in America. 2013. Available at: http://www.nhpco.org/sites/default/files/public/Statistics_Research/2013_Facts_Figures.pdf. Accessed November 2013.
12. MedPac. Report to the Congress: Medicare Payment Policy: chapter 12: hospice services. 2013.
13. Carlson MDA, Bradley EH, Du Q, Morrison RS. Geographic access to hospice in the United States. J Palliat Med. 2010;13:1331–8.
14. National Hospice and Palliative Care Organization. NHPCO facts and figures. 2011. Available at: http://www.nhpco.org/files/public/2011-facts-and-figures.pdf. Accessed May 2014.
15. Teno JM, Gozalo PL, Bynum JP, et al. Change in end-of-life care for Medicare beneficiaries: site of death, place of care, and health care transitions in 2000, 2005, and 2009. JAMA. 2013;309:470–7.
16. Jennings B, Ryndes T, D'Onofrio C, Baily MA. Access to hospice care. Expanding boundaries, overcoming barriers. Hastings Cent Rep. 2003;Suppl:S3–7, S9–13, S5–21 passim.
17. Foley K, Gelbard H, editors. Institute of Medicine report: improving palliative care for cancer. Washington, DC: National Academy Press; 2001.
18. Lynn J, Forlini JH. "Serious and complex illness" in quality improvement and policy reform for end-of-life care. J Gen Intern Med. 2001;16:315–9.
19. Last Acts. Means to a better end: a report on dying in America today. Washington, DC: Last Acts; 2002.
20. Paradis LF, Cummings SB. The evolution of hospice in America toward organizational homogeneity. J Health Soc Behav. 1986;27:370–86.
21. James N, Field D. The routinization of hospice: charisma and bureaucratization. Soc Sci Med. 1992;34:1363–75.
22. Omnibus Reconciliation Act. PL101-239, Section 6005; 1989.
23. Jones AL. Hospices and home health agencies: data from the 1991 National Health Provider Inventory. Adv Data. 1994;(257):1–8.

24. Strahan GW. An overview of home health and hospice care patients: preliminary data from the 1993 National Home and Hospice Care Survey. Adv Data. 1994:1–12.
25. Rhodes RL, Teno JM, Welch LC. Access to hospice for African Americans: are they informed about the option of hospice? J Palliat Med. 2006;9:268–72.
26. Cherlin E, Fried T, Prigerson HG, Schulman-Green D, Johnson-Hurzeler R, Bradley EH. Communication between physicians and family caregivers about care at the end of life: when do discussions occur and what is said? J Palliat Med. 2005;8:1176–85.
27. General Accounting Office. Medicare Hospice Care: modifications to payment methodology may be warranted. Washington, DC: GAO; 2004.
28. Friedman BT, Harwood MK, Shields M. Barriers and enablers to hospice referrals: an expert overview. J Palliat Med. 2002;5:73–84.
29. Wennberg JE, Fisher ES, Skinner JS. Geography and the debate over Medicare reform. Health Aff (Millwood) 2002;Suppl Web Exclusives:W96–114.
30. Virnig BA, Ma H, Hartman LK, Moscovice I, Carlin B. Access to home-based hospice care for rural populations: identification of areas lacking service. J Palliat Med. 2006;9:1292–9.
31. Virnig BA, Kind S, McBean M, Fisher E. Geographic variation in hospice use prior to death. J Am Geriatr Soc. 2000;48:1117–25.
32. Virnig BA, Moscovice IS, Durham SB, Casey MM. Do rural elders have limited access to Medicare hospice services? J Am Geriatr Soc. 2004;52:731–5.
33. Fowler K, Poehling K, Billheimer D, et al. Hospice referral practices for children with cancer: a survey of pediatric oncologists. J Clin Oncol. 2006;24:1099–104.
34. Johnson CB, Slaninka SC. Barriers to accessing hospice services before a late terminal stage. Death Stud. 1999;23:225–38.
35. Huskamp HA, Buntin MB, Wang V, Newhouse JP. Providing care at the end of life: do Medicare rules impede good care? Health Aff (Millwood). 2001;20:204–11.
36. Brickner L, Scannell K, Marquet S, Ackerson L. Barriers to hospice care and referrals: survey of physicians' knowledge, attitudes, and perceptions in a health maintenance organization. J Palliat Med. 2004;7:411–8.
37. Christakis NA. Predicting patient survival before and after hospice enrollment. Hosp J. 1998;13:71–87.
38. Zerzan J, Stearns S, Hanson L. Access to palliative care and hospice in nursing homes. JAMA. 2000;284:2489–94.
39. Christakis N. Death foretold: prophecy and prognosis in medical care. Chicago: University of Chicago Press; 1999.
40. Fox E, Landrum-McNiff K, Zhong Z, Dawson NV, Wu AW, Lynn J. Evaluation of prognostic criteria for determining hospice eligibility in patients with advanced lung, heart, or liver disease. SUPPORT Investigators Study to Understand Prognoses and Preferences for Outcomes and Risks of Treatments. JAMA. 1999;282:1638–45.
41. Simpson DA. Prognostic criteria for hospice eligibility. JAMA. 2000;283:2527.
42. Lorenz KA, Asch SM, Rosenfeld KE, Liu H, Ettner SL. Hospice admission practices: where does hospice fit in the continuum of care? J Am Geriatr Soc. 2004;52:725–30.
43. Casarett D, Van Ness PH, O'Leary JR, Fried TR. Are patient preferences for life-sustaining treatment really a barrier to hospice enrollment for older adults with serious illness? J Am Geriatr Soc. 2006;54:472–8.
44. U.S. Government Printing Office. Code of Federal Regulations 42CFR418.22, Certification of Terminal Illness; 2002.
45. U.S. Government Printing Office. Code of Federal Regulations 42CFR418.24, Election of Hospice Care; 2002.
46. Connor SR, Pyenson B, Fitch K, Spence C, Iwasaki K. Comparing hospice and nonhospice patient survival among patients who die within a three-year window. J Pain Symptom Manage. 2007;33:238–46.
47. Temel JS, Greer JA, Muzikansky A, et al. Early palliative care for patients with metastatic non-small-cell lung cancer. N Engl J Med. 2010;363:733–42.

48. Penrod JD, Deb P, Luhrs C, et al. Cost and utilization outcomes of patients receiving hospital-based palliative care consultation. J Palliat Med. 2006;9:855–60.
49. Bruera E, Neumann CM, Gagnon B, Brenneis C, Quan H, Hanson J. The impact of a regional palliative care program on the cost of palliative care delivery. J Palliat Med. 2000;3:181–6.
50. Fromme EK, Bascom PB, Smith MD, et al. Survival, mortality, and location of death for patients seen by a hospital-based palliative care team. J Palliat Med. 2006;9:903–11.
51. Center to Advance Palliative Care. Palliative care in hospitals continues rapid growth trend for 11th straight year, according to latest analysis. Available at: http://www.capc.org/news-and-events/releases/08-27-12. Accessed October 2013.
52. Morrison RS, Maroney-Galin C, Kralovec PD, Meier DE. The growth of palliative care programs in United States hospitals. J Palliat Med. 2005;8:1127–34.
53. Goldsmith B, Dietrich J, Du Q, Morrison RS. Variability in access to hospital palliative care in the United States. J Palliat Med. 2008;11:1094–102.
54. Aldridge Carlson MD, Barry CL, Cherlin EJ, McCorkle R, Bradley EH. Hospices' enrollment policies may contribute to underuse of hospice care in the United States. Health Aff (Millwood). 2012;31:2690–8.
55. Conversation with Bev Sloan President and CEO of The Denver Hospice; August 2013.
56. Thompson JW, Carlson MDA, Bradley EH. US hospice industry experienced considerable turbulence from changes in ownership, growth, and shift to for-profit status. Health Aff (Millwood). 2012;31:1286–93.
57. Deremo D. Advanced illness management: the 'missing piece' in health care reform. Presented at the Center to Advance Palliative Care National Seminar, Nov 2013.
58. Wright AA, Katz IT. Letting go of the rope–aggressive treatment, hospice care, and open access. N Engl J Med. 2007;357:324–7.
59. Medicare Payment Advisory Commission. Report to the Congress: Medicare's payment policy: reforming Medicare's Hospice Benefit. Washington, DC: Medicare Payment Advisory Commission; 2009.
60. Nicosia N, Reardon E, Lorenz K, Lynn J, Buntin MB. The Medicare hospice payment system: a consideration of potential refinements. Health Care Financ Rev. 2009;30:47–59.
61. Fitch K, Pyenson B. First and last days of hospice cost more: an actuarial evaluation of hospice benefits provided to Medicare Beneficiaries. New York: Milliman; 2003.
62. Conversation with Samira Beckwith of Hope HealthCare Services; Sept 2013.
63. Centers for Medicaid & Medicare Services. Medicare and Medicaid Programs: hospice conditions of participation; Final Rule. 42CFRPart418 2008;73.
64. Taylor DH, Steinhauser K, Tulsky JA, Rattliff J, Van Houtven CH. Characterizing hospice discharge patterns in a nationally representative sample of the elderly, 1993–2000. Am J Hosp Palliat Care. 2008;25(1):9–15.
65. Casarett DJ, Marenberg ME, Karlawish JH. Predictors of withdrawal from hospice. J Palliat Med. 2001;4:491–7.
66. Carlson MDA, Herrin J, Du Q, et al. Impact of hospice disenrollment on health care use and Medicare expenditures for patients with cancer. J Clin Oncol. 2010;28(28):4371–75.
67. Johnson KS, Kuchibhatla M, Tanis D, Tulsky JA. Racial differences in hospice revocation to pursue aggressive care. Arch Intern Med. 2008;168:218–24.
68. Carlson MDA, Herrin J, Du Q, et al. Hospice characteristics and the disenrollment of patients with cancer. Health Serv Res. 2009;44:2004–21.
69. Aldridge MD, Schlesinger M, Barry CL, et al. National hospice survey results: for-profit status, community engagement, and service. JAMA Intern Med. 2014;174(4):500–6.
70. Medicare Payment Advisory Commission. Report to the Congress: reforming the delivery system, Chap. 8: Evaluating Medicare's Hospice Benefit: Washington, DC; 2008.
71. Carlson MDA, Morrison RS, Holford TR, Bradley EH. Hospice care: what services do patients and their families receive? Health Serv Res. 2007;42:1672–90.

Chapter 6
Palliative Care in the Long-Term Care Setting

Mary Ersek, Justine S. Sefcik, and David G. Stevenson

Palliative Care in the Nursing Home Setting: Challenges and Opportunities

Approximately 1.8 million Americans live in nursing homes (NHs) [1], and this number is expected to double or triple by 2030 [2]. More than half of these NH residents require extensive assistance with, or are completely dependent on staff for bathing, dressing, toileting, and transferring needs [3]. Over 25 % of adults, age 65 and older, die in a NH and 67 % of persons with advanced dementia live their final days in this setting [4, 5].

Billions of dollars are spent every year by the state and federal governments on care for NH residents [6–8]. NH costs are as high as $136 billion per year, with Medicaid paying for the majority of residents' care. Medicare covers almost 18 % of NH costs, as well as being the major payer for the first 100 days of a NH stay [1]. Despite the billions of dollars spent, care for NH residents has long been associated with poor symptom control, burdensome transitions, and low family satisfaction with care [9, 10].

Palliative care is one approach to enhancing care for persons with progressive, life-limiting illnesses, including those in NHs. In the acute care setting, implementation

---

M. Ersek, Ph.D., R.N., F.A.A.N. (✉)
National PROMISE Center, Philadelphia Veterans Affairs Medical Center, Philadelphia, PA, USA

University of Pennsylvania School of Nursing, 3900 Woodland Avenue, Annex, Suite 203, Philadelphia, PA 19104, USA
e-mail: ersekm@nursing.upenn.edu

J.S. Sefcik, M.S., R.N.
Doctoral Student, 2012–2014 National Hartford Centers of Gerontological, Nursing Excellence Patricia G. Archbold Scholar, University of Pennsylvania School of Nursing, Philadelphia, PA, USA

D.G. Stevenson, S.M., Ph.D.
Department of Health Policy, Vanderbilt University School of Medicine, Nashville, TN, USA

of palliative care is associated with better quality of care and decreased healthcare costs [11]. Using robust statistical methods and a national sample, Kelley et al. [12] found that receipt of hospice services was also associated with decreased healthcare costs. Compared to usual care, palliative care delivered to NH residents with advanced disease is associated with improved quality and satisfaction [13–16]. Despite these documented benefits of palliative care, this approach to care has not been widely integrated into the NH industry. Moreover, there are currently no rigorous studies that have evaluated cost or resident outcomes of palliative care NH programs [17].

Several challenges impede the provision of high-quality palliative care in NHs. A major obstacle expressed by NH administrators includes knowledge deficits and attitudinal barriers among physicians, nurses, and families [18]. Additionally, staff shortages and turnover are frequently reported as challenges to providing quality palliative care to residents and their families [18, 19]. Financial barriers also hinder the ability to attract and retain quality staff members [18]. Finally, regulatory issues can threaten the integration of palliative care into the NH setting. The regulatory framework governing NHs is largely shaped by the Omnibus Budget Reconciliation Act of 1987 (OBRA-87), which emphasized that the primary goal of NH care delivered to long-term residents is to provide supportive services that maximize resident function and quality of life. Although these goals are consistent with those of palliative care, mismatches can occur, since NHs regulations and quality metrics tend to focus more on rehabilitation of function, whereas palliative care emphasizes the quality of life [20].

Despite these challenges, there are opportunities to provide excellent palliative care during long-term stays within NHs; moreover, healthcare teams in NHs often do have expertise in providing care to dying residents [21]. Daily interactions between staff members and residents foster intimate relationships as well as emotional attachments. These close relationships enable staff members to detect subtle changes in residents' clinical and emotional status. Furthermore, this kind of daily close social contact can promote an understanding about residents' personal goals and care preferences. This familiarity and consistency of personal contact is especially important among NH residents with dementia, where an effective and consistent caregiving relationship can improve residents' moods [22].

The purpose of this chapter is to describe current models for palliative care in NHs and explore healthcare system factors that hinder widespread adoption of palliative care in this setting. We then propose strategies and policies that can facilitate adoption of palliative care services for NH residents.

Current Models of Palliative Care Delivery in Nursing Homes

There are several models for incorporating palliative care into NHs, including hospice-NH partnerships, palliative care consultation with clinical teams that are external to the facility, and in-house teams or specialized palliative care units [17, 23]. The following section briefly describes the three models.

Hospice Care

The most established program for delivering palliative care in US NHs is hospice care. As detailed in other chapters, Medicare beneficiaries are eligible for the Medicare Hospice Benefit (MHB) if their physician certifies that their prognosis is a life expectancy of 6 months or less if the terminal illness runs its natural course, and if they agree to forgo treatment intended to cure the terminal illness. In the initial years of hospice, most beneficiaries electing hospice care had cancer and received care in their own homes. With the OBRA of 1989, Medicare extended the availability of the hospice benefit to NHs. Now, any NH that wants to incorporate such care can freely contract with hospice agencies, although there is no requirement that they do so. By 2004, 78 % of US NHs contracted with at least one hospice agency for services [3], a figure that has likely grown higher in recent years. Reflecting these changes, the percentage of NH decedents receiving hospice services rose from 14 % in 1999 to 33 % in 2006 [24]. At the same time, the percent of all hospice users who live in NHs has increased to more than 30 % [25].

The Medicare hospice payment is made directly to the hospice agency, regardless of the setting in which an individual lives. For individuals dually eligible for Medicare and Medicaid who reside in NHs, state Medicaid programs also pay the hospice agency at least 95 % of the NH room and board costs, which the hospice, in turn, pays to the NH. Room and board costs of NH care for private paying residents are determined by contract. Room and board payments are redirected to the hospice because it is the hospice's responsibility to professionally manage the care of the patient. The hospice agency subsequently pays NHs a negotiated rate, typically passing the NH payment to the facility in full.

When NH residents enroll in hospice, the facility continues to provide room and board and ongoing clinical care and supportive services, while the hospice agency is responsible for overseeing the plan of care for the resident's terminal illness. The hospice supplements the resources available at the NH; additional services may include expert symptom assessment and management, personal care from the hospice agency's home health aides, spiritual counseling, social work services, and volunteer and bereavement services. The hospice also pays for medical supplies and medications but only for those related to the terminal condition. The addition of hospice to usual NH care may improve the quality of care. Researchers have reported that hospice use in NHs is associated with decreased use of invasive therapies and hospitalizations, improved pain and symptom management, and higher family satisfaction with care [26–29].

Despite the potential benefits of hospice care added to routine NH care, there are several barriers to enrolling residents in hospice. One barrier is the belief by some NH administrators and staff that the acceptance of hospice services is an admission that NH care is inadequate [30]. Further, poor communication and lack of collegial relationships between NH and hospice staff can compromise care delivered to NH residents [17]. Another challenge to greater integration of hospice into NH care is the inability of most patients admitted to nursing homes under the Medicare Part A—Skilled Nursing Facility (SNF) benefit to simultaneously access hospice care.

Because reimbursement to NHs is higher under the Medicare-funded SNF benefit than the Medicaid rate for subsequent long-term NH care, there is a financial disincentive for NHs to recommend hospice for these patients, as this would require moving the patient from the better reimbursed SNF level of care to a poorly reimbursed long-term care NH bed. Equally important, the SNF payment includes room and board. If a patient and family opt for hospice they must either assume personal responsibility for their room and board in the NH, or seek Medicaid eligibility for this purpose. Finally, the 6-month prognosis requirement for hospice eligibility can be a barrier to enrollment, given the high prevalence in NHs of conditions, such as dementia and other neurological conditions, which typically have very uncertain prognoses.

A final point worth noting is that the expansion of NH hospice has not been without controversy. Hospice reimbursement involves a fixed per-diem rate creating a financial incentive for long hospice stays. Some policymakers have raised questions about the extent to which some hospices agencies are aggressively targeting more profitable (i.e., long stay) patients and whether common ownership of NHs and hospice agencies has spurred inappropriate use [25, 31].

External Consultation Teams

External palliative care consultation teams are either based within a community hospice/palliative care organization or, less frequently, associated with a hospital palliative care program. In this model, a consultation is requested by a NH administrator (most commonly Medical Director or Director of Nursing Services) or a resident's primary care provider. Residents who receive these consultations may or may not be hospice-eligible. The consultant, a physician or nurse practitioner, bills under Medicare part B; therefore, the costs for these services are not incurred by the NH.

The Bluegrass Palliative Care Consultation Service is an example of the external consultation team model. The program is part of Palliative Care Center of the Bluegrass, an affiliate of Hospice of the Bluegrass. Consultations generally are limited, focusing on symptom management, advance care planning, communication with the family, and facilitating transition to hospice, if appropriate. Although no rigorous independent evaluation has been done, the program asserts that participating NHs report high patient satisfaction, fewer emergency department visits, enhanced symptom management, and improved staff retention [17]. Program leaders emphasize several keys to success including having access to many patients in each facility to minimize travel time, maximize efficiency, and ensure financial viability, and staffing NH-focused hospice teams with clinicians who understand and appreciate the NH setting and culture [17].

A different type of consultation model is delivered by Evercare™ a division of the UnitedHealth Group®. Evercare™ is a Medicare Advantage plan that operates in a full risk capitation model without cost to the NH [32]. Evercare Nurse practitioners provide primary care services within NHs, paying particular attention to advance care planning, goal setting, and communication with family members [17]. This model is associated with fewer hospitalizations and lower costs compared to usual NH care [33].

One major challenge to the effectiveness of external palliative care consultations is that NH staff and primary care providers may be inconsistent in following the recommendations made by the palliative care consultation team [32]. Because reimbursement is typically through Medicare part B and focused on billable physician and nurse practitioner visits, it is difficult to incorporate comprehensive interdisciplinary team care. Effective in 2005, the Medicare Prescription Drug, Improvement, and Modernization Act of 2003 authorized a one-time payment to be made to a hospice for evaluation and counseling services provided by a physician who is either the medical director or an employee of a certified hospice agency. To be eligible for this consultation, a beneficiary must have a prognosis of 6 months or less if the illness runs its normal course and not have elected the MHB or received hospice pre-election evaluation and counseling services previously; however, the individual may currently be receiving potentially life-extending therapies. Adoption of this policy represents the first instance of Medicare payment specifically for palliative or hospice care for patients who have not elected hospice, and it allows patients to receive this benefit while simultaneously receiving Medicare-funded home health or Part A SNF services. To date, little is known about how this benefit is being used [20].

Internal Palliative Care Teams and Units

Internal programs generally encompass NH staff training in advance care planning and symptom management; however there are no standard elements of these programs [32]. Based on the 2004 National Nursing Home Survey data, 27 % of US NHs self-reported having a specialized program and/or staff trained in hospice or palliative care. Factors that were significantly associated with having a specialized hospice/palliative care program included nonprofit status, employing a American College of Health Care Administrators certified administrator, contracting with external hospice agencies, having mental health services internally available, and having a program or staff specially trained in pain management [34]. A notable example of an internally developed NH palliative care models is the Palliative Care for Advanced Dementia program (now re-named *Comfort First*), developed at Beatitudes Campus, a Continuing Care Retirement Community in Phoenix, Arizona.

Comfort First

The *Comfort First* model of care is radical in its simplicity—staff learn to respect resident wishes. For example, if someone wants to sleep all day and be up at night, that's okay. If another prefers to eat dinner at midnight, that's okay too.

(continued)

(continued)

People eat what they prefer and all therapeutic diets have been eliminated. Thus, if chocolate is favored by a diabetic with dementia, so be it. Responses to dementia-related behaviors have been reframed; if a person is resisting staff attempts to care for them, a root-cause analysis is conducted to determine the underlying meaning of the resistance. Staff know that often resisting care, moaning, and distress may be suggestive of pain and a pain management plan is instituted that includes analgesics and nonpharmacologic interventions as opposed to potent antipsychotics or other chemical or physical restraints. In the Comfort First model of care, staff have adopted a person-directed approach that relies on taking cues from the person with dementia for what is pleasurable and comfortable for her/him. The consequences of implementing this model of care at Beatitudes Campus has led to the elimination of physical restraints, a marked reduction in dementia-related behaviors and incontinence, significantly reduced weight loss and a reduction in the reliance on anxiolytic and antipsychotic medications. In addition to positive outcomes for people with dementia, Campus staff have also benefitted with high job satisfaction, minimal turnover, and reduced operational costs. *Comfort First* been replicated at several nursing homes in Phoenix, Arizona with support from BHHS Legacy Foundation.

The Beatitudes model of care has received substantial media attention, including the New York Times and The New Yorker. With funding from the New York City chapter of the Alzheimer's Association, a number of New York City nursing homes are receiving education and support for implementation of this approach [35–39].

Video links:

A local news story about Beatitudes Campus *Comfort First* program: (Link: http://www.beatitudescampus.org/about/news-and-press/vermilion-cliffs-neighborhood-on-channel-3/) [39]

NPR's "Here and Now" program—KJZZ (Monica Brady-Myerov)—1/21/11 (interview with Peggy Mullan and May Vance, daughter-in-law Vermilion Cliffs resident, Aline Vance regarding palliative care program practices and NYT article.)

Link: http://hereandnow.wbur.org/2011/01/21/alzheimers-beatitudes-campus

NPR Phoenix (KJZZ) "Here and Now" radio program (May 22)—Tena Alonzo represents Beatitudes Campus as panelist regarding comfort-focused dementia care on recorded show. Link: http://www.kjzz.org/content/1305/beatitudes-campuss-unique-approach-dementia-care\http://www.kjzz.org/content/1305/beatitudes-campuss-unique-approach-dementia-care/

Advantages to internal programs include the ability to infuse palliative care principles into daily NH care, especially the care for residents who have not enrolled in, or are not eligible for, hospice. Clinicians' daily interaction with residents on a palliative care program may lead to timely detection of clinical changes as well as facilitate an understanding of resident/family values, personal goals, and care preferences [23]. Internal programs also place the expertise and authority with the entity—that is, the NH itself—that is ultimately held accountable for the residents' quality of care [17, 40].

Other potential benefits following admission to a NH-based palliative care unit or service include decreased use of unnecessary medications [41]. The ability to empower NH staff to provide high quality palliative care may also have facility-wide benefits such as enhanced staff satisfaction and decreased turnover [42]. Similarly, specialized dementia "comfort care" units are associated with higher staff satisfaction, less observed resident discomfort, and lower costs than standard NH care [43].

The growth of internal NH palliative care services is challenged by the lack of financial resources and by inadequately trained staff. The relatively high reimbursement for skilled nursing care may create a financial incentive for NHs to invest in palliative care capacity, since these residents do not have access to the MHB and such consultations are billable (for doctors and nurse practitioners) under Medicare Part B. However, the need to invest in specialized training and the additional staff time required to deliver high quality palliative care constitute the major barriers to this model.

Recommendations

In this section, we propose several strategies for enhancing palliative care in NHs. These approaches are: (1) restructuring the MHB to align payment with a broader conceptualization of palliative care, (2) ensuring that palliative care is part of emerging integrated payment models, such as accountable care organizations and bundled payments, (3) infusing palliative care into ongoing efforts to enhance NH quality, (4) incorporating palliative care indicators into the state inspection process and quality measures reporting, (5) supporting a skilled palliative care workforce, and (6) rigorously evaluating the outcomes of innovative payment and care models (Table 6.1).

Realigning the Medicare Hospice Benefit to Enhance Palliative Care in NHs

Because hospice is the most widely used model of palliative care in NHs, an obvious target for payment and delivery realignment is the MHB. The MHB has changed little over its 30-year existence, despite a transformation in the populations served and the type of care that agencies provide. In particular, hospice has grown well beyond its initial intent of provision of palliative care for community-dwelling terminally ill persons with cancer [44]. More than two-thirds of Medicare hospice

Table 6.1 Recommended policy changes to enhance palliative care in nursing homes

Recommended policy changes	Examples of specific strategies
Modify the Medicare Hospice Benefit	• Allow concurrent use of the MHB and the Part A Medicare SNF benefit • Develop a case-mix adjustment for the NH setting • Modify the hospice per diem to match the NH-hospice length of stay and services
Include palliative care as part of other NH payment reforms and models	Payment models: • Accountable Care Organizations • Bundled Payments • Value Based Purchasing Care delivery models: • Culture Change model • Transitional Care models
Prepare and maintain a NH workforce that is skilled in palliative care practices and delivery	• End-of-life Nursing Education Consortium (ELNEC) Geriatric curriculum • Encourage and support palliative care certification for certified nursing assistants, licensed practical nurses (LPNs), registered nurses (RNs), and nurse practitioners (APRNs) through the National Board for Certification of Hospice and Palliative Nurses (NBCHPN®)
Test models of NH palliative care delivery	• CMS-funded demonstration projects • NIH-funded implementation projects
Monitor palliative care processes and outcomes for nursing home residents	• Incorporate palliative care practices and assessments more fully into the Minimum Data Set (MDS) • Align CMS Nursing Home Quality Indicators with palliative care outcomes
Incorporate palliative care into NH regulatory mechanisms	• Train state surveyors to recognize resident and family-centered palliative care goals as consistent with high quality care • Incorporate palliative care practices and assessments more fully into the MDS

recipients currently have had non-cancer diagnoses, and growing numbers live in NHs and assisted living facilities [31]. Reflecting both increased use and increased lengths of stay, Medicare hospice spending has more than quadrupled over the last decade to its current level of $13 billion annually [31]. Despite the scrutiny that inevitably accompanies increased government spending, a robust for-profit hospice sector has emerged, ostensibly focused on enrolling more profitable (i.e., relatively stable, long stay) patients [45, 46]. At a more fundamental level, however, the expansion of hospice and the manner in which it has grown raises deeper questions about the need to fundamentally redesign the MHB. Initially conceptualized as a benefit for those who are predictably and clearly dying and who might reasonably relinquish insurance coverage for life prolonging treatment, the MHB is no longer well suited for its current role in a fragmented health care system with a growing population of debilitated Medicare beneficiaries with multiple chronic conditions, uncertain prognoses, and continued benefit from some types of life prolonging therapies [40, 47].

Nowhere are the growing pains of the MHB more apparent than at the intersection of hospice and the NH setting. Current eligibility policies limit the potential use and effectiveness of hospice care by NH residents. In particular, requiring beneficiaries to have a prognosis of 6 months or less to live is a barrier to timely hospice enrollment for many NH residents, where less than 5 % have cancer as a primary diagnosis and the majority has multiple chronic conditions for which it is difficult to predict prognosis accurately [3, 48]. The most politically controversial manifestation of this mismatch between the design of the MHB and the needs of seriously ill Medicare beneficiaries is evidenced by the roughly 25 % of NH hospice enrollees with lengths of stay exceeding 6 months. Yet more concerning from a quality of care standpoint are the 30 % of NH hospice beneficiaries who receive hospice care for less than 1 week and the roughly 60 % of NH residents with dementia who receive no hospice care at all before they die [40, 47, 49].

Current hospice payment policies are also problematic in the NH setting. In particular, hospice's per-diem payment rewards long stays in hospice and, for some enrollees, the payments are excessively high apart from the resource-intensive beginning and end-of a hospice stay [50]. In addition, Medicare's one-size-fits all approach to payment does not adjust for case-mix or setting of care. Thus, Medicare policy ignores potential efficiencies that are, as a result, captured by agencies delivering hospice to NH residents and other resource differences that adhere more closely to individuals' diagnoses [51]. Finally, by paying hospice agencies separately for the delivery of hospice care to NH residents, Medicare policy reinforces the notion that NHs are not responsible for—or capable of—providing specialized palliative care to their residents. Although this position might be justified by pointing to well-identified deficits in the palliative care received by NH residents, carving out hospice care from the services for which we hold facilities accountable fails to improve palliative care for the majority of NH decedents who do not enroll in hospice.

Going forward, Medicare hospice policy should seek not only to address the efficiency of hospice payments (e.g., by adjusting payments for case-mix, length of stay, or setting), but it should strive to promote earlier and greater integration of palliative care into NH practice. One mechanism to achieve this is to modify hospice eligibility standards to recognize the prognostic uncertainty inherent to NH populations, by broadening the 6-month standard and adjusting payments to reflect changes in resource needs of long stay beneficiaries accordingly.

An alternative is to allow patients to access the MHB while also receiving curative care, which currently is not allowed. Although concurrent care is most often discussed in the context of pediatric and cancer care, this concept also can be applied to SNF patients upon discharge from the hospital. Under current regulations, patients who are admitted to NHs under the more highly reimbursed SNF benefit cannot simultaneously elect the MHB unless their terminal illness is different from the medical condition that made them eligible for SNF care. Miller et al. [52] reported that 40 % of non-HMO NH decedents with advanced dementia received SNF care in the last 90 days of life. Similarly, Aragon and colleagues [53] examined post-hospitalization SNF use among Medicare beneficiaries and found that 30.5 % had a SNF admission in the last 6 months of life and 9.2 % died while receiving SNF care. Further, decedents who accessed the SNF benefit during this period were much less likely to die at home (10.7 %) than beneficiaries who did not access the SNF benefit (40.4 %). Miller and colleagues reported that SNF patients with advanced dementia who also received hospice care either concurrent with or following SNF care received fewer medications and injections, less artificial nutrition and hydration, and fewer therapy services than SNF patients with no hospice. Moreover, receipt of any hospice care was associated with lower odds of dying in a hospital compared with patients who had no hospice [52]. Taken together, these two studies suggest that allowing concurrent hospice and SNF care could decrease burdensome, expensive treatments and transitions in care.

Additional research is needed to examine the quality of care and patient outcomes for concurrent hospice and SNF care. Future investigations may be supported by Section 3140 of the Patient Protection and Affordable Care Act (PPACA), which requires that Medicare fund and evaluate a 15-site concurrent care demonstration. At this writing, CMS has not yet initiated these projects; when and if they occur, it will be important to include a setting providing concurrent SNF and hospice care.

A more comprehensive reform would "carve in" hospice and palliative care into NH care more broadly. This approach could direct payments to NHs, rather than hospice agencies, thereby recognizing the primary role NHs already have in providing services and supports to their residents. NHs would then have the choice of contracting with hospice agencies and external palliative care services to deliver the care, or of providing financial support to develop and sustain their own palliative care services [40]. A bundled payment approach could also include post-acute and SNF care along with long-term and palliative care, having the potential to further reduce incentives to frequently readmit residents to the hospital and giving providers greater flexibility to meet residents' changing service needs.

Efficiencies gained through the revision of the MHB could be used to fund palliative care in NHs. Another strategy would be to use savings to Medicare resulting from reduced acute care expenditures to pay for palliative care services in NHs. The Centers for Medicare and Medicaid Innovation (CMMI) recently funded seven projects with its "Initiative to Reduce Avoidable Hospitalizations among Nursing Facility Residents." One of the seven awardees, explicitly includes palliative care interventions and training for staff and all seven awardees incorporate the Interventions to Reduce Acute Care Transfers (INTERACT) tools [54] which include early identification and management of symptoms and an advance care planning component. When the demonstration projects are completed (scheduled for 2016) there may be new options for effective, sustainable palliative care programs in nursing homes.

Including NH Palliative Care as Part of Other Payment Reforms and Models

As federal and state governments seek to integrate payments for acute, post-acute, and long-term supportive services, palliative care providers have the potential to play an important role because of their demonstrated ability to improve quality of care, and in so doing, reduce the need for emergency hospitalizations and their associated high costs [11, 12]. For example, as ACOs seek to partner with NHs in building their provider networks, they will likely seek to contract with facilities that have relatively low rates of hospital readmissions and emergency department use, while, at the same time, offering hospitals the ability to reduce inpatient lengths of stay. NHs with a strong palliative care emphasis, including collaborative relationships with hospice providers, should be strongly positioned to succeed in this context. Similarly, with state demonstration programs that seek to integrate the financing and delivery of Medicare- and Medicaid-financed services for dual-eligible beneficiaries, integrated care plans will place a premium on facilities' ability to manage residents' symptoms and acute events effectively in the NH, thus avoiding unnecessary hospitalizations. Finally, recently initiated bundled payment demonstration projects offer NHs with strong palliative care practices further opportunities to distinguish themselves, especially in the model that bundles together acute and post-acute services [55].

Infusing Palliative Care into Nursing Homes via Complementary, Innovative Care Models

Although hospice and external palliative care services hold promise for integrating palliative care into NHs, a full transformation cannot occur without addressing internal NH policies, practices, and culture. As noted above, NHs are ultimately responsible for their residents' care. Paying hospices to manage care that is focused on residents' terminal illness(es) can thwart efforts to meet the palliative care needs of other NH residents, further fragment responsibility for resident's care, and confuse residents, families, and care providers as to who is accountable for various healthcare components.

A more logical strategy is to integrate palliative care into ongoing NH workflows, regulatory requirements, and training. The culture change movement, which has gained momentum since the late 1990s, aligns well with palliative care principles and practices because of its overarching focus on resident quality of life and choice [56]. Although culture change is variously described, its key elements always include care that focuses on residents' needs and preferences in a home-like setting, rather than the typically institutional organizational routines and physical environments. Culture change NHs can readily integrate holistic, comfort care that is driven by residents' and families' goals, preferences, and needs. In a 2008 Center to Advance Palliative Care report on palliative care in NHs, the authors describe two New York City facilities that have embraced palliative care; their descriptions of these programs are barely distinguishable from culture change initiatives. Moreover, one of these facilities does not refer to its program as palliative care, explaining that "the high caliber of nursing home care they provide *is* palliative care" [17, p. 3.23].

Adoption of the culture change model is associated with several outcomes desired by NHs, such as enhanced staff satisfaction, reduced turnover, greater market share, and higher occupancy rates [56–58]. Furthermore, CMS has advanced the culture change movement by contracting with quality improvement organizations (QIOs) to train NH staff and administrators in culture change and by sponsoring meetings to bring relevant stakeholders together. CMS also supports culture change training for NH surveyors and regulators [59]. Several states have funded a range of strategies to facilitate the adoption of culture change. Most focus on workforce development to promote resident-directed care, especially for nursing assistants [59].

Although culture change initiatives are compatible with and even overlap with palliative care clinical guidelines, a quality NH palliative care program will need additional elements. Key palliative care components include providing holistic care that honors cultural and spiritual preferences and practices; addressing the needs of family as both caregiver and care recipient; ensuring prompt and effective symptom assessment and management; offering grief counseling and bereavement services before and after death of a resident; and supporting and role modeling open, respectful communication [60]. A strong argument can be made that these palliative care practices are critical to delivering resident-directed care.

Incorporating Palliative Care into Quality Reporting and the Inspection Process

Whether achieved through payment reform, additional service provision, regulatory changes, or culture change, mechanisms must be in place to assess providers' performance on measures of importance to this uniquely vulnerable patient population, to enforce expectations for care delivery, and to minimize unintended consequences. In other words, providers, policymakers, and consumers alike must be able to evaluate providers' performance and hold them accountable. A key barrier to creating greater accountability for palliative care in NHs is that the survey process and current quality measures are not well aligned with achieving high quality palliative care. Several quality measures are derived from the Minimum Data Set (MDS), which is a federally mandated assessment tool with multiple purposes—to guide care planning, determine payments to NHs, and evaluate care through the survey process and public reporting of MDS-based quality measures. Compared to earlier versions, the current iteration of the MDS (version 3.0) has new and expanded variables related to pain and other symptoms, decision-making, and goals of care [61], although palliative care-specific quality information remains limited [60, 62].

Not only are there few specific measures for evaluating palliative care, some indicators may hinder palliative care. For example, one NH quality measure is the percent of residents who lose excessive weight [63]. To date, there is no exclusion for residents whose goals are focused on comfort and end-of-life care and in whom weight loss would be expected (for example, people dying of end-stage dementia). For this reason, nursing facility administrators and staff are often concerned that allowing these natural developments among dying residents may be misinterpreted and penalized as poor quality of care, driving inappropriate hospitalizations, feeding tube placements, and burdensome transitions [64].

Quality measures are potentially powerful tools for advancing specific NH practices in palliative care. First, several key measures are publicly reported on the Nursing Home Compare website and are part of the CMS 5-star rating system. There is some evidence that better performance on publicly reported performance measures may increase NH's revenues and enhance its profit margin primarily through higher numbers of Medicare admissions [65]. Second, quality indicators can be integrated into pay for performance, of which the Federal Nursing Home Value Based Purchasing demonstration project, part of a CMS initiative to improve the quality of care delivered to Medicare beneficiaries in nursing homes, is a primary example. NHs in participating states are awarded points for performance on quality measures that include MDS quality indicators, staffing, hospitalization rates, and inspection survey deficiencies [66]. Although Werner et al. report that initial state Pay for Performance initiatives were associated with inconsistent improvement in NH quality [67], it is too early to say what effect this payment approach will have on key quality measures.

To achieve high levels of quality palliative care in NHs, the state inspection process needs to be adapted to focus on individualized, resident-centered care and culture change. Regulations should be shaped so that providing quality palliative care is supported by regulatory oversight, rather than impeded by it, as is the case at present. Additional education is needed for surveyors about palliative care practices so that they are readily able to recognize the quality of life and resident rights issues and distinguish them from facility deficiencies [68–70]. For example, residents and their families may choose not to provide artificial nutrition and hydration via a feeding tube for the anorexia and dysphagia that is the normal course of advanced Alzheimer's disease, especially since such interventions are not associated with better survival or improved quality of life. Instead of citing facilities for weight loss and dehydration, which are nearly ubiquitous for persons dying of advanced dementia, inspectors should be trained to examine actual goals of care for residents and whether the care provided is consistent with those goals. Findings such as lack of documentation of the goals of care or unmet spiritual needs should be the focus for defining deficient practices in residents with advanced dementia.

The CMS Survey and Certification Group issued a memorandum in late 2012 that confirmed their commitment to appropriate end-of-life care for nursing home residents. They directed state surveyors to evaluate nursing home quality according to palliative care standards when the goals of care focus on comfort [71]. This marks an important first step in aligning nursing home and palliative care.

Preparing and Maintaining a NH Workforce That Is Skilled in Palliative Care

As with any innovation, adoption of palliative care will require efforts at many levels—from corporate or national leadership to individual staff working with specific residents and families. Policies are needed to establish standards for conducting goals of care discussions, completing advance directives, assessing and managing pain and other symptoms, addressing family concerns, and assessing spiritual and cultural issues. An educated workforce is essential; all staff, including nursing assistants, administrators, pastoral care, recreational therapists, physical and occupational therapists, and dietary, housekeeping and maintenance personnel should have basic education in the philosophy and practice of palliative care. Particular attention should be paid to the training of certified nursing assistants who provide much of the hands-on care and have day-to-day human relationships with NH residents [72]. Education should also be extended to volunteers who, as hospice has shown, play an important role in palliative care. Training should be offered at regular intervals, both to reinforce earlier learning and to ensure that staff turnover does not lead to an unraveling of the program. Employers and others should encourage and support advanced education and certification by nursing assistants, licensed nursing staff, and primary care providers, who can serve as leaders, mentors, and experts for others. Other incentives, such as career ladders and better wages, can reduce turnover and improve care [42].

Evaluating Innovative Models of Palliative Care

Rigorous evaluation of all models of palliative care—whether comprehensive programs with multiple components or limited interventions of discreet therapeutic approaches—is needed. Little is known about the characteristics and effectiveness of the existing NH palliative care programs beyond anecdotal descriptions [17, 34]. There are few randomized controlled trials of discreet interventions [73–75] or complex multi-model interventions [76–78]. In the current climate of flat or shrinking budgets for NIH and many private foundations, there may need to be more reliance on demonstrations funded through CMS. While these programs are rarely, if ever, designed as controlled trials, they are intended to be generalizable and sustainable. Regardless of funding source, process of care variables (e.g., Is there a documented goals of care discussion among residents, families, and providers at regular intervals?), care outcomes (e.g., resident symptom experiences), and costs all should be measured and evaluated.

Conclusion

Our nation has long struggled to provide compassionate, person-centered care to frail elders with extensive care needs. Although many Americans dream of a day when the last NH closes its doors, this scenario is a fantasy, given the burgeoning population of adults who are living longer with chronic illness and disability. Society will need to intensify its commitment to caring for these individuals and their families. It is clear that enhancements in quality of care processes and outcomes lead to lesser reliance on emergency rooms and hospitals and to lower healthcare spending. Palliative care is a necessary element to achieve this goal.

References

1. Kaye HS, Harrington C, LaPlante MP. Long-term care: who gets it, who provides it, who pays, and how much? Health Aff (Millwood). 2010;29(1):11–21.
2. Administration on aging. Aging into the 21st century Department of Health and Human Services. 2011. http://www.aoa.gov/AoARoot/Aging_Statistics/future_growth/aging21/health.aspx#Nursing. Accessed 24 March 2013.
3. Jones A, Dwyer L, Bercovitz A, Strahan G. The National Nursing Home Survey: 2004 overview. National Center for Health Statistics. Vital Health Stat. 2009;13(167):1–155.
4. National Center for Health Statistics. Health United States, 2010: with special feature on death and dying. Hyattsville, MD: National Center for Health Statistics; 2011. http://www.cdc.gov/nchs/data/hus/hus10.pdf. Accessed 1 Aug 2013.
5. Mitchell SL, Teno JM, Miller SC, Mor V. A national study of the location of death for older persons with dementia. J Am Geriatr Soc. 2005;53(2):299–305.
6. Barnato AE, McClellan MB, Kagay CR, Garber AM. Trends in inpatient treatment intensity among Medicare beneficiaries at the end of life. Health Serv Res. 2004;39(2):363–75.
7. Goldfeld KS, Stevenson DG, Hamel MB, Mitchell SL. Medicare expenditures among nursing home residents with advanced dementia. Arch Intern Med. 2011;171(9):824–30.
8. Hurd MD, Martorell P, Delavande A, Mullen KJ, Langa KM. Monetary costs of dementia in the United States. N Engl J Med. 2013;368(14):1326–34.
9. Meier DE, Lim B, Carlson MD. Raising the standard: palliative care in nursing homes. Health Aff (Millwood). 2010;29(1):136–40.
10. Teno JM, Clarridge BR, Casey V, Welch LC, Wetle T, Shield R, et al. Family perspectives on end-of-life care at the last place of care. JAMA. 2004;291(1):88–93.
11. Morrison RS, Penrod JD, Cassel JB, Caust-Ellenbogen M, Litke A, Spragens L, et al. Cost savings associated with US hospital palliative care consultation programs. Arch Intern Med. 2008;168(16):1783–90.
12. Kelley A, Deb P, Du Q, Aldridge Carlson MD, Morrison RS. Hospice enrollment saves money for Medicare and improves care quality across a number of different lengths-of-stay. Health Aff (Millwood). 2013;32(3):552–61.
13. Casarett D, Pickard A, Bailey FA, Ritchie C, Furman C, Rosenfeld K, et al. Do palliative consultations improve patient outcomes? J Am Geriatr Soc. 2008;56(4):593–9.
14. Finlay IG, Higginson IJ, Goodwin DM, Cook AM, Edwards AG, Hood K, et al. Palliative care in hospital, hospice, at home: results from a systematic review. Ann Oncol. 2002;13 Suppl 4:257–64.
15. Hall S, Kolliakou A, Petkova H, Froggatt K, Higginson IJ. Interventions for improving palliative care for older people living in nursing care homes. Cochrane Database Syst Rev. 2011;(3):CD007132.
16. Berkowitz RE, Jones RN, Rieder R, Bryan M, Schreiber R, Verney S, Paasche-Orlow MK. Improving disposition outcomes for patients in a geriatric skilled nursing facility. J Am Geriatr Soc. 2011;59(6):1130–6.
17. Improving palliative care in Nursing Homes [online report]. New York: Center to Advance Palliative Care. 2008. http://www.capc.org/support-from-capc/capc_publications/nursing_home_report.pdf. Accessed 1 Aug 2013.
18. Rice KN, Coleman EA, Fish R, Levy C, Kutner JS. Factors influencing models of end-of-life care in nursing homes: results of a survey of nursing home administrators. J Palliat Med. 2004;7(5):668–75.

19. Tilden VP, Thompson SA, Gajewski BJ, Bott MJ. End-of-life care in nursing homes: the high cost of staff turnover. Nurs Econ. 2012;30(3):163–6.
20. Huskamp HA, Kaufmann C, Stevenson DG. The intersection of long-term care and end-of-life care. Med Care Res Rev. 2012;69(1):3–44.
21. Ersek M, Wilson SA. The challenges and opportunities in providing end-of-life care in nursing homes. J Palliat Med. 2003;6(1):45–57.
22. McGilton KS, Sidani S, Boscart VM, Guruge S, Brown M. The relationship between care providers' relational behaviors and residents mood and behavior in long-term care settings. Aging Ment Health. 2012;16(4):507–15.
23. Hanson LC, Ersek M. Meeting palliative care needs in post-acute care settings: "to help them live until they die". JAMA. 2006;295(6):681–6.
24. Miller SC, Lima J, Gozalo PL, Mor V. The growth of hospice care in U.S. nursing homes. J Am Geriatr Soc. 2010;58(8):1481–8.
25. Office of the Inspector General. Medicare Hospices that focus on nursing facility residents. Washington, DC: OIG; 2011.
26. Miller SC, Gozalo P, Mor V. Hospice enrollment and hospitalization of dying nursing home patients. Am J Med. 2001;111(1):38–44.
27. Miller SC, Mor V, Teno J. Hospice enrollment and pain assessment and management in nursing homes. J Pain Symptom Manage. 2003;26(3):791–9.
28. Hanson L, Ersek M. Meeting palliative care needs in post-acute care settings: "to help them live until they die." In: McPhee S, Winker M, Rabow M, Pantilat S, Markowitz A, editors. Care at the close of life: evidence and experience. New York: McGraw Hill; 2010. p. 513–21.
29. Baer WM, Hanson LC. Families' perception of the added value of hospice in the nursing home. J Am Geriatr Soc. 2000;48(8):879–82.
30. Stevenson DG, Bramson JS. Hospice care in the nursing home setting: a review of the literature. J Pain Symptom Manage. 2009;38(3):440–51.
31. MedPAC. Hospice Services. Report to the Congress: Medicare Payment Policy (March 2012). Washington, DC: The Medicare Payment Advisory Commission; 2012. p. 281–308. MedPAC has focused on the Medicare hospice benefit in its reports across several years, the most recent of which is the 2012 report.
32. Carlson MD, Lim B, Meier DE. Strategies and innovative models for delivering palliative care in nursing homes. J Am Med Dir Assoc. 2011;12(2):91–8.
33. Kane RL, Keckhafer G, Flood S, Bershadsky B, Siadaty MS. The effect of Evercare on hospital use. J Am Geriatr Soc. 2003;51(10):1427–34.
34. Miller SC, Han B. End-of-life care in U.S. nursing homes: nursing homes with special programs and trained staff for hospice or palliative/end-of-life care. J Palliat Med. 2008;11(6):866–77.
35. Belluck, P. Giving Alzheimer's patients their way, even chocolate. The New York Times; 31 Dec 2010. http://www.nytimes.com/2011/01/01/health/01care.html?_r=1&. Accessed 1 Aug 2013.
36. Mead R. The sense of an ending. The New Yorker; 20 May 2013. http://www.newyorker.com/reporting/2013/05/20/130520fa_fact_mead. Accessed 1 Aug 2013.
37. Long CO, Sowell EJ, Hess RK, Alonzo TR. Development of the questionnaire on palliative care for advanced dementia (qPAD). Am J Alzheimers Dis Other Demen. 2012;27(7):537–43.
38. Long CO. Palliative care for advanced dementia. J Gerontol Nurs. 2009;35(11):19–24.
39. Beatitudes Campus. Vermilion cliffs neighborhood on channel 3. BeatitudesCampus.org; 10 Jan 2011. http://www.beatitudescampus.org/about/news-and-press/vermilion-cliffs-neighborhood-on-channel-3/. Accessed 1 Aug 2013.
40. Huskamp HA, Stevenson DG, Chernew ME, Newhouse JP. A new medicare end-of-life benefit for nursing home residents. Health Aff (Millwood). 2010;29(1):130–5.
41. Suhrie EM, Hanlon JT, Jaffe EJ, Sevick MA, Ruby CM, Aspinall SL. Impact of a geriatric nursing home palliative care service on unnecessary medication prescribing. Am J Geriatr Pharmacother. 2009;7(1):20–5.
42. Stone R, Harahan MF. Improving the long-term care workforce serving older adults. Health Aff (Millwood). 2010;29(1):109–15.

43. Kovach C, Wilson S, Noonan P. The effects of hospice interventions on behaviors, discomfort, and physical complications of end stage dementia nursing home residents. Am J Alzheimers Dis Other Demen. 1996;11:7–15.
44. Davis FA. Medicare hospice benefit: early program experiences. Health Care Financ Rev. 1988;9(4):99–111.
45. Wachterman MW, Marcantonio ER, Davis RB, McCarthy EP. Association of hospice agency profit status with patient diagnosis, location of care, and length of stay. JAMA. 2011;305(5):472–9.
46. Waldman P. Aided by referral bonuses, hospice industry booms. The Washington Post; 7 Dec 2011.
47. Stevenson DG, Huskamp HA, Grabowski DC, Keating NL. Differences in hospice care between home and institutional settings. J Palliat Med. 2007;10(5):1040–7.
48. Bercovitz A, Decker FH, Jones A, Remsburg RE. End-of-life care in nursing homes: 2004 National Nursing Home Survey. National Health Statistics Report No. 9; 2008. p. 1–23.
49. Unroe KT, Meier DE. Quality of hospice care for individuals with dementia. J Am Geriatr Soc. 2013;61(7):1212–4.
50. MedPAC. Hospice Services. Report to the Congress: Medicare Payment Policy (March 2010). Washington, DC: The Medicare Payment Advisory Commission; 2010. p. 141–61.
51. Huskamp HA, Newhouse JP, Norcini JC, Keating NL. Variation in patients' hospice costs. Inquiry. 2008;45(2):232–44.
52. Miller SC, Lima JC, Looze J, Mitchell SL. Dying in U.S. nursing homes with advanced dementia: how does health care use differ for residents with, versus without, end-of-life Medicare skilled nursing facility care? J Palliat Med. 2012;15(1):43–50.
53. Aragon K, Covinsky K, Miao Y, Boscardin WJ, Flint L, Smith AK. Use of the medicare post-hospitalization skilled nursing benefit in the last 6 months of life. Arch Intern Med. 2012:1–7.
54. CMS Innovation Center. Initiative to reduce avoidable hospitalizations among nursing facility residents. CMS.gov. http://innovations.cms.gov/initiatives/rahnfr/index.html. Accessed 1 Aug 2013.
55. http://innovation.cms.gov/initiatives/BPCI-Model-2/index.html.
56. Doty M, Koren M, Sturla E. Culture change in nursing homes: how far have we come? Findings from the Commonwealth Fund 2007 National Survey of Nursing Homes: The Commonwealth Fund; 2008. Available http://www.commonwealthfund.org/Publications/Fund-Reports/2008/May/Culture-Change-in-Nursing-Homes--How-Far-Have-We-Come--Findings-From-The-Commonwealth-Fund-2007-Nati.aspx.
57. Yeatts DE, Cready CM. Consequences of empowered CNA teams in nursing home settings: a longitudinal assessment. Gerontologist. 2007;47(3):323–39.
58. Yeatts DE, Seward RR. Reducing turnover and improving health care in nursing homes: the potential effects of self-managed work teams. Gerontologist. 2000;40(3):358–63.
59. Bryant N, Stone R, Barbarotta L. State investments in culture change: case study of how states supported culture change initiatives in nursing homes. Washington, DC: American Association of Homes and Services for the Aging and the Institute for the Future of Aging Services; 2009.
60. National Consensus Project for Quality Palliative Care. Clinical practice guidelines for quality palliative care; 2013.
61. Centers for Medicare and Medicaid Services. RAI version 3.0 manual. 2011. Https://www.cms.gov/NursingHomeQualityInits/45_NHQIMDS30TrainingMaterials.asp#TopOfPage. Accessed 1 Aug 2013.
62. National Quality Forum. Preferred practices and performance measures for measuring and reporting care coordination: a consensus report 2010. http://www.qualityforum.org/Publications/2010/10/Preferred_Practices_and_Performance_Measures_for_Measuring_and_Reporting_Care_Coordination.aspx.Accessed 1 Aug 2013.
63. RTI International. MDS 3.0 Quality Measures USER'S MANUAL 2012. http://www.cms.gov/Medicare/Quality-Initiatives-Patient-Assessment-Instruments/NursingHomeQualityInits/Downloads/MDS-30-QM-Users-Manual-V60.pdf. Accessed 1 Aug 2013.
64. Kapp MB. Legal anxieties and end-of-life care in nursing homes. Issues Law Med. 2003;19(2):111–34.

65. Park J, Konetzka RT, Werner RM. Performing well on nursing home report cards: does it pay off? Health Serv Res. 2011;46(2):531–54.
66. Centers for Medicare and Medicaid Services. Nursing Home Quality Initiative: quality measures. 2012. http://www.cms.gov/Medicare/Quality-Initiatives-Patient-Assessment-nstruments/NursingHomeQualityInits/NHQIQualityMeasures.html. Accessed 6 March 2013.
67. Werner RM, Konetzka RT, Polsky D. The effect of pay-for-performance in nursing homes: evidence from State Medicaid Programs. Health Serv Res. 2013.
68. Guo KL, McGee D. Improving quality in long-term care facilities through increased regulations and enforcement. Health Care Manag. 2012;31(2):121–31.
69. Koren MJ. Person-centered care for nursing home residents: the culture-change movement. Health Aff (Millwood). 2010;29(2):312–7.
70. Miller SC, Miller EA, Jung HY, Sterns S, Clark M, Mor V. Nursing home organizational change: the "Culture Change" movement as viewed by long-term care specialists. Med Care Res Rev. 2010;67(4 Suppl):65S–81.
71. Centers for Medicare and Medicaid Services. Revisions to appendix pp—"interpretive guidelines for long-term care facilities F tag 309 quality of care". https://www.cms.gov/Medicare/Provider-Enrollment-and-Certification/SurveyCertificationGenInfo/Downloads/Survey-and-Cert-Letter-12-48.pdf. Accessed 2 Dec 2013.
72. Ersek M, editor. Core curriculum for the hospice and palliative care nursing assistant. Pittsburgh, PA: Hospice and Palliative Nurses Association; 2009.
73. Hanson LC, Carey TS, Caprio AJ, Lee TJ, Ersek M, Garrett J, et al. Improving decision-making for feeding options in advanced dementia: a randomized, controlled trial. J Am Geriatr Soc. 2011;59(11):2009–16.
74. Loeb M, Carusone SC, Goeree R, Walter SD, Brazil K, Krueger P, et al. Effect of a clinical pathway to reduce hospitalizations in nursing home residents with pneumonia: a randomized controlled trial. JAMA. 2006;295(21):2503–10.
75. Volandes AE, Paasche-Orlow MK, Barry MJ, Gillick MR, Minaker KL, Chang Y, et al. Video decision support tool for advance care planning in dementia: randomised controlled trial. BMJ. 2009;338:b2159.
76. Kovach CR, Logan BR, Noonan PE, Schlidt AM, Smerz J, Simpson M, et al. Effects of the Serial Trial Intervention on discomfort and behavior of nursing home residents with dementia. Am J Alzheimers Dis Other Demen. 2006;21(3):147–55.
77. Ersek M, Polissar N, Pen AD, Jablonski A, Herr K, Neradilek MB. Addressing methodological challenges in implementing the nursing home pain management algorithm randomized controlled trial. Clin Trials. 2012;9(5):634–44.
78. Jones KR, Fink R, Vojir C, Pepper G, Hutt E, Clark L, et al. Translation research in long-term care: improving pain management in nursing homes. Worldviews Evid Based Nurs. 2004;1 Suppl 1:S13–20.

Part III
Measuring Quality and Paying for the Care of the Seriously Ill

Chapter 7
Quality and Outcome Measures

Laura C. Hanson, Anna P. Schenck, and Helen Burstin

What Distinguishes High Quality Care for Older Adults with Serious Illness?

Value is the new healthcare imperative for the USA—improving quality while controlling costs. Americans spend almost twice what other developed countries spend for healthcare services, yet the return on our investment is poorer health outcomes, including higher rates of preventable death [1]. High quality care, defined in 1990 by the Institute of Medicine, is care that "*increases the likelihood of the desired health outcomes and is consistent with current professional knowledge*" [2]. In subsequent reports the Institute of Medicine has synthesized what is known and what we still need to know about measuring quality of care in order to improve patient safety and health outcomes [3, 4].

The greatest opportunity to enhance value in US healthcare is to improve quality of care for older adults with serious illness. Elders with advanced stage chronic illness or life-threatening acute illness use the majority of services, yet receive poor quality care [5]. Serious illness—illness from which patients are unlikely to be cured, recover, or stabilize—is life-altering for patients and family caregivers. It includes advanced, symptomatic stages of diseases such as congestive heart failure, chronic lung disease, cancer, kidney failure, and dementia. Serious illness

L.C. Hanson, M.D., M.P.H. (✉)
Division of Geriatric Medicine and Center for Aging and Health, University of North Carolina School of Medicine, 5003 Old Clinic Building, CB 7550, Chapel Hill, NC 27599, USA
e-mail: laura_hanson@med.unc.edu

A.P. Schenck, Ph.D.
Public Health Leadership Program, Gillings School of Global Public Health,
University of North Carolina, Chapel Hill, NC, USA

H. Burstin, M.D., M.P.H.
National Quality Forum, Washington, DC, USA

also results from the cumulative effects of multiple chronic conditions causing functional decline or frailty, a large population which accounts for up to 80 % of Medicare expenditures [6].

Patients with serious illness and their families value patient-centered care which promotes function, comfort, and shared decision-making. When medical treatment for cure is not possible, most patients desire healthcare that balances the goal of life prolongation with patient-centered outcomes of independent function, pain relief, physical comfort, and attention to family, emotional, and spiritual needs. Healthcare priorities shift in serious illness, and patients value control over goals of care and treatment through shared decision-making [7–10]. In serious illness, the way we define quality of care must respect the outcomes prioritized by patients and their families [11].

Is There Evidence for Healthcare Interventions to Improve Outcomes in Serious Illness?

Best research evidence supports three interventions to improve outcomes for older adults with serious illness—(1) expert pain and symptom treatment, (2) communication eliciting patient preferences for treatment decisions, and (3) interdisciplinary palliative care services.

In a 2008 systematic review, Lorenz examined treatment for specific symptoms in serious illness and found strong evidence for improved outcomes with systematic expert assessment and treatment of pain or depression for cancer patients, and assessment and treatment of dyspnea from chronic lung disease [12, 13]. This review also found evidence for improved care quality with structured communication to elicit patient treatment preferences. When this body of evidence was addressed in a major report to the Agency for Healthcare Research and Quality in 2012, investigators found the strongest research evidence supports expert treatment to improve pain and communication interventions to engage patient and family values in treatment decisions [14].

Palliative care teams provide specialized medical care for people with serious illness to improve quality of life for patients and families. Palliative care is usually delivered by interdisciplinary teams who combine expertise in pain and symptom management with support for shared decision-making. Research on palliative care services, or similar complex case management or hospice interventions show this innovative service model improves patient and family satisfaction with care in serious illness [15, 16]. Numerous studies—including 12 randomized trials—provide evidence that interdisciplinary palliative care improves patient and family satisfaction while reducing patients' use of intensive and acute care services [17–25]. Patients receiving palliative care live as long or longer than those receiving traditional medical care. The timing and intensity of palliative care interventions may be essential to maximize benefit [26]. While some palliative care interventions have not been able to improve patients' quality of life, involving the palliative care team early and continuously for patients with advanced lung cancer does improve quality of life, decrease depression, and prolong survival while reducing the intensity and cost of treatment [27].

Are There Practice Guidelines to Promote Quality Healthcare for Seriously Ill Older Adults?

National Consensus Project Guidelines for Quality Palliative Care are unique in addressing the universal needs of seriously ill patients. Many disease-specific practice guidelines do not apply in serious illness because they focus on early stage disease or omit patients with multiple chronic conditions. In recognition of the unique needs of seriously ill patients, the Institute of Medicine recommended developing new guidelines and quality measures for palliative care, which is specialized medical care for patients and families facing serious illness [28, 29]. In 2004, 2009, and 2013, the National Consensus Project for Quality Palliative Care (NCP) defined practice guidelines and preferred practices for palliative care [30]. The NCP framework reflects domains of healthcare quality considered important by seriously ill patients, including physical symptoms, emotional, spiritual, and family caregiver needs, and patient control over treatment decisions.

The National Quality Forum (NQF) is a voluntary organization established to build consensus standards among healthcare stakeholders, as defined by the National Technology Transfer and Advancement Act [31]. In 2007 the NQF reviewed and endorsed NCP guidelines and an associated list of 38 preferred practices, establishing them as the definitive statement of standards of care for serious illness [32, 33].

How Do We Currently Measure Quality of Healthcare for Older Adults with Serious Illness?

Guidelines describe ideal standards for healthcare, but quality measures are needed to understand how often real world care lives up to these ideals. Quality measures report the frequency of a desired care process or outcome for a group of patients for whom that measure matters. Data are generally pulled from claims or clinical records. A few quality measures are structural—such as reports of clinician qualifications or presence or absence of critical patient safety strategies. To understand and improve healthcare quality, clinicians need quality measures which are feasible (not too costly to collect), actionable (under the control of clinicians and health systems), reliable (easily measured the same way by different data collectors), and valid (meaningfully connected to person-centered outcomes).

Quality measures show gradual improvement in care for older adults. Since 2003 the Agency for Healthcare Research and Quality has published a summative report on healthcare quality using data from Medicare and other sources [34]. Quality measures are removed from this core measure set when practice is uniformly high, and new measures are added in response to new evidence. Longitudinal hospital data on process of care measures for acute myocardial infarction, congestive heart failure, pneumonia, immunization, and other preventive services has shown slow but consistent improvements in care for Medicare enrollees [35]. Progress is slow but real—in 2011 small improvements were recorded for 60 % of quality measures tracked. Access to care and disparities by race, ethnicity, and income are generally not improving. In 2011, disparities by age were added to this report, demonstrating that older adults have better access to services but receive poorer quality of care than young adults on 39 % of measures being tracked. This comprehensive report primarily relies on disease-specific measures, but includes a few cross-cutting concerns important in serious illness such as functional status preservation and, beginning in 2010, access to supportive and palliative care.

Which Quality Measures Are Ready for Systematic Use in the Care of Seriously Ill Patients?

Work is underway to develop and test quality measures for serious illness. Over 100 published quality measures address domains of potential relevance to palliative care and serious illness—yet few have been implemented and tested with adequate rigor to justify use [36–38]. The voluntary University Health System Consortium (UHC) palliative care benchmarking study was an important early effort to examine the feasibility and meaningful use of systematic quality measurement in serious illness [39]. Thirty-five academic hospitals abstracted quality data for $n = 1,596$ patients with serious illness diagnoses (heart failure, cancer, HIV infection, and respiratory failure) and recent readmissions. Benchmarking across sites was feasible, and care processes were consistently good for symptom assessments. Opportunities for improvement were identified in symptom control, communication of prognosis, determining and implementation of patient preferences for care, and attention to psychosocial needs. Only 13 % of patients received specialty palliative care.

In 2011 NQF recognized the need for quality measures unique to hospice and palliative care patients and in early 2012 endorsed 14 such measures [40]. One approach to quality measurement in serious illness is to survey family caregivers, and three major after-death family surveys have been endorsed by NQF (Table 7.1). After-death surveys use surrogates looking back in time, focus on the final phase of illness, and are limited to the subset of families who choose to respond. However, they capture the important family perspective and offer insights into

Table 7.1 Quality measures designed for adults with serious illness

Name	Measure type	Target population and setting	Domains included	NQF measures
NHPCO Family Evaluation of Hospice Care (FEHC)	After death survey of family caregivers	Patients who died in hospice care	In hospice— Caregiver support Caregiver information Coordination of care Physical and emotional comfort Overall satisfaction	0208 FEHC—Family Evaluation of Hospice Care
CARE Survey	After death survey of family caregivers	Patients who died after receiving care for at least 48 h from home health agency, nursing homes, hospice, or acute care hospital	In the last days of life— Physical comfort Emotional comfort Advance care planning Decision-making Respect, dignity Closure Caregiver support Caregiver efficacy	1632 CARE—Consumer Assessments and Reports of End of Life
VA Bereaved Family Survey	After death survey of family caregivers of Veterans	Veterans who died in any setting	In the last month of life— Well-being Communication Decision-making Emotional and spiritual distress Physical symptoms Facility choice Care in active dying Access	1623 Bereaved Family Survey
NHPCO Comfortable Dying	Patients with pain on admission whose are comfortable within 48 h	Patients who died in hospice	Physical symptoms	0209 Comfortable dying
RAND ACOVE Opioid bowel regimen	Patients who are prescribed opioids who are also given a bowel regimen	Vulnerable elders in outpatient or hospital settings	Physical symptoms	1617 Patients treated with an opioid who are given a bowel regimen

(continued)

Table 7.1 (continued)

Name	Measure type	Target population and setting	Domains included	NQF measures
RAND ACOVE ICU Care preferences	Patients admitted in the ICU who have care preference documented	Vulnerable elders in intensive care	Communication	1626 Patients admitted to ICU who have care preferences documented
RAND ACOVE ICD deactivation	Hospitalized patients who die an expected death who have an ICD deactivated, or documentation of why it was not deactivated	Patients with expected death in hospital	Communication	1625 ICD deactivation
RAND ASSIST Cancer pain assessment	Clinic patients with advanced cancer who are assessed for pain	Patients with advanced cancer in outpatient settings	Physical symptoms	1628 Patients with advanced cancer assessed for pain
PEACE Pain Screening Assessment	Patients in hospice/palliative care who are screened for pain Patients in pain who are assessed	Hospice and palliative care patients	Physical symptoms	1634 Pain screening 1637 Pain Assessment
PEACE Dyspnea Screening Assessment	Patients in hospice/palliative care who are screened for dyspnea Patients with dyspnea who are assessed	Hospice and palliative care patients	Physical symptoms	1638 Dyspnea Screening 1639 Dyspnea Assessment
PEACE Treatment preferences	Patients in hospice/palliative care who have chart documentation of treatment preferences	Hospice and palliative care patients	Communication	1641 Treatment preferences
DEYTA Spiritual assessment	Hospice patients with a documented discussion of spiritual/religious concerns or desire not to discuss	Hospice patients	Spiritual care	1647 Hospice patients with spiritual assessment

multiple domains of serious illness care. The National Hospice and Palliative Care Organization, working in collaboration with investigators from Brown University, has developed process of care metrics and an after-death family survey to measure quality of care for hospice patients. This survey—the Family Evaluation of Hospice Care—has been widely accepted. Thousands of hospice family caregivers report good quality of care; some respondents indicate unmet needs for family support (18 %), communication (10–29 %), and care coordination (22 %) [41–43]. The broader CARE survey has been used to address quality of care in the final days of life in multiple healthcare settings, with demonstration that the site of care may strongly influence aspects of care quality at the end of life [44–46]. The Bereaved Family Survey is a similar, cross-setting after-death survey covering multiple domains of quality of care in the Veterans Affairs (VA) system during a patient's final month of life [47, 48]. A newer short form may become especially useful, relieving some response burden and perhaps permitting a broader group of family caregivers to provide feedback [49]. Applied in a national study in 77 VA medical centers, results found consistent improvements in family satisfaction with care when Veterans had access to specialty palliative care [50].

Process and outcome quality measures capture discrete aspects of care for patients with serious illness from medical records (Table 7.1). Quality measurement research initiatives have led to NQF-endorsed quality measures of this type. First, the Assessing Care of Vulnerable Elders (ACOVE) project, with leadership from the RAND Corporation, has carefully developed and tested quality of care measures for vulnerable elders—older adults who self-report poor health with functional limitations [51, 52]. The ACOVE project has generated over 200 quality measures in domains of preventive care, disease-specific care, and geriatric syndromes; many ACOVE measures are relevant to seriously ill older adults in outpatient clinics [53]. A specific subset of 16 ACOVE quality measures addresses physical symptoms and communication of treatment preferences for vulnerable elders in hospital. NQF has endorsed three ACOVE quality measures for use in hospice and palliative care—use of bowel regimen with opioids, communication of treatment preferences, and ICD deactivation decisions [54]. Investigators from RAND and Johns Hopkins have also validated Cancer Quality ASSIST measures specifically focused for patients with advanced stage cancer in outpatient and hospital settings [55–57]. A third study to test quality measures for patients with serious illness, the PEACE Project, was led by investigators at the University of North Carolina and the federal Quality Improvement Organization for North and South Carolina. Existing or proposed quality measures for settings of hospice and hospital-based palliative care were reviewed by an expert panel for feasibility, actionability, reliability, and validity, and 17 PEACE measures have been validated in hospice and hospitalized palliative care patient populations [36, 58]. Measures for care for pain, dyspnea, and for communication of treatment preferences have also been endorsed by NQF [40]. However, none have yet been incorporated into Medicare's value-based purchasing or ACO quality measure requirements.

How Does US Policy Promote High Quality Care for Seriously Ill Older Adults?

Federal regulations first addressed quality standards for patients with serious illness by addressing the quality of care for older adults in nursing home care and hospice. Nursing home regulatory changes in 1987 led to the implementation of a nationwide dataset used to measure and improve quality of care for residents [59]. Data on key quality measures are publically available on the Nursing Home Compare website, and used for regulatory oversight and payment incentives. Quality improvement initiatives have had demonstrable positive effects on pain management and reduced use of physical restraints [60–62]. Nursing home quality data has been recently revised to incorporate more resident-centered outcomes and preferences [63].

In 2010, President Obama signed the Patient Protection and Affordable Care Act (ACA), mandating a new emphasis on healthcare quality. The law requires the Department of Health and Human Services to create a National Strategy on Quality Improvement in Health Care. Legislative provisions include creation and testing of new approaches to quality measurement, and implementation of quality measures for the Medicare and Medicaid populations. Beginning in 2012, quality measurement is reinforced by the value-based purchasing power of the federal Medicare and Medicaid programs. Acute care hospitals in the USA will see 1 % of federal payments at risk based on performance on clinical care quality measures and patients' reports in Hospital Consumer Assessment of Healthcare Providers and Systems (HCAHPS) surveys. Following hospitals, end-stage renal disease programs, outpatient physicians, long-term care hospitals, inpatient rehabilitation hospitals, hospice programs, and cancer hospitals will then be required to submit data on quality measures. Financial risk incentives will be followed by more comprehensive value-based purchasing [64].

In 2008, revised Conditions of Participation for hospices were published by the Centers for Medicare and Medicaid Services (CMS). Section 418.58 of the Final Rule requires hospices to create procedures for quality assessment and performance improvement (QAPI) addressing important domains of patient care quality, with measures to track and improve practices [65]. With funding from CMS, the Research Triangle Institute is pilot testing six quality measures to ascertain the feasibility and burden of standardized data elements for hospice. This hospice bundle may be used to modify hospice payment using NQF-endorsed measures beginning in 2016 [66].

What Are Future Opportunities—and Essential Strategies—to Improve Quality and Outcomes for Seriously Ill Older Adults?

Scientifically sound and clinically meaningful quality measures are available for the care of seriously ill older adults. Implementation of these measures poses future challenges, but also great opportunities to ensure care is consistently person centered (Box 7.1). To ensure high quality healthcare for seriously ill older adults, private and public organizations should target seven key opportunities.

Box 7.1 Opportunities and Strategies to Improve Quality of Care for Serious Illness

1. Identify patients with serious illness as a unique population in all healthcare settings

    - Create documentation of disease stage and function in electronic health records
    - Require disease stage modifiers for major diagnoses
    - Require functional status modifiers
    - Develop modifiers for multi-morbidity, frailty syndrome
    - Link access to payment for enhanced services to codes indicating serious illness

2. Measure what matters to patients with serious illness, including patient- and family-reported outcomes

    - Focus quality measures on pain and symptom control, function and shared decision-making
    - Exclude patients with serious illness from other measures
    - Fund research on feasible patient- and family-reported outcomes for serious illness

3. Respect patient preferences; promote shared decision-making

    - Implement quality measures for shared decision-making
    - Implement time-based payment for decision-making
    - Fund dissemination research for decision aids, structured communication
    - Promote education in communication skills

4. Assist hospice organizations to improve care using quality measurement and benchmarking

    - Implement quality measures in hospices
    - Provide technical assistance for implementation and quality improvement from QIOs

5. Coordinate care for seriously ill patients across healthcare settings

    - Review best practices in case management and care coordination
    - Identify programs improving patient outcomes in serious illness
    - Create a "glide path" to provide payment for case management and care coordination

6. Improve access to clinicians with expertise in serious illness—geriatrics, palliative care, and hospice care

    - Incentivize training for physicians, nurses, and social workers in these fields
    - Fund demonstration projects to extend expertise to underserved populations and settings

1. *Identify patients with serious illness as a unique population in all healthcare settings.* To be eligible for unique quality measures and enhanced services, patients with serious illness need to become a distinct population in healthcare. Routine identification of advanced stage disease and of functional impairments are the place to begin. Most major chronic diseases have defined staging systems, and several widely accepted measures of functional status are reliable, valid and feasible for clinical application. Beyond hospice, seriously ill patients are found in all other healthcare settings. Electronic health record vendors can create this opportunity now, and clinicians can demand these modifications to enable effective targeting of this population for quality improvement. Conditions of multi-morbidity and frailty syndrome clearly contribute to serious illness, but clear operational definitions remain an essential area for research. The NQF has begun this work, by creating a framework for multi-morbidity quality metrics—an essential first step [67]. Until patients with serious illness are identified as a unique population in all settings, quality measurement may result in imposition of unwanted tests or treatments while omitting what patients want and need. Key strategies are to—

    (a) Create documentation of disease stage and functional status in electronic health records, allowing health systems to identify patients with serious illness
    (b) Require disease stage coding modifiers for major diagnoses in all healthcare settings
    (c) Require functional status coding modifiers in all healthcare settings
    (d) Develop and test new modifiers for multi-morbidity and frailty syndrome, low literacy and other markers of vulnerability
    (e) Link access to payment for enhanced services—geriatric team care, palliative care, chronic care management—to identification of serious illness

2. *Measure what matters to patients with serious illness, including patient- and family-reported outcomes.* Quality measures should focus on the top priorities of patients with serious illness—relief from pain and other distressing symptoms, independent function, and shared decision-making for major treatments. The logic for patient-reported outcomes is particularly powerful when life expectancy is short [68, 69]. To avoid burdening this vulnerable population, research on feasible implementation strategies is needed to explore family reporting, shortened instruments, and combined use of patient reported measures with chart-based process measures.

    A corollary to this recommendation is that quality measures emphasizing prevention or disease-specific processes of care are less relevant, and may be harmful. For example, tightly controlled diabetes or timely cancer screening tests are high quality care for healthy older adults, but are poor quality of care for persons with advanced or incurable progressive diseases [70]. Neither patients nor their healthcare providers should be included in these metrics [71]. A major opportunity to improve quality for seriously ill older adults will be realized when metrics uniquely tailored to serious illness are the only ones applied in the care of these patients. Key strategies are to—

   (a) Implement quality measures for serious illness focused on priority domains of pain and symptom control, support of function, and shared decision-making for major treatments
   (b) Exclude these same patients with serious illness from other disease-specific quality measures
   (c) Fund research to implement feasible patient- and family-reported outcome measures for serious illness

3. *Respect patient and family preferences and promote shared decision-making.* Many preference-sensitive decisions emerge during the care of patients with serious illness. Research evidence supports the use of decision aids, structured clinical communication, and intensive clinician training to improve shared decision-making. These effective interventions are rarely disseminated in practice. Clinicians may be responsive to incentives for use of validated decision aids and effective clinical communication, so that seriously ill patients can consider the pros and cons of major medical treatment decisions. Key strategies are to—

   (a) Implement quality measures for documentation of shared decision-making
   (b) Implement time-based billing for shared decision-making
   (c) Fund research to test feasible dissemination strategies for decision aids and structured communication interventions
   (d) Promote education in shared decision-making skills in medical, nursing, and social work training

4. *Assist hospice organizations to improve care using quality measurement and benchmarking.* Hospices have been relatively slow to adopt electronic health records and data tracking [72]. The Quality Assessment and Performance Improvement regulations for hospice providers are promoting hospice growth in electronic health records and quality measurement. Smaller and nonprofit hospice organizations may require greater technical assistance to make these changes [73]. Key strategies are to—

   (a) Implement quality measures and benchmarking in hospice organizations
   (b) Provide technical assistance from Quality Improvement Organizations to allow effective implementation and quality improvement

5. *Coordinate care for older patients with serious illness across settings.* Current approaches to quality measurement are setting specific, yet seriously ill patients experience a multitude of providers and sites of care. The use of quality measures must be consistent and meaningful across provider hand-offs and transitions in site of care [74]. Reducing the number of transitions will help. However, quality care will only become meaningful when a single healthcare system or medical home provides continuity and coordination across all settings. Innovative insurers and healthcare organizations are testing these models, and CMS has

funded demonstration projects. However, the translation of these models to universal practice remains uncertain [75]. Key strategies are to—

   (a) Review best practice case management and care coordination programs from private sector innovators, and from funded demonstration projects
   (b) Identify case management and care coordination models that improve patient-centered outcomes such as pain control, satisfaction with care, care transitions
   (c) Create a rapid policy "glide path" to implement payment for proven models of case management and care coordination

6. *Improve access to clinicians with expertise in the care of seriously ill older adults.* Diffusion of new norms in medicine is a complex social process, mediated by peer leaders who adopt best practices, and influence other clinicians through education and demonstration. Peer leaders with expertise in care of seriously ill older adults are largely clinicians in geriatric care, palliative care, and hospice—they include physicians, nurses, and social workers, as well as other disciplines. Profound workforce shortages for physicians, nurses and other healthcare providers in both specialties may slow diffusion of good care for seriously ill patients [76]. For example, in 2012 there were approximately 6,000 palliative medicine physicians and just over 7,000 geriatricians in the USA to serve millions of seriously ill older adults [77, 78]. Expertise is less available in smaller, rural, or primary access hospitals. Key strategies are to—

   (a) Incentivize training in geriatric care, hospice, and palliative care through loan repayment, mid-career certification programs, and expansion of fellowship funds
   (b) Fund demonstration projects to extend expertise to underserved populations, geographic areas, and sole community provider hospitals [79]

References

1. The Commonwealth Fund Commission on a High Performance Health System. Why not the best? Results from the National Scorecard on US Health System Performance. 2011. http://www.commonwealthfund.org/Publications/Fund-Reports/2011/Oct/Why-Not-the-Best-2011.aspx. Accessed 10 Feb 2013.
2. Institute of Medicine. Medicare: a strategy for quality assurance, K.N. Lohr, ed. Washington, DC: National Academy Press; 1990.
3. Quality of Health Care in America Committee of the Institute of Medicine. Crossing the quality chasm: a new health system for the 21st century. Washington DC: Academy; 2001.
4. Committee on Identifying Priority Areas for Quality Improvement. Priority areas for national action: transforming health care quality. Washington, DC: National Academy Press; 2003.
5. The Commonwealth Fund Commission on a High Performance Health System. The performance improvement imperative: utilizing a coordinated, community-based approach to enhance care and lower costs for chronically Ill patients. 2012. http://www.commonwealthfund.org/Publications/Fund-Reports/2012/Apr/Performance-Improvement-Imperative.aspx. Accessed 10 Feb 2013.

6. Working Group on Health Outcomes for Older Persons with Multiple Chronic Conditions. Universal health outcome measures for older persons with multiple chronic conditions. J Am Geriatr Soc. 2012;60:2333–41.
7. Singer PA, Martin DK, Kelner M. Quality end-of-life care: patients' perspectives. JAMA. 1999;281(2):163–8.
8. Steinhauser KE, Christakis NA, Clipp EC, et al. Factors considered important at the end of life by patients, family, physicians, and other care providers. JAMA. 2000;284(19):2476–82.
9. Hanson LC, Danis M, Garrett J. What is wrong with end of life care? Opinions of bereaved family members. J Am Geriatr Soc. 1997;45:1339–44.
10. Teno JM, Clarridge BR, Casey V, et al. Family perspectives on end-of-life care at the last place of care. JAMA. 2004;291(1):88–93.
11. Teno JM, Casey VA, Welch JC, Edgman-Levitan S. Patient-focused, family-centered end-of-life care: views of the guidelines and bereaved family members. J Pain Symptom Manage. 2001;22(3):738–51.
12. Lorenz KA, Lynn J, Dy SM, Shugarman LR, Wilkinson A, Mularski RA, Morton SC, Hughes RG, Hilton LK, Maglione M, Rhodes SL, Rolon C, Sun VC, Shekelle PG. Evidence for improving palliative care at the end of life: a systematic review. Ann Intern Med. 2008; 148:147–59.
13. Qaseem A, Snow V, Shekelle P, et al. Evidence-based interventions to improve the palliative care of pain, dyspnea, and depression at the end of life: a clinical practice guideline from the American College of Physicians. Ann Intern Med. 2008;148:141–6.
14. Dy SM, Aslakson R, Wilson RF, Fawole OA, Lau BD, Martinez KA, Vollenweider D, Apostol C, Bass EB. Improving health care and palliative care for advanced and serious illness. Closing the quality gap: revisiting the state of the science. Evidence report no. 208. (Prepared by Johns Hopkins University Evidence-based Practice Center under Contract No. 290-2007-10061-I.) AHRQ publication no. 12(13)-E014-EF. Rockville, MD: Agency for Healthcare Research and Quality. 2012. www.effectivehealthcare.ahrq.gov/reports/final.cfm. Accessed 15 Feb 2013.
15. Dy SM, Shugarman LR, Lorenz KA, Mularski RA, Lynn J, RAND-Southern California Evidence-Based Practice Center. A systematic review of satisfaction with care at end of life. J Am Geriatr Soc. 2008;56:124–9.
16. Dy SM, Apostol C, Martinez KA, Aslakson RA. Continuity, coordination and transitions of care for patients with serious and advanced illness: a systematic review of interventions. J Palliat Med. 2013;16(4):436–45.
17. Gade G, Venohr I, Conner D, et al. Impact of an inpatient palliative care team: a randomized controlled trial. J Palliat Med. 2008;11:180–90.
18. Ringdal GI, Jordhoy MS, Kaasa S. Family satisfaction with end of life care for cancer patients in a cluster randomized trial. J Pain Symptom Manage. 2002;24:53–63.
19. Engelhardt JB, McClive-Reed KP, Toseland RW, Smith TL, Larson DG, Tobin DR. Effects of a program for coordinated care of advanced illness on patients, surrogates, and health care costs: a randomized trial. Am J Manag Care. 2006;12:93–100.
20. Jordhoy MS, Fayers P, Saltnes T, Ahlner-Elmqvist M, Jannert M, Kaasa S. A palliative care intervention and death at home: a cluster randomized trial. Lancet. 2000;356:888–93.
21. Smith TJ, Coyne P, Cassel B, Penberthy L, Hopson A, Hager MA. A high-volume specialist palliative care unit and team may reduce in-hospital end-of-life care costs. J Palliat Med. 2003;6:699–705.
22. O'Mahoney S, Blank AE, Zallman L, Selwyn P. The benefits of a hospital-based inpatient palliative care consultation service: preliminary outcome data. J Palliat Med. 2005;8:1033–9.
23. Elsayem A, Smith ML, Palmer JL, Jenkins R, Reddy S, Bruera E. Impact of a palliative care service on in-hospital mortality in a comprehensive cancer center. J Palliat Med. 2006; 9:894–902.
24. Gelfman LP, Meier D, Morrison RS. Does palliative care improve quality? A survey of bereaved family members. J Pain Symptom Manage. 2008;36f:22–8.
25. Goldsmith B, Dietrich J, Du Q, Morrison RS. Variability in hospital access to palliative care in the US. J Palliat Med. 2008;11(8):1094–102.

26. Casarett D, Pickard A, Bailey FA, Ritchie C, Furman C, Rosenfeld K, Shreve S, Chen Z, Shea JA. Do palliative consultations improve patient outcomes? J Am Geriatr Soc. 2008;56:593–9.
27. Temel JS, Greer JA, Muzikansky A, Gallagher ER, Admane S, Jackson VA, Dahlin CM, Blinderman CD, Jacobsen J, Pirl WF, Billings JA, Lynch TJ. Early palliative care for patients with metastatic non-small cell lung cancer. N Engl J Med. 2010;363:733–42.
28. Field MJ, Cassel CK, editors. Approaching death: improving care at the end of life. Washington, DC: National Academy Press; 1997.
29. Lunney JR, Foley KM, Smith TJ, Gelband H. Describing death in America: what we need to know. Washington, DC: National Academy Press; 2003.
30. National Consensus Project for Quality Palliative Care. Clinical practice guidelines for quality palliative care, National Consensus Project, Pittsburgh, PA. http://www.nationalconsensus-project.org. Accessed 15 May 2013.
31. National Technology Transfer and Advancement Act of 1995. PL 104-113, 15 USC 3701. 1996.
32. National Quality Forum (NQF). National priorities for healthcare quality measurement and reporting: a consensus report. Washington, DC: NQF; 2004.
33. National Quality Forum (NQF). National framework and preferred practices for palliative and hospice care. Washington, DC: NQF; 2007.
34. 2012 National Healthcare Quality Report. Rockville, MD: Agency for Healthcare Research and Quality; 2013. Available from: http://www.ahrq.gov/research/findings/nhqrdr/nhqr12/.
35. Jencks SF, Huff ED, Cuerdon T. Change in the quality of care delivered to Medicare beneficiaries, 1998-1999 to 2000-2001. JAMA. 2003;289(3):305–12.
36. Schenck AP, Rokoske FS, Durham DD, Cagle JG, Hanson LC. The PEACE Project: identification of quality measures for hospice and palliative care. J Palliat Med. 2010;13:1451–9.
37. Pasman HRW, Brandt HE, Deliens L, Francke AL. Quality indicators for palliative care: a systematic review. J Pain Symptom Manage. 2009;38:145–56.
38. Lorenz KA, Lynn J, Dy S, Wilkinson A, Mularski RA, Shugarman LR, Hughes R, Asch SM, Rolon C, Rastegar A, Shekelle PG. Quality measures for symptoms and advance care planning in caner: a systematic review. J Clin Oncol. 2006;24:4933–8.
39. Twaddle ML, Maxwell TL, Cassel JB, Liao S, Coyne PJ, Usher BM, Amin A, Cuny J. Palliative care benchmarks form academic medical centers. J Palliat Med. 2007;10:86–98.
40. NQF Endorses Palliative and End-of-Life Measures. http://www.qualityforum.org/News_And_Resources/Press_Releases/2012/NQF_Endorses_Palliative_and_End-of-Life_Care_Measures.aspx. Accessed 21 Feb 2013.
41. Connor SR, Teno J, Spence C, Smith N. Family evaluation of hospice care: results from voluntary submission of data via Website. J Pain Symptom Manage. 2005;30(1):9–17.
42. Rhodes RL, Teno JM, Connor SR. African American bereaved family members´ perceptions of the quality of hospice care: lessened disparities, but opportunities to improve remain. J Pain Symptom Manage. 2007;34(5):472–9.
43. Rhodes RL, Mitchell SL, Miller SC, Connor SR, Teno JM. Bereaved family members' evaluation of hospice care: what factors influence overall satisfaction with services? J Pain Symptom Manage. 2008;35(4):365–71.
44. Teno JM, Casey VA, Welch L, Edgman-Levitan S. Patient-focused, family-centered end-of-life medical care: views of the guidelines and bereaved family members. J Pain Symptom Manage. 2001;22(3):738–51.
45. Teno JM, Clarridge B, Casey V, Edgman-Levitan S, Fowler J. Validation of toolkit after-death bereaved family member interview. J Pain Symptom Manage. 2001;22(3):752–8.
46. Teno JM, Clarridge BR, Casey V, et al. Family perspectives on end-of-life care at the last place of care. JAMA. 2004;291(1):88–93.
47. Casarett D, Pickard A, Bailey FA, Ritchie CS, Furman CD, Rosenfeld K, Shreve S, Shea J. A national VA palliative care quality measure: the family assessment of treatment at the end of life. J Palliat Med. 2008;11(1):68–75.
48. Finlay E, Shreve S, Casarett D. Nationwide Veterans Affairs quality measure for cancer: the family assessment of treatment at the end of life. J Clin Oncol. 2008;26(23):3838–44.
49. Casarett D, Shreve S, Luhrs C, Lorenz K, Smith D, De Souse M, Richardson D. Measureing families' perceptions of care across a health care system: preliminary experience with the

Family Assessment of Treatment at End of Life Short Form (FATE-S). J Pain Symptom Manage. 2010;40:801–9.
50. Casarett D, Johnson M, Smith D, Richardson D. The optimal delivery of palliative care: a national comparison of the outcomes of consultation teams vs inpatient units. Arch Intern Med. 2011;171:649–55.
51. Saliba D, Elliott M, Rubenstein LZ, et al. The Vulnerable Elders Survey: a tool for identifying vulnerable older people in the community. J Am Geriatr Soc. 2001;49:1691–9.
52. Shekelle PG, MacLean CH, Morton SC, Wenger NS. ACOVE quality indicators. Ann Intern Med. 2001;135:653–67.
53. Wenger NS, Solomon DH, Roth CP, MacLean CH, Saliba D, Kamberg CJ, Rubenstein LZ, Young RT, Sloss EM, Louie R, Adams J, Change JT, Venus PJ, Schnelle JF, Shekelle PG. The quality of medical care provided to vulnerable community-dwelling older patients. Ann Intern Med. 2003;139:740–7.
54. Lorenz KA, Rosenfeld K, Wenger N. Quality indicators for palliative and end-of-life care in vulnerable elders. J Am Geriatr Soc. 2007;55:S318–26.
55. Lorenz KA, Dy SM, Naeim A, Walling AM, Sanati H, Smith P, Shanman R, Roth CP, Asch SM. Quality measures for supportive cancer care: the Cancer Quality-ASSIST Project. J Pain Symptom Manage. 2009;37:943–64.
56. Dy SM, Lorenz KA, Oneill SM, Asch SM, Walling AM, Tisnado D, Antonio AL, Malin JL. Cancer Quality-ASSIST supportive oncology quality indicator set: feasibility, reliability and validity testing. Cancer. 2010;116:3267–75.
57. Dy SM, Asch SM, Lorenz KA, Weeks K, Sharma RK, Wolff AC, Malin JL. Quality of end-of-life care for patients with advanced cancer in an academic medical center. J Palliat Med. 2011;14:451–7.
58. Hanson LC, Rowe C, Wessell K, Caprio A, Winzelberg G, Beyea A, Bernard SA. Measuring palliative care quality for seriously ill hospitalized patients. J Palliat Med. 2012;15: 798–804.
59. Hawes C, Mor V, Phillips CD, Fries BE, Morris JN, Steele-Friedlob E, Green AM, Nennstiel M. The OBRA-87 nursing home regulations and implementation of the Resident Assessment Instrument: effects on process quality. J Am Geriatr Soc. 1997;45:977–85.
60. Nursing Home Compare Website. http://www.medicare.gov/nursinghomecompare/. Accessed 22 May 2013.
61. Rollow W, Lied TR, McGann P, Poyer J, LaVoie L, Kambic TR, Bratzler DW, Ma A, Huff ED, Ramunno LD. Assessment of the Medicare Quality Improvement Organization program. Ann Intern Med. 2006;145:342–53.
62. Horner JK, Hanson LC, Wood D, Silver AG, Reynolds KS. Using quality improvement to address pain management practices in nursing homes. J Pain Symptom Manage. 2005;30: 271–7.
63. Saliba D, Buchanan J. Making the investment count: revision of the Minimum Data Set for nursing homes, MDS 3.0. J Am Med Dir Assoc. 2012;13:602–10.
64. VanLare JM, Conway PH. Value-based purchasing—national programs to move from volume to value. N Engl J Med. 2012;367:292–5.
65. Centers for Medicare and Medicaid Services. Hospice conditions of participation final rule. Federal register vol. 73 no. 109. 2008. http://www.nhpco.org/sites/default/files/public/regulatory/Medicare_COPS_Updated_072911.pdf. Accessed 4 March 2011.
66. Federal Register. Medicare Program; FY 2014 Hospice Wage Index and Payment Rate Update; Hospice Quality Reporting Requirements; and Updates on Payment Reform, A Proposed Rule by the Centers for Medicare & Medicaid Services. https://www.federalregister.gov/articles/2013/05/10/2013-10389/medicare-program-fy-2014-hospice-wage-index-and-payment-rate-update-hospice-quality-reporting#h-38
67. National Quality Forum. Multiple chronic conditions measurement framework: final report. 2012. http://www.qualityforum.org/Publications/2012/05/MCC_Measurement_Framework_Final_Report.aspx. Accessed 11 Aug 2013.

68. Berenson RA, Provonost PJ, Krumholz HM. Achieving the potential of health care performance measures. Robert Wood Johnson Foundation with the Urban Institute; 2013. http://www.rwjf.org/content/dam/farm/reports/reports/2013/rwjf406195. Accessed 11 Aug 2013.
69. National Quality Forum. Patient-reported outcomes (PROs) in performance measurement. http://www.qualityforum.org/Publications/2012/12/Patient-Reported_Outcomes_in_Performance_Measurement.aspx. Accessed 11 Aug 2013.
70. Boyd CM, Darer J, Boult C, Fried LP, Boult L, Wu AW. Clinical practice guidelines and quality of care for older patients with multiple comorbid diseases: implications for pay for performance. JAMA. 2005;294:716–24.
71. Lee EO, Emanuel EJ. Shared decision making to improve care and reduce costs. N Engl J Med. 2013;368:6–8.
72. Cagle JG, Rokoske FS, Durham D, Schenck AP, Spence C, Hanson LC. Use of electronic documentation for quality improvement in hospice. Am J Med Qual. 2012;27:282–90.
73. Hanson LC, Schenck AP, Rokoske FS, Abernethy AP, Kutner JS, Spence C, Person JL. Hospices' preparation and practices for quality measurement. J Pain Symptom Manage. 2010;39:1–8.
74. Pham HH, Schrag D, O'Malley AS, Wu B, Bach PB. Care patterns in Medicare and their implications for pay for performance. N Engl J Med. 2007;356:1130–9.
75. "The nurse's house call: If this were a pill, you'd do anything to get it." Washington Post; 2013. http://files.parsintl.com/eprints/77000.pdf. Accessed 8 Aug 2013.
76. Kovner CT, Mezey M, Harrington C. Who cares for older adults? Workforce implications of an aging society. Health Aff. 2002;21:78–89.
77. Morrison RS, Augustin R, Souvanna P, Meier DE. America's care of serious illness: a state-by-state report card on access to palliative care in our nation's hospitals. J Palliat Med. 2011;14:1094–6.
78. Bragg EJ, Warshaw GA, Meganathan K, Brewer DE. The development of academic geriatric medicine 2005 to 2010: and essential resource for improving the medical care of older adults. J Am Geriatr Soc. 2012;60:1540–5.
79. Center to Advance Palliative Care Website. http://www.capc.org/reportcard/findings. Accessed 8 Aug 2013.

Chapter 8
Palliative Care's Impact on Utilization and Costs: Implications for Health Services Research and Policy

J. Brian Cassel

Introduction

The fundamental ethos of palliative care and hospice services is to improve quality of life and quality of care for those with serious and chronic illnesses as well as those approaching their death. The clinical innovators in hospice and palliative care—starting with Cicely Saunders herself—responded to the unmet needs of patients, focusing on the relief of suffering and creating the ability to provide for a "good death" when death is inevitable and imminent. The sole motivation of these innovators has been to reduce pain and suffering, and to cease futile interventions that create more burden than benefit for the patient [1].

A secondary outcome of higher quality care for patients with serious diseases, however, is reduced costs of care. Through improving responsiveness to patient and family needs, namely expert symptom management, improved communication, and linking with available community health resources, specialist palliative care reduces costs. By informing patients and families about what to expect in the future, explaining the pros and cons of available treatment options and helping patients and families set their priorities for how best to use their time in the context of progressive disease, palliative care teams help clarify the patient and family goals of care and the treatment plan that meets these goals. These goals and treatment plan can then be communicated to all clinicians and specialists involved in the patient's care. The result is a clear, well-communicated plan that mobilizes the necessary community supports, manages distressing symptoms, helps family caregivers, and provides these services

J.B. Cassel, Ph.D. (✉)
Hematology/Oncology and Palliative Care, Virginia Commonwealth University, Richmond, VA, USA
e-mail: jbcassel@vcu.edu

in concert with the primary treating physician. This approach markedly reduces the incidence of symptom crises and family caregiver exhaustion, both of which are common reasons for Emergency Department (ED) visits and hospitalization. Thus, it is better quality of care and quality of life that results in an epiphenomenon or side effect of lower costs. Studies demonstrate that through these mechanisms palliative care consultation routinely leads to cessation of futile, burdensome treatments and tests and makes ED visits and hospitalizations unnecessary through better management of symptoms and prevention of crises at home or community settings. These outcomes have been demonstrated by both inpatient palliative care programs [2], and home- or outpatient-based palliative care interventions [3, 4].

While economic outcome analyses were not needed for creation of the first hospice and palliative care programs, they have proven useful for widespread adoption of specialized palliative care, defined as care focused on relief of the symptoms, pain and stress of a serious illness for both patients and their families. Indeed, economic outcomes of those efforts are now widely used to make the "business case" for palliative care, justifying further expansion of programs and the field as a whole both in the US and abroad [5]. When giving a presidential award to a financial consultant at the annual assembly of the American Academy of Hospice and Palliative Medicine in 2011, Dr. Sean Morrison described the financial model for hospital-based palliative care as the most important factor in the growth of the field since the creation of the Medicare Hospice Benefit 30 years ago.

Where Financial Outcomes Fit into the Specialist Palliative Care Measurement Model

It is crucial to begin with a consideration of how the impact of *specialist palliative care* involvement should be evaluated, and where cost-avoidance should be situated in a comprehensive outcomes measurement model for this field. As shown in Fig. 8.1, the primary outcomes of *specialist palliative care* involvement are person-centered, including improved symptoms, improved quality of life, and even improved survival [4, 6, 7]. Secondarily, people surrounding the patient in both the short-term (clinicians) and long-term (family, friends) social sphere are positively affected [8]. As a further "ripple effect" of the improved bedside and home and community-based care for the patient, beneficial institutional outcomes may also be measured—such as changes in efficiency, quality, standardization, appropriate utilization, total costs of care, and revenues.

It must be emphasized that cost reduction is *the consequence* of better quality care, and is not the motivating factor or purpose of palliative care interventions for persons living with serious or advanced, chronic illness. However, the reduced spending enabled by improving patient quality of life is valued sufficiently by institutions (hospitals, health systems, Accountable Care Organizations [ACOs], payers) to motivate them to invest in the education, training, employment, payment, and capacity of *specialist palliative care* teams.

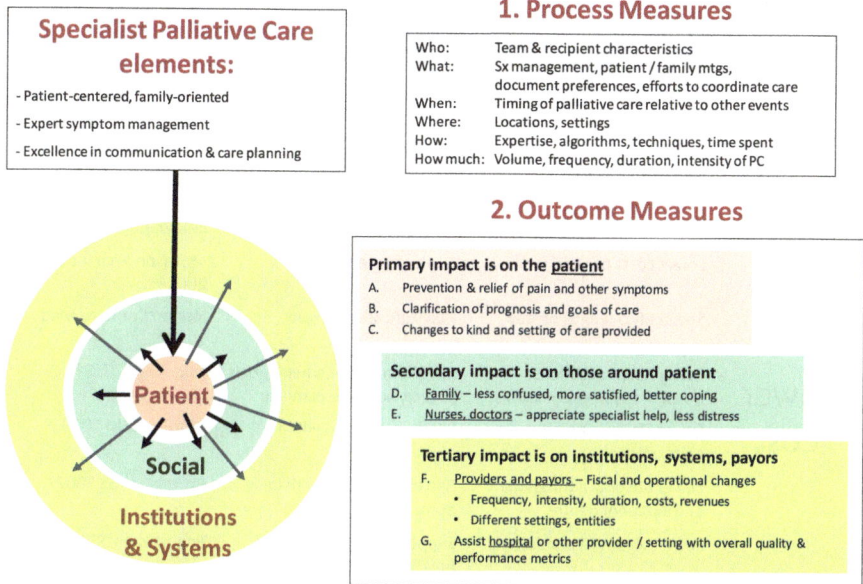

Fig. 8.1 The Specialist Palliative Care Measurement Model. In this model, financial impacts (e.g., reduced costs) are among those tertiary outcomes that accrue to institutions. The primary and secondary outcomes accrue to individuals. Adapted from Cassel (2013) [50]

Implicit to achievement of this higher value care is that the specialist palliative care program can only achieve impact on quality of care or utilization if it is actually able to identify and care for patients who can benefit; has adequate staff capacity to provide services to the number in need; and is trained and supported in provision of quality palliative care concordant with national guidelines described in the National Consensus Project for Quality Palliative Care Clinical Practice Guidelines (www.nationalconsensusproject.org).

Numerous studies have evaluated the impact of specialist palliative care in a variety of settings with a range of research designs and methods. A summary of the outcome measures evaluated is provided in Fig. 8.2, which mirrors the specialist palliative care measurement model provided in Fig. 8.1.

Following from the specialist palliative care Measurement Model (Fig. 8.1), the outcomes listed begin with what matters directly to patients (symptoms, quality of life, survival) and families (satisfaction), which together comprise the quality measures. These are followed by the institutional outcomes such as costs, intensive care unit (ICU) utilization, ED visits, hospital admissions and 30-day readmissions, and inpatient deaths, which together comprise the cost measures. Together these two sets of measures produce the so-called "value equation" [9] in which value is defined as the ratio of quality over cost.

Value equation	Outcome	How does PC help?	Best Evidence
Higher Quality	Patients live longer with higher QoL	More communication, symptoms, improved	Temel NEJM 2010 [4]
	Greater family satisfaction with quality of care	More communication, greater comfort, preferences met	Casarett Arch Int Med 2011 [8]
	Improved pain, symptoms and satisfaction with care	Symptom management and multidisciplinary team	Higginson JPSM 2003 [6]; El-Jawahri JSO 2011 [7]
Lower Cost	Lower costs per day	Goals of care changed	Morrison Arch Int Med 2008 [10]
	Shorter ICU length of stay	Goals of care changed	Norton Crit Care Med 2007 [2]
	Fewer hospitalizations, hospital days, readmissions	Symptom management, goals of care, adv care planning	Lukas JPM 2013 [11]
	Fewer ED visits and hospital admissions	Better symptoms with in-home PC	Brumley JPM 2003 [12]
	Fewer hospital admissions and inpatient deaths	Better symptoms with in-home PC	Brumley JAGS 2007 [3]
	Fewer 30-day re-admissions	Support with home PC or hospice	Enguidanos JPM 2012 [13]

Fig. 8.2 Examples of the kinds of outcomes evaluated in studies of specialist palliative care, categorized by improved quality or decreased utilization and costs

Methods and Results of Studies Assessing Specialist Palliative Care Impact on Utilization and Costs

Randomized controlled trials (RCTs). In the past 5 years, three major reviews of specialist palliative care cost impact have been published [10–12], citing 13 purported RCTs of specialist palliative care [3, 13–24]. Close examination, however, reveals that only 3 of the 13 studies are true RCTs describing non-hospice specialist palliative care [3, 13, 14]. The others were either not truly randomized [15], never actually published as a peer-reviewed journal article [16], or studied related models such as case management, hospice, education sessions, or other interventions that do not meet NCP criteria for specialist palliative care interventions [17–24]. The three studies that are true RCTs of specialist palliative care interventions and evaluated cost impact are summarized as follows:

- Brumley [3] compared palliative home care ($n=145$ for an average of 196 days) to usual home care ($n=152$ for an average of 242 days) for home-bound patients with chronic obstructive pulmonary disease (COPD), congestive heart failure (CHF), or cancer. PC patients had greater satisfaction, were more likely to die at home, and had lower healthcare costs (net difference of \$7,552 per patient) due to fewer ED visits and hospitalizations.
- Gade [13] compared inpatient PC consultation ($n=275$) to usual inpatient care ($n=237$) among patients hospitalized with a life-limiting disease; utilization and costs were assessed across the 6 months following discharge. PC patients had greater satisfaction, were readmitted at the same rate as control patients but used

the ICU less if readmitted to hospital, and had lower healthcare costs (net difference of $6,766 per patient) following discharge.
- Higginson [14] compared fast-tracked PC ($n=25$) to PC delivered after a delay of 3 months ($n=21$) for patients with severe multiple sclerosis. PC was delivered in home, community (clinic), and hospital settings. PC patients' caregivers reported lower burden, and lower total costs of care (net difference of £1,789 per patient, 2005) [approximately $3,256 USD in 2005] after 12 weeks; notably these analyses encompassed both formal healthcare system costs as well as informal (family out-of-pocket) caregiving costs.

These three RCTs of specialist palliative care are notable for a number of reasons. First, they were conducted using longitudinal assessments of healthcare costs in the 3–8 months following introduction of the specialist palliative care intervention (not just cost reduction during an index hospitalization). They were conducted in the context of a non-fee-for-service system: a health maintenance organization [3, 13] or England's National Health Service [14]. All three showed significant reductions in healthcare costs, owing primarily to a reduction in hospital costs—in contrast to Zimmerman's [10] summary.[1]

Note that at the time of preparing this chapter, the financial results of the RCT of early palliative care for patients with non-small-cell lung cancer [4] which demonstrated better quality of life and survival in the intervention group, were presented in abstract form [25], but not yet published in a peer-reviewed article.

Non-RCT Studies

A much larger number of non-randomized studies have been published regarding palliative care interventions and cost or utilization outcomes (Box 8.1). The recent review by Smith [12] which covers 10 years of publications describes 41 such studies: 2 non-randomized controlled trials, 34 cohort studies, and 5 others. Twenty-seven (65 %) were conducted in the US, of which nine focused on hospice care. The remaining 18 studies include a broad variety of outcome measures. Utilization measures include ED visits, hospital admissions, hospital bed days, intensive care use, hospice use, and duration. Cost measures included costs from providers' perspective (charges, direct hospital costs, total hospital costs), from consumers' perspective (informal and out-of-pocket costs), and from payers' perspective (expenditures). The wide variety of specialist palliative care interventions and settings, combined with a variety of utilization and cost measures used[2] makes it difficult to summarize the effects. Generally the introduction of specialist palliative care is

---

[1] Zimmerman's review, published in JAMA, summarized its main cost finding as "There was evidence of significant cost savings of specialized palliative care in only 1 of the 7 [RCT] studies that assessed this outcome" (Zimmerman 2008, p. 1698) [10]. In fact most of those 7 were either not specialist palliative care interventions or were not RCTs.

[2] In Teno's 2013 JAMA article on trends in end-of-life care, there were 18 distinct measures of healthcare utilization analyzed and described (exclusive of costs of care) [51].

associated with reduced hospital utilization and costs, as well as increased hospice utilization (and costs). Smith [12] summarized the findings from 24 cohort studies this way: "9 out of 11 studies [with *multivariate* analyses of costs] found evidence of significantly lower costs in the palliative care intervention relative to the control group" (p. 17); and "10 of the 13 cohort studies with *univariate* analyses found partially or consistently that the palliative intervention group's care was less costly than the control group's" (p. 18).

> **Box 8.1 Quality assessment of research to date**
>
> All three RCTs [3, 13, 14] and the majority of non-randomized studies (see Smith 2013) [12] have found that specialist palliative care reduces costs, especially hospitalization costs. However the dearth of RCTs of specialist palliative care (excluding hospice and pseudo-palliative) interventions, and the preponderance of cohort studies, is a limitation of this body of research.
>
> Quasi-experimental studies have used pre-intervention periods as baseline [2, 26, 27]. Simon and Higginson [28] reviewed the use of such "before-and-after" studies in palliative care research and made recommendations for strengthening such studies in the absence of randomization. Observational studies have included efforts to strengthen internal validity, such as the use of propensity score [29, 30] or instrumental variable techniques [31] to reduce selection bias [32].
>
> Different research designs and approaches are needed for assessing various utilization and cost outcomes. The hypothesis that inpatient specialist palliative care reduces cost per day during that hospitalization requires within- and between-patient analyses of daily direct (or variable) costs that are analyzed relative to the date of specialist palliative care appearance [29, 33–35]. The hypothesis that inpatient specialist palliative care reduces ICU bed days requires between-patient analyses and a quasi-experimental design [2, 26, 27]. The hypothesis that inpatient specialist palliative care reduces total duration of that hospitalization (length of stay) has not been adequately tested to date [11, 36] owing in part to the relatively infrequent use of specialist palliative care at the very beginning of a hospitalization. The hypothesis that inpatient specialist palliative care or community-based specialist palliative care reduces readmissions, 30-day mortality admissions or other utilization weeks or months following intervention requires an RCT or strong quasi-experimental design and longitudinal assessment of utilization including duration of survival [3, 13, 37, 38].
>
> *Barriers to high quality research on palliative care outcomes*
>
> The strongest forms of research on palliative care outcomes would be randomized controlled trials and large-scale health services research. As indicated above, few RCTs in palliative care have incorporated outcome measures

(continued)

(continued)

such as costs and other measures of utilization. Large-scale evaluations of the timing and impact of specialist palliative care on costs is challenging because there is no reliable, detectable "signal" of PC provision in claims data that can be distinguished easily amidst all the "noise" of hospital and physician services. It cannot be determined reliably and validly from physician identifiers or any form of billing or administrative coding:

- While the American Boards of Medical Specialties (ABMS) approved the Hospice & Palliative Medicine (HPM) subspecialty in 2006, many HPM-certified physicians working in hospitals also continue other clinical work (such as primary care, or specialty practice). Thus, even if claims or expenditure data were linked to HPM certification it would be impossible to discern which patient encounters were for palliative care services and which were for oncology services, for example.
- While there is a "palliative care encounter" ICD-9-CM (International Classification of Diseases, Ninth Revision, Clinical Modification) diagnosis code, it is a non reimbursable V- code and is hence used inconsistently by hospital coders when PC is involved in hospital care; furthermore its use is not exclusive to specialist PC services and may be employed by coders when any physician documents end-of-life care, hospice care, or terminal care [39, 40].
- There are no PC-specific procedures and thus no CPT-4 (Current Procedural Terminology) codes that are specific to PC.
- There are no PC-specific inpatient grouping codes (such as Medicare Severity Diagnosis Related Groups (MS-DRGs) or All Patient Refined Diagnosis Related Groups (APR-DRGs)).
- There is no widespread palliative care "benefit" available from major payers that would provide dates of PC enrollment and specialist PC encounters, as does the Medicare Hospice Benefit for hospice care.

For these reasons most health services research on PC cost impact in the US has relied on the availability of institution-specific billing and administrative data, typically in the form of an electronic spreadsheet or database of PC encounters that is maintained by the PC service. While this does provide the specialist palliative care "signal" it generally limits the utilization data to the same institution at which the specialist palliative care was provided (which would not capture emergency visits and admissions at other hospitals), nor does it typically capture any costs other than hospitalizations. This could be resolved in several ways. One approach is to create a pooled regional registry for specialist palliative care delivery. Another approach is to purchase and link payer data (e.g., Medicare data) with identifiers that could link the timing of specialist palliative care at a specific institution with later use of healthcare services of all types for those same patients. Yet another method is to conduct analyses within a closed system (e.g., an HMO) that has standardized documentation for specialist palliative care involvement.

Translating Research Methods into Practice

Researchers are not the only ones who are interested in measuring cost and utilization impact of specialist palliative care. It is common in the US for hospital administrators and specialist palliative care program leaders to evaluate (or try to evaluate) program cost impact. Thus it has been necessary to translate research methods into palliative care business analytics for use in clinical settings, a process that has been scaled nationwide through the *Palliative Care Leadership Center* training of over 1,000 hospitals, sponsored by the Center to Advance Palliative Care (www.capc.org) for the past 10 years for inpatient specialist palliative care (www.capc.org/pclc), and has been started as part of the Palliative Care Action Community in California for community-based specialist palliative care (http://www.chcf.org/projects/2013/pcac).

Whose Costs Are Saved?

Whose costs are saved when specialist palliative care reduces utilization and costs of care? Are hospital costs merely shifted to other settings, or does specialist palliative care result in a reduction in total spending across all settings, models of care, and payers? The answer to this question is critically important for understanding the potential link between specialist palliative care and health policy. Assessment of this question depends on three factors: the *form and timing of specialist palliative care* (inpatient versus community-based), the *mix of payers* whose members actually receive specialist palliative care, and the *structure of reimbursement* for hospital care from all or at least the predominant payers.

The majority of specialist palliative care, *inpatient* care, occurs after a week or more of hospitalization. According to Morrison [29], in a study of eight hospitals with well-established inpatient palliative care programs, palliative care patients' payer mix was 69 % Medicare, 11 % Medicaid, and about 20 % all other—commercial, HMO, PPO, Tricare, self-pay, indigent, etc. Medicare and most states' Medicaid reimbursement for inpatient hospital care is paid through DRGs or similar per-case mechanisms [41]. An inpatient palliative care intervention on day 8 of a 12-day hospitalization cannot affect the costs occurring on the first 7 days, and the DRG designation and reimbursement is not changed by specialist palliative care interventions from day 8 forward. Therefore the cost-savings that a hospital sees are real for the hospital (because the payment is already fixed regardless of actual costs). Conversely, in such a scenario, savings are not passed on to government payers or others who pay on a per-case basis, because their payment or expenditure was prospectively determined and is not linked to the details of the services rendered.

In contrast, *community-based* palliative care (CBPC) may help to avoid hospitalization altogether through early involvement and better management of care, preventing the symptom and distress crises that typically lead to 911 calls, ED visits, and hospital admissions [3, 37, 38, 42]. For a hospital, this would reduce both variable costs and reimbursement (i.e., income). For payers, however, an avoided hospitalization results in avoided or reduced expenditures as presumably less expensive community-based services are provided instead. This latter point is of great importance as the nation slowly moves from the traditional fee-for-service reimbursement model (which rewards providers for high utilization) to a population health management payment model (which rewards low utilization).

Thus the financial model for inpatient and community-based specialist palliative care is simple (higher quality care for a serious illness also costs less). Delivery of longitudinal palliative care is aimed not just at improved care for those sick enough to be in the hospital or nearing death, but also improved care for patients with debilitating chronic diseases with which they may live for months or years prior to death. Earlier outpatient palliative care will be provided concurrently with disease-focused care—for example, alongside chemotherapy rather than instead of it [4]. In terms of utilization metrics, increased outpatient-based and home-based palliative care will reduce ED visits and hospitalizations, particularly 30-day readmissions [38], admissions within 30 days of death [43] and those hospitalizations that do occur will be less prolonged and less costly if specialist palliative care is involved [44].

Porter's seminal article [9] on the value equation is instructive; as he says, "Today, health care organizations measure and accumulate costs around departments, physician specialties, discrete service areas, and line items such as drugs and supplies—a reflection of the organization and financing of care. Costs, like outcomes, should instead be measured around the patient. Measuring the total costs over a patient's entire care cycle and weighing them against outcomes will enable truly structural cost reduction, through steps such as reallocation of spending among types of services, elimination of non–value-adding services, better use of capacity, shortening of cycle time, provision of services in the appropriate settings, and so on." (p. 2481).

In the short term, hospital and health system administrators will need to be convinced that outpatient palliative care is better for their bottom line, not only better for patients and payers, if they are going to invest in it and promote its use. Incentives for such investment by hospitals and health systems include participation in shared risk or full risk payment models such as Pioneer and Shared Savings Accountable Care Organizations, and, importantly, new Medicare penalties tied to 30-day readmissions, hospital mortality rates, and poor patient satisfaction.

Payers will need to recognize the re-tooling that is necessary for hospitals and health systems to create or adopt a new culture of care for such patients, and will need to reward incremental steps toward that goal. Metrics endorsed by the NQF (http://www.qualityforum.org) such as ICU use or ED visits in the final 30 days of life, could be part of quality incentives offered by payers. Such metrics can be self-evaluated by hospitals [43, 44] and by payers. The focus should be on quality and performance metrics such as these, rather than direct costs per se, in the development of this new financial model. Currently Medicare has been penalizing hospitals for high 30-day readmission rates for three conditions (http://www.cms.gov/Medicare/Medicare-Fee-for-Service-Payment/AcuteInpatientPPS/Readmissions-Reduction-Program.html), and as of FFY2014 has incorporated 30-day mortality rates for three

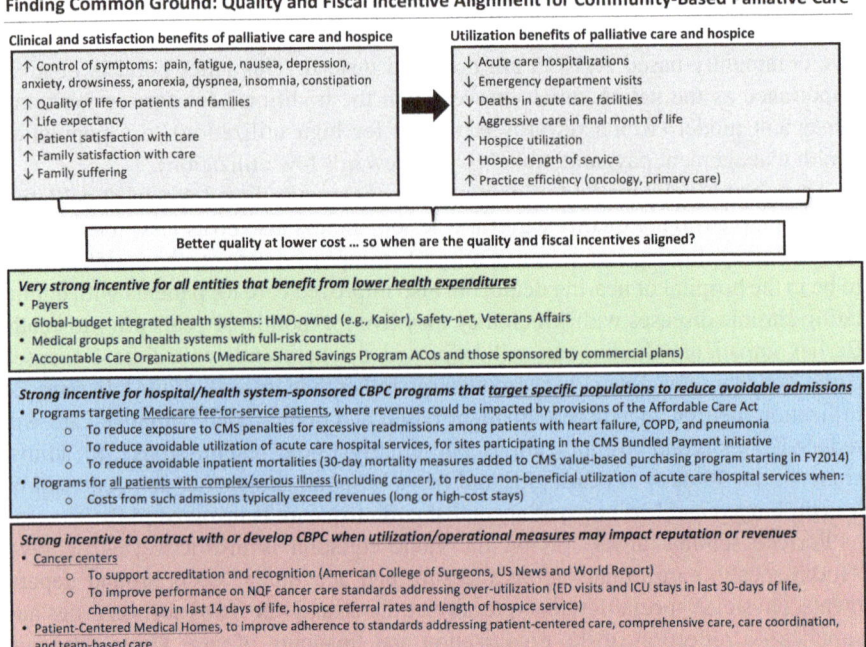

Fig. 8.3 Finding common ground between patient-focused and business-focused interests relevant to best possible care for patients with progressive, life-limiting diseases. Developed by Kathleen Kerr & J. Brian Cassel, August 2013. http://coalitionccc.org/documents/CBPC_business_case_Aug_2013_000.pdf

conditions into its computation of total scores used in its separate Value-Based Purchasing program (http://www.cms.gov/Medicare/Quality-Initiatives-Patient-Assessment-Instruments/hospital-value-based-purchasing/index.html).

To aid in understanding how CBPC could be involved in this transition away from traditional fee-for-service and toward a culture of rewarding quality rather than quantity of care, we have developed a summary figure (Fig. 8.3). This describes the clinical and satisfaction benefits of palliative care, followed by changes in utilization that typically occur when palliative care is involved. Below that, we describe three scenarios that provide greater or lesser degrees of alignment between the clinical and financial imperatives for providing better care to patients with serious or complex illness. This schematic was first disseminated by the Coalition for Compassionate Care of California and can be found at their website, http://coalitionccc.org/documents/CBPC_business_case_Aug_2013_000.pdf.

As shown in Fig. 8.3, if financial support of such models become feasible, both specialist palliative care teams and other clinicians caring for the seriously ill will be enabled to respond to the clinical imperative and quality incentives linked to provision of CBPC—(see Box 8.2: Veterans Health Administration: Transformation of hospice and palliative care, an interview with Dr. Scott Shreve). The *financial* imperative would be felt most keenly by those who are most at-risk for avoidable costs in the last months of life (the box with green shading in Fig. 8.3)—such as payers, globally budgeted or shared savings health systems accepting risk, and accountable care organizations. For health systems not yet experimenting with risk-bearing contracts, CBPC may help to prevent 30-day readmissions, and reduce hospital mortality, both of which now result in significant financial penalties for all hospitals (blue-shaded box). Many health systems (orange box), seek to achieve higher marks of quality for accreditation, public reporting such as US News & World report scores and rankings, and rising recognition of over-utilization as inappropriate and poor quality care.

> **Box 8.2 The transformation of hospice & palliative care in the Veterans' Affairs medical system: Financial impact not required**
>
> *Dr. Scott Shreve is the national director of Hospice & Palliative Care within the Veterans Health Administration (VHA) system. Here he describes the VHA efforts to transform its care for patients with advanced, life-limiting diseases and how these lessons may be translated to other health systems in the US.*
>
> **(Q1) Could you please briefly describe the Comprehensive End-of-Life Initiative and the evolution of the national palliative care and hospice efforts within the VHA in the past 5 years?**
>
> Dr. Shreve: Transforming the Department of Veterans Affairs (VA) into a high-performing 21st century organization is a central tenant of our commitment to serve our nation's Veterans. Within the VHA, the Hospice and Palliative Care (HPC) program, through its 4-year Comprehensive End of Life Care (CELC) initiative, has followed the guiding principles of being people-centric, results-driven, and forward-looking. Over the past 4 years (2009 through 2012), HPC has integrated these principles into its mission to "honor Veterans' preferences for care at the end of life" and achieved innovative, sustainable changes in the way palliative and end-of-life care is being delivered. As a result, the VHA has improved quality, expanded access and disseminated expertise throughout the VHA and across the nation. Key accomplishments through FY 2012 include:
>
> - Access to inpatient hospice services has grown substantially to a national average of 48 % of all inpatient deaths now occurring in hospice bed sections, as compared to 30 % in FY 2008, largely as a result of 54 new hospice and palliative care units;
> - Specialized palliative care is now [FY13] delivered to 70 % of all inpatient decedents nationwide, as compared to 47 % in FY 2008. Every VA Medical Center now has an active and trained interdisciplinary palliative care team;
> - The quality of care delivered to Veterans at the end of life is being measured by a National Quality Forum endorsed measure, the Bereaved Family Survey (BFS), as part of VA's quality improvement plan for all inpatient deaths [8]; and
>
> (continued)

(continued)

- Establishing the "We Honor Veterans" campaign through innovative partnering to improve hospice care of Veterans outside VA. More than 2,026 community hospices have committed to improved care of Veterans as part of the We Honor Veterans campaign.

(Q2) To what extent has change & improvement in end-of-life care been driven from the "ground up" (frontline staff in each facility), and/or driven from the "top down" (from the national HPC office & CELC initiative)?

Dr. Shreve: Clearly the combination of "top down" and "bottom up" approach to organizational change was necessary to make the substantial changes in VHA's culture of caring for seriously ill Veterans. Senior VHA leaders were central to aligning the mission of the CELC initiative with existing VHA strategic plans. Our HPC program office then used competitively awarded funding to stimulate targeted areas of program development at facilities that were deemed "ready for change."

VHA exemplifies many of the qualities that healthcare reform aspires to in its integrated structure and patient-focused system. The CELC initiative experience serves as an example of the magnitude of change possible through a combination of engaging leadership in accountability for the care delivered and grassroots empowerment of staff as a model for improving palliative care services in other health systems.

(Q3) What have been the primary drivers of changes in hospice & palliative care across the VA—clinical quality? Patient or family satisfaction? Other?

Dr. Shreve: VHA's strategic plan calls for Veteran-centric care. The CELC initiative and its sweeping cultural changes in the end-of-life care were aligned with VHA's strategic plan; however they were likely "driven" by the passion of VHA's palliative care regional leaders and palliative care teams. As the mission statement for the HPC program "honoring Veterans' preferences for care at the end of life" states, these palliative care teams at every medical center and regional leaders became the nucleus for promoting identification of Veterans' goals of care, educating non-palliative care staff, transitioning Veterans to their desired venue of care and assisting administrative leaders in implementing interventions to improve satisfaction with care. As only regional leaders can do, Palliative Care Program Managers were able to "connect the dots" in terms of sharing success stories among facilities in their VISN. To support these regional palliative care managers, our HPC program office provides each region with detailed reports on indicators of program development, process measures associated with quality care and Veteran/family satisfaction with the care delivered. In addition to these reports, Program Managers are provided assistance in interpreting these reports and in preparing briefing documents for administrative leaders.

(continued)

(continued)

As opposed to other performance measurement plans, VHA's CELC initiative focused on successes and sharing of best practices, not identifying deficiencies. This focus on "what's working" as opposed to low performers seemed to create an atmosphere of safety while generating momentum for change. With modest amounts of seed money, facilities determined how and to what extent they would improve their programs knowing that core metrics as described below would be available but not necessarily represent the "drivers."

(Q4) What metrics are used to evaluate end-of-life care within the VA?

Dr. Shreve: There is no better indicator of the success of the CELC initiative than the Bereaved Family Survey (BFS) conducted by the Performance Reporting and Outcomes Measurement to Improve the Standard of care at End-of-life (PROMISE) Center. And, there is no other system nationally that routinely measures outcomes of palliative and end-of-life care on such a large scale. In building on Secretary Shinseki's vision, the HPC program has identified the "Strive for 65" goal as part of its strategic plan. This plan aims to achieve a national mean of 65 % of bereaved family members rating care as "excellent" for Veterans who died in VA inpatient settings (current average is 64 %, up from 57 % in 2010) with 83 % of bereaved families rating care as "excellent" or "very good" ($n = 11,004$).

Other important indicators of program effectiveness included; (1) percentage of inpatient deaths that received a palliative care consult prior to death, (2) the venue of inpatient deaths and use of designated hospice and palliative care beds, (3) use of community hospice services and (4) training for palliative care staff in both program development and clinical content. More than 10,000 VA staff received Veteran-specific palliative care training as part of this initiative.

(Q5) What lessons can be drawn from the VA's experience with expanding and improving hospice and palliative care, that could be useful for other large health systems within or outside the US?

Dr. Shreve: The CELC initiative established a coordinated plan to increase access to hospice and palliative care services by addressing policy issues, program and staff development, collaboration with community hospices, outcomes measurement, and proving value to the organization. To determine progress and monitor resource allocation, workload and outcome measures were established in all settings [45]. Much of VA's success in delivering quality healthcare has come about as a result of accountability in achieving meaningful outcomes. For example, once we had the BFS functioning nationally, local VHA administrators' pay (not that of individual providers) was tied in part to family satisfaction scores [46]. Administrators also received quotes from families about their experiences with care, and reading about families' experiences in their own words is very powerful.

(continued)

(continued)

We found that competitive financing of HPC projects, and identification of people who were ready and eager for change were key factors in the success of the CELC initiative. Regional palliative care leaders have been empowered to enact system level change by building on the individual facility strengths within their regions. Palliative care teams at each facility look to these regional leaders for guidance on policy and practice and in turn these regional leaders collaborate with other regional leaders and our HPC program office. As a result, the organizational layers between frontline staff and program office leadership are minimized with regular opportunities for dialogue and aligning of efforts.

(Q6) In contrast to other countries with well-developed health care infrastructures, the US lacks a national mandate, strategy, policy, or office to improve end-of-life care universally across the US. From the VA perspective, what value could such a national strategy or initiative add?

Dr. Shreve: As the largest integrated healthcare system, VHA has been a model for ensuring quality care for patients (Veterans) in a fixed budget system. The absence of perverse fee-for-service incentives, the extensive electronic medical record infrastructure and more specifically leadership's commitment to improved care of seriously ill Veterans through expansion of hospice and palliative care as well as other innovative programs (e.g., Home-Based Primary Care, Patient Aligned Care Teams, and Medical Foster Home, to name a few) have established VA as a leader in promoting health for the seriously ill population we serve. As performance measurement evolves and healthcare resources become scarce, VA's focus on the health of the population while improving the experience of the patient within budget constraints provides a vision for national strategies. Vladeck does a good job of articulating the need for medical care that is driven by dignity, where the patient experience is paramount, which we believe is exactly what we are doing in the VHA today [47].

Cost Studies and Health Policy Recommendations

Health services research demonstrating positive economic outcomes resulting from higher quality of care linked to palliative care may influence the further growth and development of specialist palliative care in several ways:

- Payers could expand access to CBPC by assuring coverage for a defined set of services such as a number of specialist palliative care outpatient visits and/or home-based visits. The financial value would be derived from encouraging use of low-cost CBPC services to reduce high-cost ED visits and hospitalizations during the last months to year of life through better symptom management, family caregiver support, mobilization of community support services, and earlier referral to hospice (already covered under specific benefits from all major payers).

- Federal and state governments could increase funding for education and training in palliative care for medicine, nursing and allied health with a long-term goal of increasing the workforce capacity for palliative care to handle the increasing demands of aging and long-term chronic disease populations. Sufficient well-trained generalist and specialist palliative care workforce is necessary to serve the growing population of persons with serious and chronic long-term illnesses (such as frailty, dementia, multimorbidity, and functional impairment) so that patients and families receive the care and support they need in the home and community instead of using hospitals as the safety net of last resort—in other words, better quality outcomes, much lower costs.
- Payers could increase incentives for palliative care principles and practices (such as promotion of goals of care conversations, family caregiver needs assessment, standardized symptom assessment and treatment) combined with disincentives for inappropriate and preventable hospitalizations for patients with serious chronic illness, multimorbidity, frailty, and functional and cognitive dependencies. Motivation for such investment may result from specific metrics such as 30-day hospital readmissions and death within 30 days of an admission (30-day mortality) as well as the spread of accountable care organizations and other entities that assume risk for costs of care, in exchange for capitation or shared savings revenues.
- Payers (of all sorts) and the federal government could fund further health services research and development in palliative care delivery models and the translation of specialist palliative care principles and practices into the core competencies of generalist or "primary" palliative care providers (such as dialysis nurses, nursing home staff, community and home care staff, oncologists, geriatricians, cardiologists, general medicine, etc.), and fund the rigorous testing and measurement of quality and utilization outcomes. Innovative payers such as BCBS of Michigan, Aetna, and United Healthcare have already developed delivery and payment models for CBPC, demonstrating better clinical outcomes and reduced need for hospitalizations [48, 49].

Conclusions

The goal of palliative care is to help seriously ill patients and families determine what matters most to them, and then to help them achieve these goals. Research demonstrates the beneficial impact of palliative care services on quality of life, survival, family caregiver outcomes, and symptom burden. As an epiphenomenon or side effect of the improved quality resulting from these models, multiple studies demonstrate lower intensity and costs of healthcare. Palliative care can make enormous contributions to healthcare value because by improving patient and family-centered outcomes, it leads to reduced costs, for both payers and providers. The earlier the access to palliative care the higher the likelihood that revolving door ED visits and hospitalizations will be avoided. Payers and policy makers can encourage early access to quality palliative care in community and office settings in a variety of ways, including innovative payment models, quality measurement linked to payment, accreditation and certification, and workforce training and demonstration of key competencies. Much work remains to be done in producing high-quality research on palliative care interventions including quality and utilization outcomes, as well as in translating and implementing the results of research to routine and standardized delivery of higher quality care for the sickest and most vulnerable members of our society.

References

1. Seymour JE. Looking back, looking forward: the evolution of palliative and end of life care in England. Mortality. 2012;7(1).
2. Norton SA, Hogan LA, Holloway RG, Temkin-Greener H, Buckley MJ, Quill TE. Proactive PC in the MICU: effects on LOS for selected high-risk patients. Crit Care Med. 2007;35:1530–5.
3. Brumley RD, Enguidanos S, Jamison P, Seitz R, Morgenstern N, Saito S, et al. Increased satisfaction with care and lower costs: results of a randomized trial of in-home palliative care. J Am Geriatr Soc. 2007;55:993–1000.
4. Temel JS, Greer JA, Muzikansky A, Gallagher ER, Admane S, Jackson VA, Dahlin CM, Blinderman CD, Jacobsen J, Pirl WF, Billings JA, Lynch TJ. Early palliative care for patients with metastatic non-small-cell lung cancer. N Engl J Med. 2010;363:733–42.
5. Murray E. How advocates use health economic data and projections: the Irish experience. J Pain Symptom Manage. 2009;38(1):97–104.
6. Higginson IJ, et al. Is there evidence that palliative care teams alter end-of-life experiences of patients and their caregivers? J Pain Symptom Manage. 2003;25(2):150–68.
7. El-Jawahri A, Greer JA, Temel JS. Does palliative care improve outcomes for patients with incurable illness? A review of the evidence. J Support Oncol. 2011;9(3):87–94.
8. Casarett D, Johnson M, Smith D, Richardson D. The optimal delivery of palliative care: a national comparison of the outcomes of consultation teams vs. inpatient units. Arch Intern Med. 2011;171(7):649–55.
9. Porter ME. What is value in health care? N Engl J Med. 2010;363(26):2477–81.
10. Zimmermann C, Riechelmann R, Krzyzanowska M, Rodin G, Tannock I. Effectiveness of specialized palliative care: a systematic review. JAMA. 2008;299(14):1698–709.
11. Smith TJ, Cassel JB. Cost and non-clinical outcomes of palliative care. J Pain Symptom Manage. 2009;38(1):32–44.
12. Smith S, Brick A, O'Hara S, Normand C. Evidence on the cost and cost-effectiveness of palliative care: a literature review. Palliat Med. 2014 Feb; 28(8):130–150.
13. Gade G, Venohr I, Conner D, McGrady K, Beane J, Richardson RH, et al. Impact of an inpatient palliative care team: a randomized control trial. J Palliat Med. 2008;11:180–90.
14. Higginson IJ, McCrone P, Hart SR, Burman R, Silber E, Edmonds PM. Is short-term palliative care cost-effective in multiple sclerosis? A randomized phase II trial. J Pain Symptom Manage. 2009;38(6):816–26.
15. Rabow MW, Dibble SL, Pantilat SZ, McPhee SJ. The comprehensive care team. Arch Intern Med. 2004;164(1):83–91.
16. Finn J, Pienta K, Parzuchowski J. Bridging cancer treatment and hospice care. Proc Am Soc Clin Oncol. 2002;21:1452.
17. Kane RL, Wales J, Bernstein L, Leibowitz A, Kaplan S. A randomised controlled trial of hospice care. Lancet. 1984;1(8382):890–4.
18. Zimmer JG, Groth-Juncker A, McCusker J. A randomized controlled study of a home health care team. Am J Public Health. 1985;75(2):134–41.
19. Hughes SL, Cummings J, Weaver F, Manheim L, Braun B, Conrad K. A randomized trial of the cost effectiveness of VA hospital-based home care for the terminally ill. Health Serv Res. 1992;26(6):801–17.

20. Addington-Hall JM, MacDonald LD, Anderson HR, et al. Randomised controlled trial of effects of coordinating care for terminally ill cancer patients. BMJ. 1992;305(6865):1317–22.
21. Raftery JP, Addington-Hall JM, MacDonald LD, et al. A randomized controlled trial of the cost-effectiveness of a district co-ordinating service for terminally ill cancer patients. Palliat Med. 1996;10(2):151–61.
22. Moore S, Corner J, Haviland J, et al. Nurse led follow up and conventional medical follow up in management of patients with lung cancer. BMJ. 2002;325(7373):1145.
23. Engelhardt JB, McClive-Reed KP, Toseland RW, et al. Effects of a program for coordinated care of advanced illness on patients, surrogates, and healthcare costs: a randomized trial. Am J Manag Care. 2006;12:93–100.
24. Bakitas M, Lyons KD, Hegel MT, et al. Effects of a palliative care intervention on clinical outcomes in patients with advanced cancer: the project ENABLE II randomized controlled trial. JAMA. 2009;302:741–9.
25. Greer J, McMahon P, Tramontano A, et al. Effect of early palliative care on health care costs in patients with metastatic NSCLC. J Clin Oncol. 2012;30 Suppl:abstr 6004.
26. Campbell ML, Guzman JA. Impact of a proactive approach to improve EOL care in a medical ICU. Chest. 2003;123:255–71.
27. Campbell ML, Guzman JA. A proactive approach to improve end-of-life care in a medical intensive care unit for patients with terminal dementia. Crit Care Med. 2004;32:1839–43.
28. Simon S, Higginson IJ. Evaluation of hospital palliative care teams: strengths and weaknesses of the before-after study design and strategies to improve it. Palliat Med. 2009;23(1):23–8.
29. Morrison RS, Penrod JD, Cassel JB, Caust-Ellenbogen M, Litke A, et al. Cost savings associated with hospital-based palliative care consultation programs. Arch Intern Med. 2008;168(16):1783–90.
30. Penrod JD, Deb P, Luhrs C, Dellenbaugh C, Zhu CW, Hochman T, et al. Cost and utilization outcomes of patients receiving hospital-based PC consultation. J Palliat Med. 2006;9:855–60.
31. Penrod JD, Deb P, Dellenbaugh C, Burgess JF, Zhu CW, Christiansen CL, et al. Hospital-based palliative care consultation: Effects on hospital cost. J Palliat Med. 2010;13:973–9.
32. Starks H, Diehr P, Curtis JR. The challenge of selection bias and confounding in palliative care research. J Palliat Med. 2009;12(2):181–7.
33. Smith TJ, Coyne P, Cassel B, Penberthy L, Hopson A, Hager MA. A high volume specialist palliative care unit and team may reduce in-hospital end of life care cost. J Palliat Med. 2003;6:699–705.
34. Cassel JB, Webb-Wright J, Holmes J, Lyckholm L, Smith TJ. Clinical and financial impact of a palliative care program at a small rural hospital. J Palliat Med. 2010;13(11):1339–443.
35. Albanese TH, Radwany SM, Mason H, Gayomali C, Dieter K. Assessing the financial impact of an inpatient acute palliative care unit in a tertiary care teaching hospital. J Palliat Med. 2013;16(3):289–94.
36. Cassel JB, Kerr K, Pantilat S, Smith TJ. Palliative care consultation and hospital length of stay. J Palliat Med. 2010;13(6):761–7.
37. Lukas L, Foltz C, Paxton H. Hospital outcomes for a home-based palliative medicine consulting service. J Palliat Med. 2013;16(2):179–84.
38. Enguidanos S, Vesper E, Lorenz K. 30-day readmissions among seriously ill older adults. J Palliat Med. 2012;15(12):1356–61.
39. Cassel JB, Jones AB, Meier DE, Smith TJ, Spragens LH, Weissman D. Hospital mortality rates: how is palliative care taken into account? J Pain Symptom Manage. 2010;40(6):914–25.
40. Olmsted MG, Drozd EM, Murphy J. Exclusion of palliative care from hospital mortality rates: not ready for prime time. J Pain Symptom Manage. 2010;40(6):926–8. discussion 930–1.
41. Quinn K. New directions in Medicaid payment for hospital care. Health Aff (Millwood). 2008;27(1):269–80.
42. Brumley RD, Enguidanos S, Cherin DA. Effectiveness of a home-based palliative care program for end-of-life. J Palliat Med. 2003;5:715–24.
43. Cassel B, Coyne PJ, Skoro N, Kerr K, del Fabbro E. Evaluating the impact of early versus late inpatient palliative care consultation for cancer patients. ASCO: Chicago IL; 2013.

44. Cassel JB, Shickle L, Skoro N, Kerr K, Coyne P, Del Fabbro E. The business case for integrated palliative care. Center to Advance Palliative Care National Seminar: Miami, FL; 2012.
45. Edes T, Shreve S, Casarett D. Increasing access and quality in Department of Veterans Affairs care at the end of life: a lesson in change. J Am Geriatr Soc. 2007;55(10):1645–9.
46. Kizer KW, Kirsch SR. The double edged sword of performance measurement. J Gen Intern Med. 2012;27(4):395–7.
47. Vladeck BC, Westphal E. Dignity-driven decision making: a compelling strategy for improving care for people with advanced illness. Health Aff. 2012;31(6):1269–76.
48. Sweeney L, Halpert A, Waranoff J. Patient-centered management of complex patients can reduce costs without shortening life. Am J Manag Care. 2000;13:84–92.
49. Krakauer R, Spettell CM, Reisman L, Wade MJ. Opportunities to improve the quality of care for advanced illness. Health Aff (Millwood). 2009;28(5):1357–9. doi:10.1377/hlthaff.28.5.1357.
50. Cassel JB. The importance of following the money in the development and sustainability of palliative care. Palliat Med. 2013;27(2):103–4.
51. Teno JM, Gozalo PL, Bynum JP, Leland NE, Miller SC, Morden NE, Scupp T, Goodman DC, Mor V. Change in end-of-life care for Medicare beneficiaries: site of death, place of care, and health care transitions in 2000, 2005, and 2009. JAMA. 2013;309(5):470–7.

Chapter 9
Long-term Services and Supports: A Necessary Complement to Palliative Care

Judy Feder, Harriet L. Komisar, and Robert A. Berenson

As well described throughout this book, palliative care is an approach to providing care that addresses patients' and caregivers' quality of life and well-being, assures preference-concordant care across settings and over time, provides timely professional expertise for the seriously ill, and focuses on pain and symptom relief while offering the potential to moderate high spending [1]. Under current law, Medicare only offers a palliative care benefit as part of the hospice benefit for people with a predictably terminal illness during their last 6 months of life. Proposals have been made to expand the use of palliative care for Medicare beneficiaries, including providing a Medicare palliative care benefit [2].

Whatever the fate of proposals to strengthen coverage of activities related to palliative care services, palliative care and other practitioners will continue to face challenges in mobilizing *long-term services and supports* (LTSS), that is, personal assistance to those unable to perform basic tasks of daily living on their own. No matter how well a care plan is designed to honor the wishes of people with serious or complex illness and their families, without access to LTSS, patients may end up in emergency departments or hospitals unnecessarily. These LTSS, therefore, have the potential both to improve patients' quality of life and to prevent unnecessary ED visits, hospitalizations, or nursing home admissions. That said, identifying, accessing, and coordinating long-term care services are not easy. Further, financing to support these services is beyond the scope of standard insurance. Few people have private long-term care insurance, and Medicare does not cover LTTS. Its home health and nursing home benefits are limited in a variety of ways and are typically

---

J. Feder (✉) • R.A. Berenson
Urban Institute, 2100 M Street NW, Washington, DC, USA
e-mail: federj@georgetown.edu

H.L. Komisar
AARP, Washington, DC, USA
e-mail: rberenson@urban.org

associated with an episode of acute care. Medicaid does cover these services; indeed, about a third of Medicaid spending finances long-term care [3]. Medicaid's protections, however, vary considerably across states and are only available to people who are impoverished or who become impoverished as a result of medical or long-term care spending.

In this chapter, we examine the way in which Medicaid and Medicare provide benefits to persons whose complex illnesses or chronic conditions create functional impairments, and the different program structures that inhibit the coordination of medical and long-term supports and services. We next explore proposed strategies, including demonstration initiatives being launched by the Centers for Medicare and Medicaid Services, to improve care and reduce costs specifically for dually eligible Medicare and Medicaid beneficiaries, as well other program innovations designed to improve care for vulnerable populations. Finally, we make the case that Medicare should take the primary initiative in developing care models that better serve beneficiaries with serious illness and/or multiple chronic conditions and functional limitations, presenting the core elements of these models, including a commitment to the principles and practices of palliative care.

How Current Benefits and Program Operations Impede Coordination of Long-term Care

The Medicare statute explicitly prohibits Medicare payments for "custodial" (or personal) care, a provision in the law intended to assuage concerns that the establishment of health insurance for the elderly population would create uncontrollable financial obligations. Consistent with that concern, Medicare's benefits for skilled nursing facilities (SNFs) and home health care have been closely tied to episodes of acute care and their associated "skilled" care needs. Medicare pays for care in SNFs following a hospital stay for beneficiaries who require skilled nursing or rehabilitation care, but not for those whose needs are for long-term assistance with the activities of daily living (such as bathing or dressing). The first 20 days of a SNF stay are paid in full, but beneficiaries pay substantial cost-sharing for subsequent days ($148 per day for days 21–100 in a benefit period in 2013, and all costs for each day after day 100 in a benefit period) [4]. Though originally contingent on a hospital stay, under current law Medicare's home health benefits are generally available to beneficiaries requiring skilled nursing, therapy, or other professional (not personal care) services. These benefits are subject to limits—beneficiaries must not only have skilled needs, but must also be "homebound" and in need of only "intermittent" not full-time care—and only beneficiaries who satisfy all these requirements are eligible to receive part-time personal aide services to assist with daily activities [5].

Restricted Medicare benefits have, for the most part, produced limited coverage. In 2011, the average length of a Medicare-covered stay in a nursing home facility was 27.2 days [6]. Home aide visits accounted for 15.0 % of total home health visits or about five visits per home health user per year [7]. A recent legal settlement has required CMS to clarify that home health coverage is not contingent on evidence of patient improvement. But the skilled care requirement and other conditions on coverage remain intact to limit Medicare's coverage [8].

In contrast, Medicaid is the nation's primary source of public financing for long-term care, available to Medicare beneficiaries and other people who are either poor or exhaust all their resources in purchasing medical and long-term care services. In 2009, Medicaid financed 61.5 % of national long-term care spending ($203.2 billion) and paid in part or in full the costs of about two-thirds of the nation's 1.5 million nursing home residents [9].

Challenges in Care for Dual Eligibles

In theory, Medicare and Medicaid have different and potentially complementary responsibilities for beneficiaries participating in both programs (or dual eligibles), including the 30 % of dual eligibles who receive Medicaid-financed long-term care [10]. In practice, however, the two programs have overlapping responsibilities. As a result, neither program assumes accountability for assuring quality care, and providers have powerful incentives to shift costs from one program to the other.

Research shows that dually eligible nursing home residents experience higher rates of preventable hospital admissions than Medicare or private-pay patients with similar health status, that lower Medicaid payment rates to nursing homes are associated with higher rates of hospitalization, that potentially preventable admission rates are close to 40 %, and that potentially avoidable rehospitalization rates range from 18 to 40 % [11, 12].

Two-thirds of these potentially avoidable hospital admissions came from nursing homes, where the incentives to avoid or shift costs are particularly strong. Nursing homes serve both short-term Medicare patients and long-term Medicaid patients. But Medicare payment rates are significantly higher than Medicaid's. Nursing homes therefore benefit financially when they transfer Medicaid patients to hospitals—substituting treatment in the hospital for their own investment in care and gaining from Medicare's higher payment rates at the start of the patient's return stay. These transfers are further encouraged by nursing homes' incentives to avoid high-cost Medicaid patients (given the way Medicaid rates are set) and by Medicaid "bed-hold" policies, under which states guarantee the readmission of transferred patients by paying nursing homes a daily rate to hold their beds [13].

How to Improve Coordination of Care and Reduce Costs for Dual Eligibles

For dual eligibles—almost half of the Medicare population who needs long-term care—the potential for better coordination across health and long-term care services for people who need both is enhanced by the creation of the Medicare-Medicaid Coordination Office within CMS. Since its establishment, this office has moved aggressively to improve the delivery of primary, acute, behavioral health and long-term services and supports for Medicare-Medicaid enrollees, and to better align and integrate the financing of these two programs [14].

Through demonstrations, negotiated between states and the federal government, CMS will allow states to rely on managed care or other mechanisms, to which Medicare and Medicaid will both contribute to provide both acute and long-term care to dual eligibles. Per capita contributions to financing from each program must be lower than projected per capita spending—a requirement justified largely on assumptions about reductions in unnecessary, expensive hospital services that care management is supposed to produce. In 2012, more than 26 states submitted proposals to the State Demonstrations to Integrate Care for Dual Eligible Individuals Initiative, and CMS is working with states on Memoranda of Understanding (MOUs) to implement demonstrations [15]. As of early 2013, nine states had signed MOUs with CMS, almost all of which are moving forward with capitated program. Only one state, Massachusetts, with a capitated program has actually begun to enroll beneficiaries in its demonstration [16]. Although others are scheduled to begin enrollment in the near future, they have not yet begun negotiating contracts with managed care plans—a task that has proved challenging, given the effort both to reduce spending and assure access to care.

Consolidating Medicare and Medicaid payment streams into a single, capitated payment that has the potential to decrease current perverse incentives to shift costs between programs, as well as to provide greater flexibility to clinicians to do what is in the patient's best interest rather than do what conforms to payment specifications. But capitation's powerful incentives to spend less can also reduce access to quality care. This concern is heightened by the inexperience of health plans in general, and of Medicaid managed care plans in particular, in caring for the complex social and medical needs of the dual eligible population. Patients dually eligible for both Medicare and Medicaid present unique clinical challenges requiring both specialized clinical expertise and a commitment to care coordination across providers and community-based resources. Further, the dual eligible population is extremely heterogeneous, with specific and complex health problems with which most health plans and providers may not have experience. Dually eligible patients are poorer and sicker than their non-dual Medicare contemporaries: 86 % live below 150 % of the Federal Poverty Level (versus 22 %), and 50 % report that they are in fair to poor health (versus 22 %). Dual eligible beneficiaries are also more likely to report limitations in activities of daily living (44 % versus 26 %), reside in a long-term care facility (13 % versus 1 %), suffer from dementia and/or serious and persistent mental illness (58 % versus 25 %), and more frequently experience multiple chronic conditions (55 % versus 44 %) [17].

Accordingly, although conceptually advantageous to dual eligible beneficiaries, these demonstrations could fundamentally alter financing and delivery for as many as two million people nationwide, based on assumptions—not evidence—that the proposed arrangements will generate better care at lower cost. Efforts to engage such large populations and reduced funding up front distinguish these dual eligible demonstrations from most other payment and delivery reforms CMS is pursuing under the Medicare program. Typically, these and other demonstrations are relatively small scale, with savings shared between Medicare and participating provider organizations if they emerge. By contrast, both Medicare and Medicaid payments will be reduced from the outset of these demonstrations, despite the inexperience of both Medicare and Medicaid managed care plans with this vulnerable high risk population and the dearth of evidence on their ability to provide quality care at lower costs. Given this inexperience, taking savings up front raises concerns that plans may seek to reduce expenses by limiting both provider payments and access to care, rather than promoting efficiency. In theory, these state initiatives are time-limited demonstrations, with continued operation and expansion contingent on demonstrable evidence of reduced costs and/or improved quality at equal costs. However, past experience with negotiated demonstrations or waivers in state Medicaid programs raises questions about the ability of policymakers to unwind large scale financial and delivery arrangements to which states are administratively and financially committed [18].

Regardless of the merits and eventual findings from this integrated Medicare and Medicaid payment demonstration, major delivery reform aimed only at the dual eligible population excludes roughly half the Medicare beneficiaries who have impairments, but are not Medicaid-eligible, whose care would also be improved by better coordination across acute and long-term care services. Moreover, it shifts to states responsibility for better coordination of Medicare-financed care for dually eligible beneficiaries at high risk of hospitalization—an objective that is at the heart of Medicare payment and delivery reforms promoted by the Affordable Care Act (ACA).

Why Medicare Should Focus on Care Coordination for Medicare Beneficiaries with Functional Impairments [19]

The Medicare payment and delivery reform agenda, initiated by the ACA, aims to improve quality and save money by reducing provision of unnecessary and expensive care. Although CMS is well underway in pursuit of this goal, its initiatives have focused overwhelmingly on people whose chronic conditions generate a need for complex medical care, without regard to the need for assistance with routine activities of life (such as bathing, dressing, and toileting), that is, the need for LTTS.

This approach reflects unfortunate myopia. The 15 % of Medicare beneficiaries who have both chronic illness(es) and personal care needs account for about a third of all Medicare spending (Fig. 9.1). In comparison, enrollees with substantial chronic illness—as indicated by the presence of three or more chronic conditions, but without functional impairment—represent roughly equal shares of the Medicare population and Medicare spending. Thus, it is the high cost associated with enrollees with the combination of chronic illness and functional limitations—and not the cost of those with multiple chronic conditions alone—that drives the disproportionate share of Medicare spending associated with enrollees with multiple chronic conditions.

Average Medicare spending for chronically ill beneficiaries with functional limitations is twice as high as for beneficiaries with three or more chronic conditions and

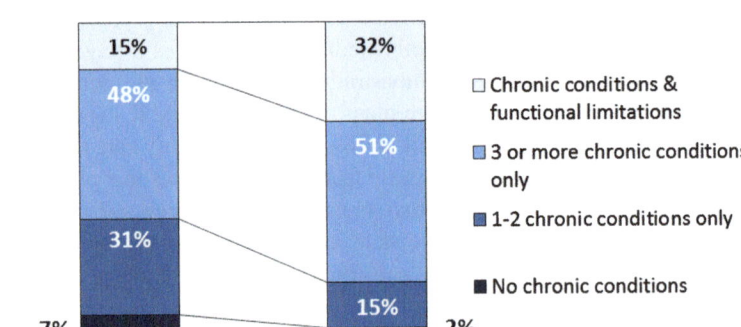

Fig. 9.1 Chronic conditions and functional limitations, not chronic conditions alone, explain high per person Medicare costs. *Source*: Komisar HL, Feder J. "Transforming Care for Medicare Beneficiaries with Chronic Conditions and Long-Term Care Needs: Coordinating Care Across All Services." (Washington, DC: Georgetown University, October 2011)

no functional limitations—about $15,800 compared with $7,900 in 2006. While about a quarter of Medicare beneficiaries with chronic conditions and functional limitations reside in nursing homes, the majority do not—and for both groups, Medicare spending is significantly higher than for beneficiaries with three or more chronic conditions and no functional limitations. The pattern of higher spending for chronically ill people with limitations, as compared to chronically ill people without limitations holds true no matter what the number of chronic conditions. Among enrollees with chronic conditions and no functional limitations, average annual spending in 2006 ranged from $2,800 (for people with one chronic condition) to $10,200 (for those with five or more chronic conditions). In comparison, the amount for those with functional limitations ranged from about $13,000 for those with one to three chronic conditions to nearly $19,000 for those with five or more chronic conditions—more than twice as high as those without functional limitations at every level of chronic illness.

Not surprisingly, beneficiaries with functional limitations and long-term care needs are among Medicare's highest spenders (Fig. 9.2). Nearly half the beneficiaries in the top 20 % of Medicare spenders have functional limitations as well as chronic conditions. Among Medicare's top five percent of spenders, the proportion is even higher. Three out of five of these highest-cost Medicare beneficiaries are chronically ill people who need long-term care.

Enrollees with the combination of chronic conditions and long-term care needs are far more likely than other beneficiaries to use hospital inpatient and emergency department services. As a result, average spending per person on hospital services was nearly double for enrollees with chronic conditions and functional limitations, compared to those with three or more chronic conditions only ($4,600 versus $2,500 in 2006). Higher hospital and post-acute spending are the largest sources of the overall difference in average spending between these groups.

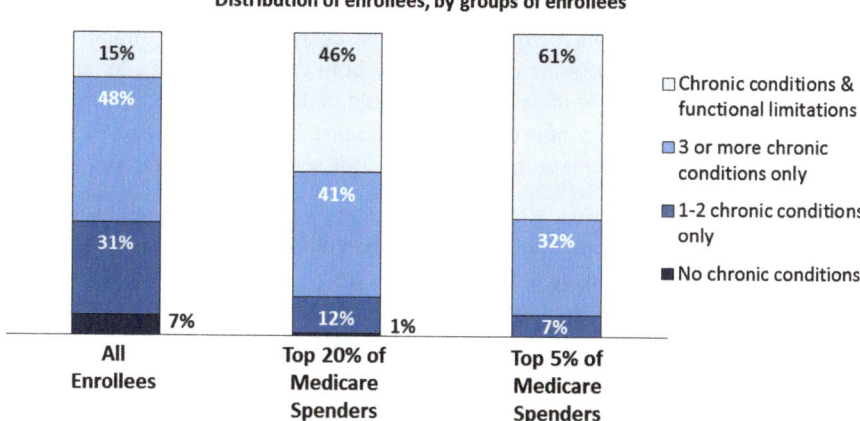

Fig. 9.2 Medicare enrollees with chronic conditions and functional limitation are over half of Medicare's highest spenders. *Source*: Komisar HL, Feder J. "Transforming Care for Medicare Beneficiaries with Chronic Conditions and Long-Term Care Needs: Coordinating Care Across All Services." (Washington, DC: Georgetown University, October 2011)

Improving Medicare's Care Coordination: Innovations and Reforms Under the Affordable Care Act [20]

The Centers for Medicare and Medicaid Services are actively engaged in using new authority for innovation under the ACA to promote Medicare delivery innovations, aimed largely at reducing unnecessary hospital costs. Past experience demonstrates that in the absence of targeting beneficiaries at high risk of inappropriate and high-cost hospital use, care coordination is unlikely to produce significant savings [21]. Targeting innovations to people with chronic conditions and functional limitations—and coordinating the full range of their service needs—offers a path to achieving the cost savings and quality improvements that policymakers aim to achieve.

Although limited in number, programs with these characteristics have shown promise in reducing hospital use, nursing home admissions, and costs for selected patient groups while improving quality of care. Key elements of these models include:

- A core of comprehensive primary medical care
- Assessment of patients' long-term service and support needs, plus caregiver capabilities and support needs
- Coordination of long-term care as well as medical care (same person or team involved in coordinating both)
- Ongoing collaboration and relationship among care coordinators, physicians, patients, and families, with attention to supporting patients during transitions between care settings
- Monthly per-person payments to cover coordination costs Medicare does not cover

CMS can build on these delivery reform initiatives to create a Medicare platform that encourages innovations focused on beneficiaries with functional limitations and coordinating services across the continuum for both their long-term care and their medical needs. Adoption of these practices would be facilitated by accommodating the varied size and capacity of primary and specialist-level physician practices, and by improving upon, but not eliminating, the fee-for-service payment system. These interventions would:

- Target: Zero in on people most at risk of preventable hospital use to maximize impact on reducing unnecessary and costly care
- Customize: Allow different approaches—both networks that hire and manage care coordinators and coordinators employed by physicians' practices—in order to maximize provider participation
- Pay for coordination: Pay monthly amounts per enrolled patient, sufficient to support currently uncovered care coordination services
- Hold providers accountable: Hold participating providers accountable for savings that offset these care coordination payments and pay providers—who satisfy quality standards—a share of savings if spending is less than projected
- Make states accountable: Encourage state participation for dual eligibles provided states, like participating providers, actually invest in delivery

Investment in policies and programs aimed directly at patients with chronic conditions and functional limitations can generate much needed lessons on how to improve their care. But these initiatives should not be designed to isolate the functionally impaired population in tailored delivery or to limit lessons learned only to this patient group. The ultimate goal of targeting delivery reforms to Medicare beneficiaries with chronic conditions and functional impairments is to assure that we learn as quickly as possible what it will take to assure the whole system's capacity to serve people with functional limitations as well as medical care needs appropriately and effectively, wherever and whenever these needs arise.

Conclusion

Detailing potential new models to improve care for people with chronic conditions and functional impairments reveals that their objectives and approach are complementary to what many envision for broadening the role of palliative care for the same target population. Specific elements of palliative care, such as vigilant attention to symptom relief and developing and following a person-and family-determined care plan, should be core elements of the care models being tested. Indeed, more interaction between palliative care practitioners and designers and implementers of these new models of care can assure that core elements of palliative care are incorporated into service design.

The other, perhaps less optimistic, message of this chapter is to emphasize that, currently, a core element of what is needed to support both palliative care and ongoing chronic care management are LTTS to help patients and their caregivers get through the day and remain safely in their preferred place—at home. The Medicare pilot test we propose would assess the need for LTTS—for patients and caregivers—and would coordinate these services and supports with the acute care services for these complex patients. But the pilot test model we propose does not contemplate actually financing long-term care on a Medicare platform. Financing remains a private and Medicaid responsibility. The absence of broader financing clearly remains a challenge to the achievement of equitable and accessible high value health care for Medicare beneficiaries and to the achievement of palliative care for Medicare beneficiaries—care that is first and foremost person and family centered and determined; is based on a care plan defined by what matters most to the patient and their family; provides effective symptom management to prevent crises; and ensures consistent and coordinated communication of care across settings and over time.

Acknowledgments The authors received valuable research support from Anna Spencer.

References

1. Meier DE. Improving health care value through increased access to palliative care issue brief. Washington, DC: National Institute for Health Care Management; 2012.
2. Meier DC. Increased access to palliative care and hospice services: opportunities to improve value in health care. Milbank Q. 2011;89(3):343–80.
3. Kaiser Commission on Medicaid and the Uninsured. The Medicaid Program at a glance. Washington, DC: Kaiser Commission on Medicaid and the Uninsured; 2013. http://www.kff.org/medicaid/7235.cfm
4. Centers for Medicare and Medicaid Services. Medicare: costs at a glance. http://www.medicare.gov/your-medicare-costs/costs-at-a-glance/costs-at-glance.html#collapse-4660. Accessed March 2013.
5. O'Brien E. Medicare and long-term care. Washington, DC: Georgetown University Health Policy Institute; 2007.
6. The Medicare Payment Advisory Commission. Skilled nursing facility services, Chap. 8. A report to Congress: Medicaid Payment Policy. Washington, DC: MedPAC; March 2013. p. 167.
7. The Medicare Payment Advisory Commission. Home health care services, Chap. 9. A report to Congress: Medicaid Payment Policy. Washington, DC: MedPAC; 2013. p. 190.
8. Center for Medicare Advocacy. Improvement standard and Jimmo news. http://www.medicareadvocacy.org/medicare-info/improvement-standard/. Accessed March 2014.
9. Feder J, Komisar HL. The importance of federal financing to the nation's long-term care safety net. Washington, DC: Georgetown University; 2012.
10. Feder J, Clemans-Cope L, Coughlin T, et al. Refocusing responsibility for dual eligibles: why medicare should take the lead. Washington DC: The Urban Institute; 2011. http://www.urban.org/UploadedPDF/412418-Refocusing-Responsibility-For-Dual-Eligibles.pdf.
11. Medicare Payment Advisory Commission. Coordinating the care of dual-eligible beneficiaries, Chap. 5. A report to the Congress: aligning incentives in Medicare. Washington, DC, Medicare Payment Advisory Commission; 2010.
12. Walsh EG, Freiman M, Haber S, et al. Cost drivers for dually eligible beneficiaries: potentially avoidable hospitalizations from nursing facility, skilled nursing facility, and home and community-based services waiver programs, final task 2 report. Washington, DC: Centers for Medicare and Medicaid Services; 2010.

13. Grabowski D. Medicare and Medicaid: conflicting incentives for long-term care. Milbank Q. 2007;85(4):579–610.
14. Centers for Medicare and Medicaid Services. Financial alignment services. http://www.cms.gov/Medicare-Medicaid-Coordination/Medicare-and-Medicaid-Coordination/Medicare-Medicaid-Coordination-Office/FinancialModelstoSupportStatesEffortsinCareCoordination.html. Accessed March 2013.
15. Musumeci M. State demonstrations to integrate care and align financing for dual eligible beneficiaries: a review of the 26 proposals submitted to CMS. Washington, DC: Kaiser Commission on Medicaid and the Uninsured; 2012.
16. Kaiser Family Foundation. Financial and administrative alignment demonstrations for dual eligible beneficiaries compared; 2013. http://kaiserfamilyfoundation.files.wordpress.com/2013/11/8426-05-financial-and-administrative-alignment-demonstrations-for-dual-eligible-beneficiaries-compared1.pdf. Accessed March 2014.
17. Jacobson G, Neuman T, Damico A. Medicare's role for dual eligible beneficiaries, issue brief. Washington, DC: Kaiser Family Foundation; 2012.
18. Berenson RA. Examining Medicare and Medicaid coordination for dual-eligibles. Testimony before the U.S. Special Committee on Aging, Hearing; 26 July 2012.
19. This section and next draw heavily from: Komisar HL, Feder J. Transforming care for Medicare Beneficiaries with chronic conditions and long-term care needs: coordinating care across all services. Washington, DC: Georgetown University; 2011. Findings reflect the collaboration with colleagues at Avalere Health on an extension of an analysis conducted by Avalere of data from the Medicare Current Beneficiary Survey, Cost and Use file for 2006. The analysis defined individuals as having functional limitations (and therefore to need long-term care) when they receive hands-on or standby assistance from another person with at least 1 of 5 activities of daily living or ADLs (bathing, dressing, eating, transferring from bed or chair, and using the toilet) or at least 3 of 5 instrumental activities of daily living or IADLs (light housework, managing medications, managing money, preparing meals, and using the telephone). Individuals were considered to have chronic conditions when they indicated that they had ever been diagnosed with any of the following conditions: arthritis, Alzheimer's Disease, broken hip, cancer (excluding skin), congestive heart failure, depression, diabetes, hypertension, mental illnesses (excluding depression), myocardial infarction, osteoporosis, Parkinson's Disease, pulmonary diseases (such as emphysema, asthma, and Chronic Obstructive Pulmonary Disease), stroke, and other heart conditions. The figures exclude Medicare beneficiaries with functional limitations and no chronic conditions; they represent just under 0.5 % of all Medicare beneficiaries. http://www.thescanfoundation.org/sites/default/files/Georgetown_Trnsfrming_Care.pdf.
20. This section draws heavily from Komisar and Feder, "Transforming Care for Medicare Beneficiaries with Chronic Conditions and Long-term Care Needs: Coordinating Care Across All Services."
21. Brown R, Mann DR. Best bets for reducing medicare costs for dual eligible beneficiaries: assessing the evidence issue brief. Washington, DC: Kaiser Family Foundation; 2012.

Chapter 10
The Manifest Destinies of Managed Care and Palliative Care

Richard H. Bernstein and Karol K. DiBello

Introduction

Two unremitting forces are shaping changes in the US health care system: (1) the graying of America or "silver tsunami," in which 10,000 individuals are now turning age 65 each day [1] and (2) the cost trends associated with caring for seniors and those with multiple chronic and often life-limiting conditions. Medicare expenditures are crowding out other national priorities and threatening the financial stability of this country [2]. Healthcare experts have identified palliative care and managed care as essential ways to address the special needs of an aging population and for providing care that can lower the rate of national health expenditures [3].

Twenty-seven percent of Medicare beneficiaries are now enrolled in Medicare Advantage plans [4]. Enrollment should accelerate as "boomers," who have been accustomed to employer-sponsored managed care plans, seamlessly age into their commercial insurer's Medicare Advantage plans. To effectively and cost-efficiently manage the complex set of clinical demands of this growing wave of Medicare members, Managed Care Organizations (MCOs) must address the special needs of the most expensive segment of this group of seniors, including multimorbidity, frailty, and functional/cognitive decline. These medical management challenges are compounded for dual eligibles, that is, those with both Medicare and Medicaid. This group has a higher prevalence of medical literacy issues, comorbid psychiatric

R.H. Bernstein, M.D. (✉)
Department of Geriatrics and Palliative Medicine, Icahn School of Medicine at Mount Sinai, 10th Floor, Annenberg Building, One Gustave L. Levy Place, Box 1070, New York, NY 10029, USA
e-mail: rhb1@aol.com

K.K. DiBello, D.N.P
Lawrence Medical Associates, New York-Presbyterian/Lawrence Hospital,
Bronxville, NY, USA
e-mail: kkdibello@gmail.com

and behavioral health problems, substance abuse, social and socioeconomic resource limitations, and dementia [5]. MCOs often employ risk stratification of their population and intensive care management programs, including palliative care, for those individuals with greatest need who are expected to cost the most.

This chapter will review the 30-year history of efforts to demonstrate the inherent synergies of MCOs and palliative care which have driven their conjoint destinies. As important, this collaboration has also shown that effective palliative care interventions can reduce MCO costs and secure a foundation for palliative care program funding.

Managed Healthcare Terminology

Managed care began with models of Prepaid Group Practices (PPGPs) in 1910. These were company sponsored and employed salaried groups of physicians. The model evolved over the next few decades to include multi-specialty groups and even hospital systems. Today the latter would be called integrated delivery systems, the paradigm of which is the Kaiser Health Plan with its hospitals and Permanante Medical Groups. To compete with these PPGPs, medical foundations were established in the mid-1950s to enfranchise individual practitioners and small practices into an independent practice association model (IPA). Insurers could contract directly or through an umbrella organization with this "group practice without walls." Fee for service (FFS) was the dominant reimbursement form in the early IPAs, although larger and mature organizations were able to accept per member per month payment, called capitation, with its attendant risk related to potential overutilization and unexpected costs. PPGPs and IPAs were labeled Health Maintenance Organizations with the HMO Act in 1973.

The early literature about managed care and palliative care describes HMOs as relying on salaried and capitated groups. However, since the 1950s, the landscape of organizational structures and reimbursement arrangements became more complex. PPGPs and IPAs could be reimbursed by health plans on a fixed per member per month basis or as a percent of the total premium. Clinicians participating in these organizations could be salaried, paid a "draw" or percent of the medical group's sub-capitation, or paid FFS. Thus, descriptions of potential ethical conflicts affecting HMOs with incentives to under-serve and doctors with divided loyalties may have oversimplified the impact of these diverse reimbursement arrangements. HMOs were often identified as "capitated," but this did not accurately describe the variety of actual arrangements and incentives affecting clinician decision makers.

All forms of MCOs are characterized by their accountability for cost, quality, and access for a defined population enrolled in the health plan. MCOs integrate the financing and delivery system and use a defined network of contracted providers, facilities, and other vendors. MCOs provide and pay for all services within a defined set of plan benefits [6]. Limiting access to contracted providers and facilities for non-emergencies is a feature of closed model plans. Open-access models, which now dominate, do not have these limits but impose higher cost sharing when non-network providers are used. This open-access feature is also a feature of the most prevalent model of MCO, the preferred provider organization (PPO).

The Program of All-Inclusive Care for the Elderly (PACE) is a "unique capitated managed care benefit for the frail elderly provided by a not-for-profit or public entity. The PACE program features a comprehensive medical and social service delivery system using an interdisciplinary team approach in an adult day health center that is supplemented by in-home and referral services in accordance with participants' needs." It is for dual eligibles, age 55 years and older, who can safely live in the community [7]. In the 1970s On Lok Senior Health Services in San Francisco was the first demonstration model for subsequent PACE programs. A trial of risk based, capitation was started in 1983, proved successful and established PACE as a special type of MCO. Unlike other MCOs, PACE programs have very limited membership (several hundred to fewer than 3,000 enrollees). There are currently 91 PACE models in the USA [8].

Accountable Care Organizations (ACOs), as defined by the Patient Protection and Accountability Care Act (PPACA), are limited to FFS Medicare beneficiaries and do not involve formal enrollment into a health plan. Although such ACOs are not MCOs, the term "accountable care organization" has been adopted by some health plans to describe a capitated or partial risk sharing arrangement with a large group or IPA. Finally, the Patient Centered Medical Home (PCMH), stipulated by PPACA, is not an MCO but a medical practice with enhanced care management, electronic health records, and a team of nonphysicians to provide more comprehensive, culturally, and linguistically sensitive care along with many standards for quality and access.

The balance of this chapter will discuss MCO in the delimited context of health plans with a prepaid premium, paid for by employers, individuals, the Department of Defense (Tri-Care), Medicaid, and Medicare. The discussion will exclude PCMHs and ACOs that are not part of MCOs.

1980–1990s: Relationship of MCOs and Palliative Care— "Important, Mysterious, and Interesting" with Opportunities and Concerns

In 1983, research began to show the value and potential savings resulting from palliative care in an MCO. The On Lok PACE was able to achieve hospital utilization rates 30 % lower than the general Medicare population by using elements of palliative care in its intensive care management approach [9].

In a different PACE program, Wieland et al. [10] found that, despite greater disease burden and disability among the PACE population, bed-days per 1,000 members were not significantly higher. Only 8 % of deaths for PACE enrollees were in hospital, and fewer than one-third of decedents were hospitalized during the last 6 months of life. These studies and others [11] suggested that a capitation program could allocate resources for palliative care and support such value added programs from hospital savings, especially given traditional Medicare's use of costly hospital services in the last few months of life [12].

The EverCare™ Program, developed by United Healthcare (UHC), began in 1986 and was an unusual form of managed care which enrolled residents in long-term care facilities who were not in hospice and not suffering from end stage renal disease. The capitation by Medicare provided flexible funding for physician/geriatric nurse practitioners teams to promote care management and treatment in place when possible. It also incorporated key features of palliative care. Its financial viability has depended on successfully managing its risk for all professional services and all acute and subacute facility costs. The program has documented a one-third reduction in acute care admissions and a 30 % decrease in costs compared with FFS Medicare [11].

In the mid-1990, the relationship between MCOs and palliative care was characterized by Steve Miles et al. as "important, mysterious, and interesting" [13]. Its importance derived from MCOs as the dominant form of health care in this country. MCOs now cover two-thirds of all Americans [14] including over a quarter of Medicare beneficiaries and about 75 % of Medicaid beneficiaries [15].

There was some "mystery" about managed care, since little research had been done on its impact on quality of care for the severely ill. MCOs were also "interesting" because their broad range of providers, incentives, and their provision of care across the continuum promoted integrated care, with accountability both for quality and efficient use of health resources. These factors were an important environment in which palliative care could thrive.

Despite these attractive attributes, MCOs harbored potential ethical perils: divided loyalty, conflicts of interest about patient vs. health plan advocacy, system savings garnered at the expense of patient needs, suppression of discussions about expensive but effective alternative treatments and devaluation of the most frail and vulnerable, who could not advocate for themselves [16, 17].

A cautionary, qualitative study was conducted in 1996–1997 at Harvard Pilgrim Health Care, a non-profit staff (salaried) model HMO. It found "concerns about the impact of cost containment on the quality of care, reflecting the conflict between the dual roles of MCOs as both insurers and providers of care." Nonetheless, this MCO continued to promote the development of palliative care programs [18].

Other authors agreed that managed care systems could not only support quality palliative care but also recognized the potential ethics conflicts inherent in such systems where financial concerns might complicate medical judgment and compromise the mission of palliative care to meet the needs of the most vulnerable [19–22].

Kuczewski and DeVita [23] expressed their reservations with clarity:

> The very mention of the term *managed care* can carry negative ethical connotations to those committed to patient care and the fiduciary model of the physician-patient relationship. It suggests travesties, including the unwarranted denial of necessary services and the pitting of the physician's interest in making a living against the needs of the patient. Perhaps most strikingly, it may evoke an image of the physician as gagged and prevented from telling the patient about beneficial treatments that are not covered by the plan or about fiscal arrangements that will lead to the demise of the patient.

At the same time, other researchers began to document MCO's benefits for the elderly, including a lower rate of potentially ineffective care among HMO vs. FFS Medicare beneficiaries [24]. In 1998, Lynn, Wilkinson et al. [25] described the potential for "capitated or salaried managed care systems...to provide high quality, cost-effective end-of-life care." They outlined the advantages of capitated managed care, including care coordination for a stable, enrolled population, robust data availability, the ability to develop innovative models for care, measure quality and evaluate outcomes. However, this opportunity was qualified by the strong incentive to avoid high risk populations. The authors recognized the deficiencies of FFS practices related to inadequate pain and symptom management, the lack of long-term supports and services, and care coordination. They proposed a model, MediCaring, to provide comprehensive and ideal palliative care within an MCO. They expected that a combination of capitation for teams and equipment along with salary or FFS for professionals could provide incentives compatible with managed care's goals while fostering excellence in caring for those with serious and complex illnesses.

Kane [26] echoed the potential that MCOs had for caring for the elderly with multiple chronic illnesses, but stressed that this would only work if Medicare risk-adjusted payments for the most costly beneficiaries among the Medicare population. Fortunately, Medicare (at that time called the Health Care Financing Administration or HCFA) recognized this concern and worked with actuaries to develop a reimbursement model for health plans to risk adjust capitation based on the mix of diagnoses in the prior years, weighted proportionately to their expected impact on overall costs in the following year [27]. This predictive model was needed to encourage continued participation by health plans in the Medicare program, especially after many such plans had threatened to exit the Medicare market in 1998 [28].

As was noted by Kuttner [29], risk adjusted payments were also a crucial development to address potentially perverse incentives affecting the health plan and individual providers. As he stated:

> First, health plans that receive the same payments may have sicker or healthier populations. Second, capitated payments to groups of doctors that contract with health plans are adjusted only partly, if at all, to reflect differences in the health of their patients. And finally, unadjusted capitation payments may ultimately be passed along to individual doctors treating dissimilar groups of patients.
>
> Thus, failure to adjust compensation for patients' health status reinforces two of the more worrisome trends in the present health care system. First, it rewards plans for a business strategy of "risk selection," in which they deliberately market their services to relatively healthy populations and avoid relatively sick ones. This strategy, in turn, punishes plans and physicians that do a good job of treating the sick, thus reinforcing the incentive to stint on care that is already present in a system that increasingly relies on payments by means of capitation rather than on fee-for-service reimbursement. Second, as risks are shifted to the individual physician, doctors with sicker patients must work longer hours or receive a reduced income or make unethical or clinically dangerous decisions to withhold necessary care.

At the end of the 1990s, an important monograph was published by the National Task Force on End-of-Life Care in Managed Care [30]. It codified 12 recommendations for improving and promoting palliative care within MCOs, including improved access, accountability for quality, and the study of reimbursement alternatives. The Task Force outlined an ambitious agenda for managed care leaders and governmental policy makers as well as for public and private purchasers. This document was emblematic of the national recognition being given to MCOs as a vehicle to promote palliative care.

2000 to the Present: Synergies Between MCOs and Palliative Care; Documenting Improved Care and Savings to Support Palliative Care

Fowler and Lynn outlined the complexity and inadequacy of Medicare reimbursement for palliative care when managing the frail elderly with complex medical needs [31]. Their research documented that most palliative care programs were sustained by philanthropy and institutional cross-subsidies and not by Medicare FFS. This created a challenge facing most non-hospice programs providing palliative care in the community, namely, the need to find more sustainable financing mechanisms to support the interdisciplinary team, a core and necessary feature of quality for palliative care across the continuum of care [32].

Another outcome of MCOs compared with FFS Medicare was the higher use of hospice [33]. This pattern reflected more appropriate end of life care and also supported funding of palliative care and end of life counseling by MCOs.

Champions of quality end of life care, such as Ira Byock, soon began examining best practices of palliative care within MCOs and recognized in 2001 that "the goals of managed care and palliative care are already well aligned…[and]can address the needs and preferences of dying patient and families, while increasing public trust in managed care" [34].

In 2002, a pivotal research paper was published by Brumley [35] at Kaiser Permanente on the value of a community-based palliative care program which integrated curative and comfort care. The study home health care-based population had chronic obstructive pulmonary disease, congestive heart failure, or cancer; two or more emergency department visits or hospitalizations in the prior year and a prognosis of less than 24 months to live. They were compared with a matched home care population at Kaiser. Two hundred and ninety-six patients enrolled in the study: 145 in the Palliative Care Program and 151 in the home-health comparison group. After 8 months of follow-up, there was a statistically significant drop in the cost for physician, emergency department, acute and skilled nursing facility, and home health costs in the intervention group. This group showed higher palliative home care costs, as expected. The cost of decedents was almost $5,000 less in the palliative care group. Satisfaction with care was maintained in the intervention group. The result substantiated the feasibility of supporting innovative palliative care programs within MCOs by net savings.

In the next year, Brumley et al. [36] reported a full 2 years' experience at Kaiser, and the program showed persistence of the pattern of cost savings and patient satisfaction among their total enrollment of 558 individuals. They documented a 45 % decrease in cost compared with usual care. In addition, an in-home palliative care program at Kaiser later showed high satisfaction and cost reduction [37]. Noteworthy in this study was the ability of Permanente Medical Group to flex the standard benefits to incorporate all the key elements of a quality palliative care program within their pre-defined capitated budget.

At this time, palliative care and managed care experts identified few references to palliative care in specialty textbooks and disease management guidelines. They saw the potential for MCOs to be a vehicle for encouraging and adopting clinical practice guidelines that incorporated referral to palliative care at certain inflection points in the trajectory of common, progressive chronic illnesses [38].

Palliative care programs were soon being tested in MCO settings outside of the large integrated systems like Kaiser and Harvard. A small plan in New York, Elderplan, with 14,000 frail elderly members, developed a palliative care program for those with advanced illness needs but who were not enrolled in hospice. While net savings during the 2-year study period were not reported, they did show high satisfaction with pain and other symptom management and reduced use of ICU compared with a control group [39].

Additional research was published on clinical subsets of the population and the effects of palliative care programs within MCOs. In PhoenixCare, members with COPD and CHF with a 2-year prognosis were assigned to a demonstration program involving intensive home-based palliative care case management [40]. Compared with controls, the intervention group showed lower symptom distress, better physical functioning, and higher self-rated health. Emergency department utilization was not significantly affected.

That the MCO environment can be fertile ground for the rapid development of an inpatient palliative care unit was documented at Kaiser in 2009 [41]. The authors felt this innovation was adopted rapidly in this complex institutional setting because their model employed organizational "push" strategies and grassroots-level pull. The authors felt this approach might be applicable to other settings. Kaiser has also shown the effectiveness of inpatient palliative care with subsequent palliative care follow-up in reducing readmissions among the seriously ill elderly [42, 43].

Other MCO populations which have benefited from palliative care advanced care management include Medicaid recipients. One study [44] found improved utilization of medical services, hospice, and member satisfaction.

Despite concerns about perverse incentives affecting providers who care for the seriously ill in MCOs, a recent, large satisfaction survey among 402,593 Medicare Advantage (MA) beneficiaries employed a standardized instrument (the Consumer Assessment of Healthcare Providers and Systems). It adjusted results for age, sex, race, ethnicity, education, Medicaid status, geographic region, and health status. While it was not designed to evaluate palliative care interventions per se, the survey found that those who died within a year of taking the survey rated their care as good as or better than other MA members, indicating that Medicare MCOs appeared to be meeting the needs of their members in the last stage of their life [45].

An unexplored area for MCOs and palliative care is for pediatric and neonatal patients with life limiting conditions. Several medical center-based pediatric palliative care programs have been described, and the complexities of palliative care funding are well documented [46]. Financing is even more difficult in pediatric and neonatal palliative care due to the variation in natural history of some of the subacute and chronic conditions benefiting from palliative care and the mix of dominant conditions. The difficulty using Medicaid and Medicare hospice financing models becomes quickly apparent when considering the need for decade-long palliative care for neurodegenerative and other chronic pediatric diseases.

One pediatric and neo-natal palliative care group [47] has analyzed several hundred of its cases and noted a significant reduction in readmissions and emergency department use compared with usual care. The sponsoring organization, Circle of Life Children's Center of New Jersey, has proposed a case rate to a Medicaid managed care plan to fund its pediatric palliative care team. Reimbursement would be based on four categories of conditions with four distinct intensity levels of team involvement: (1) Perinatal (e.g., fetal loss, nonviable live births), (2) Neonates expected to survive less than 1 year (e.g., trisomy 13, birth weight less than 2.2 lbs), (3) Neonatal survivors with chronic illness (e.g., cerebral palsy, intraventricular hemorrhage, necrotizing enterocolitis, bronchopulmonary dysplasia), and (4) Children/Adolescents with life limiting acute and chronic illnesses (e.g., traumatic brain injury, motor vehicle accidents, meningitis, cancer, cystic fibrosis, sickle cell anemia, HIV/AIDS). While the model has not been adopted by any Medicaid plan to date, it has received interest from the State of New Jersey and some private foundations as an alternative to FFS payment for palliative care.

Another opportunity for MCOs is to evaluate the impact of palliative care on quality and cost for an HIV/AIDs population. Several studies of palliative care in HIV/AIDS in non-MCO settings have demonstrated better quality and reduced costs [46, 48, 49]. At least one HIV Special Needs MCO [50] will begin offering palliative care for its 5,500 members.

VNSNY SPARK: An MCO-Palliative Care Program for a Medicare Special Needs Population

The Visiting Nurse Service of New York (VNSNY) is a 120-year-old home health agency and the largest non-profit certified home health agency in the USA. VNSNY has its own hospice and palliative care service and several managed care insurance programs (under the VNSNY CHOICE name) serving special needs populations (a Medicaid HIV/AIDs special needs plan, a partial capitation plan for nursing home eligibles living at home, a Medicare dual eligible special needs plan, and a Medicare Advantage plan for non-duals).

The agency also started a professional corporation, ESPRIT Medical Care, PC, to allow private billing of clinical programs that could serve MCOs. With support from VNSNY Hospice and Palliative Care and product development specialists within VNSNY, a palliative care management model was created to provide services through Esprit. A clinical team of nurse practitioners (NPs) and licensed clinical social workers (LCSWs) along with medical consultants and hospice team members formed a palliative care team within Esprit in 2010 for home and telephonic care management. The program was called SPARK©. Its acronym stands for Self-care, Pain and symptom control, Additional care, Respect needs and Kindness.

In the SPARK care management model, each NP/LCSW team shares the responsibility of managing a caseload of patients through both telephonic contact and home visits. Consistent with many care management programs, SPARK coordinates care across settings and providers to achieve quality, cost-effective, non-duplicative care over time [51]. With this goal, SPARK teams work in collaboration with community health care providers such as primary care providers, specialists, public health nurses, and social workers. SPARK care coordination is an added benefit for the MCO and may provide value over what a more consultative palliative care model which focuses on episodic symptom management.

Traditional care management programs may focus on disease management for members with multiple chronic illnesses. By contrast, SPARK care management focuses on the symptoms, psychosocial, and spiritual burdens, and advance care planning needs of both patients with serious illness and their caregivers' related concerns. Through this approach, the program is able to combine the benefits of both the care management model and palliative care principles.

In risk stratifying its most complex members, VNSNY CHOICE Medicare's clinical team [52] noticed the need to help members with advanced care management needs that were not benefiting from repeated acute care hospitalizations. An agreement between CHOICE Medicare and SPARK began in April 2010, with the following aims:

- Understanding the goals of care for the sickest 2–3 % of the Medicare members and providing options to better meet those needs to improve the quality of life
- Reducing futile care and hospitalizations that were not consistent with member and families' wishes
- Improving member satisfaction, quality of life indicators, and completion rates of advance directives
- Developing program support for the SPARK team that would be financially self-sustaining by demonstrating reduced overall costs compared to expected costs for this very high risk cohort
- Better diagnostic coding of illness to provide more accurate Medicare plan risk scores and reimbursement
- Collecting data to document Medicare Quality Star measures such as those related to the Care of Older Adults.

The initial monthly case rate was set at over $1,000.

From April 2010 to December 2012 over 600 members have been referred to SPARK. Seventy percent were enrolled[1] following a comprehensive initial assessment.

---

[1] Reasons for not enrolling after referral included: unwillingness to participate by member and family after the program was explained, unwillingness by the member's primary physician to support and communicate with SPARK staff, direct referral to hospice more appropriate, profound behavior issues that would undermine the ability to help after multiple attempts to enlist cooperation.

Their average Medicare risk score was almost three times that of an average Medicare beneficiary. Most had multiple hospital admissions within the prior 12 months and had a condition with less than 24 months life expectancy as well as a high symptom burden. In addition, over one-third had a diagnosis of significant comorbid mental health or substance abuse (i.e., Medicare Hierarchical Condition Categories 51–55).

After over 2½ years, SPARK outcomes have been favorable. Ninety-three percent of SPARK members had advance directives and a similar percent had quality of life responses indicating that members felt their quality of life was maintained or improved under the program. Almost 99 % of family and member respondents were either satisfied or very satisfied with care with the SPARK team. One in five members has met Hospice criteria and of those around 50 % were referred by SPARK to hospice. They had an average Hospice length of stay of 73 days. Compared with prior hospitalization rates before enrollment, there was a reduction of almost 40 %, using members as their own controls from a year before to a year or more following enrollment. Including the cost of the SPARK case rate, the net savings were over $250 per member per month to VNSNY CHOICE Medicare.

Remaining Challenges: Difficulty Proving Savings to Skeptics and Risk Stratifying Advanced Care Management

While the reported benefits met the health plan's goals, there were issues raised about how real the savings were. What role did regression to the mean have in showing reduced hospitalizations and cost avoidance? How effective was the method of using patients as their own control to demonstrate program effectiveness? Is the model scalable, that is, will the cost of over $1,000 per month be attractive to other MCOs if they were not guaranteed savings?

VNSNY's research unit identified a control group from among other patients of VNSNY programs. Matching on age, gender, risk score, and mental health/substance abuse frequency, the research group identified a propensity score matched control group to better compare outcomes. One hundred and twenty-eight individuals in SPARK and the same number in the control group were studied. The results included inpatient cost saving over $1,500 ($p<0.01$) for the SPARK group. While professional, outpatient, prescription (Part B and Part D), home health, and skilled nursing facility costs were somewhat higher in SPARK patients, total costs remained over $700 per member per month lower in the SPARK group for the 6 months post-intervention period. Due to the relatively low numbers of patients studied, this difference did not reach statistical significance.

Most noteworthy, however, was that after 3 months of enrollment, only 5 % of the SPARK group died while the control group lost 23 % to death. The cumulative death rate after 6 months was 21 % in the SPARK population and 32 % in the control group.

These observations suggest that the usual methodologies to evaluate the impact of health program models on utilization may be more difficult to apply to palliative care. The high death rates and difficulty finding "matched controls" to determine actual to expected costs make it challenging to fully allay skeptics' concerns.

VNSNY Medicare and SPARK will be modifying the program in the future. To increase the value of the program to MCOs, the referred population will be stratified into three groups with corresponding levels of intensity of team intervention. The revised program will customize the proportion of in-home and telephonic contact to match the level of patient stability and need. The mix of care managers (nurse practitioners, social workers, and RNs) will be deployed to match the risk level.

These changes should allow the program to significantly reduce the MCO's case rate without adversely affecting program outcomes. Substantiating these expectations will remain an important next step for VNSNY CHOICE Medicare and SPARK to establish for both advocates and skeptics the value of similar programs in small- and medium-sized MCOs throughout the country.

Conclusion

MCOs have initiated or incorporated palliative care programs for over 30 years and increasingly recognize the crucial contribution these programs can make to address the special needs of many of their most vulnerable, complex, and expensive members. The synergy between MCO and palliative care derives from their shared goals of improving access and quality of care in a manner that effectively prevents and manages predictable crises and emergencies, and in doing so, reduce reliance on emergency services and hospital care.

Models for delivering palliative care need further experimentation to assure that quality standards and desired outcome metrics are maintained while programs define the most appropriate mix of resources to achieve long term and sustainable funding. Successful models already exist in some large integrated health systems. For palliative care to be available to broader segments of the population, programs need to be adapted to more typical health plans and ACOs, which may not have the resources and infrastructure of the largest MCOs. Community-based palliative care programs should become more readily available as more data establish their return on investment.

References

1. http://www.agingresearch.org/content/article/detail/826/. Accessed 23 Feb 2013.
2. http://www.commonwealthfund.org/~/media/Files/Publications/Issue%20Brief/2012/May/1595_Squires_explaining_high_hlt_care_spending_intl_brief.pdf. Accessed 23 Feb 2013.
3. AHRQ Health Care Innovations Exchange Team. Effective Palliative Care Programs require health system change. Update: 24 Oct 2012. http://www.innovations.ahrq.gov/content.aspx?id=3742. Accessed 23 Feb 2013.

4. http://www.kff.org/medicare/upload/8323.pdf. Accessed 23 Feb 2013.
5. http://www.commonwealthfund.org/Publications/Issue-Briefs/2008/Feb/Medicare-Advantage-Special-Needs-Plans-for-Dual-Eligible---Primer.aspx and http://www.kff.org/medicare/upload/8138-02.pdf. Accessed 23 Feb 2013.
6. Iglehart JK. The American health care system. Managed care. N Engl J Med. 1992;327(10):742–7.
7. http://www.cms.gov/Medicare/Health-Plans/pace/downloads/pacefactsheet.pdf. Accessed 23 Feb 2013.
8. http://www.npaonline.org/website/article.asp?id=12&title=Who,_What_and_Where_is_PACE? Accessed 27 April 2013.
9. Cheng SSW. On Lok SeniorHealth: a national model of community-based long-term care in the USA. Asian J Gerontol Geriatr. 2006;1:101–6.
10. Wieland D, Lamb VL, Sutton SR, Boland R, Clark M, Friedman S, Brummel-Smith K, Eleazer GP. Hospitalization in the Program of All-Inclusive Care for the Elderly (PACE): rates, concomitants, and predictors. J Am Geriatr Soc. 2000;48(11):1373–80.
11. Wilkinson AM, Harrold JK, Kopits I, Ayers E. New endeavors and innovative programs in end of life care. Hosp J. 1998;13(1–2):165–80.
12. Lubitz J, Prihoda R. The use and costs of medicare services in the last two years of life. Health Care Financ Rev. 1984;5:117–31.
13. Miles SH, Weber EP, Koepp R. End-of-life treatment in managed care. The potential and the peril. West J Med. 1995;163(3):302–5.
14. http://www.mcol.com/current_enrollment. Accessed 16 Feb 13.
15. http://facts.kff.org/chart.aspx?ch=180. Accessed 16 Feb 2013.
16. Sulmasy DP. Managed care and managed death. Arch Intern Med. 1995;55:133–6.
17. Loewy EH, Loewy RS. Ethics and managed care: restructuring a system and refashioning a society. Arch Intern Med. 1998;158:2419–22.
18. Gazelle G, Buxbaum R, Daniels E. The development of a palliative care program for managed care patients: a case example. J Am Geriatr Soc. 2001;49(9):1241–8.
19. Morrison RS, Meier DE. Managed care at the end of life. Trends Health Care Law Ethics. 1995;10(1–2):91–6.
20. Fade A, Kaplan K. Managed care and end of life decisions. Trends Health Care Law Ethics. 1995;10(1–2):97–100.
21. Meier DE, Morrison RS, Cassel CK. Improving palliative care. Ann Intern Med. 1997;127(3):225–30.
22. Rousseau P. Palliative care in managed Medicare: reasons for hope–and for concern. Geriatrics. 1998;53(11):59–65.
23. Kuczewski MG, DeVita M. Managed care and end-of-life decisions: learning to live ungagged. Arch Intern Med. 1998;158(22):2424–8.
24. Cher DJ, Lenert LA. Method of Medicare reimbursement and the rate of potentially ineffective care of critically ill patients. JAMA. 1997;278(12):1001–7.
25. Lynn J, Wilkinson A, Cohn F, Jones SB. Capitated risk-bearing managed care systems could improve end-of-life care. J Am Geriatr Soc. 1998;46(3):322–30.
26. Kane RL. Managed care as a vehicle for delivering more effective chronic care for older persons. J Am Geriatr Soc. 1998;46(8):1034–9.
27. Iezonni L, Ayanian J, Bates D, Burstin H. Paying more fairly for Medicare capitated care. N Engl J Med. 1998;339:1933–8.
28. Pear R. HMOs are retreating from Medicare, citing high costs. New York Times; 2 Oct 1998. p. A18.
29. Kuttner R. The risk-adjustment debate. N Engl J Med. 1998;339:1952–6.
30. Mildred ZS. Meeting the challenge: twelve recommendations for improving end-of-life care in managed care. A national task force of the Educational Development Center, Inc. 1999. p. 3–10.
31. Fowler N, Lynn J. Potential medicare reimbursements for services to patients with chronic fatal illnesses. J Palliat Med. 2000;3:165–80.

32. Wiener JM, Tilly J. End-of-life care in the United States: policy issues and model programs. Int J Integr Care. 2003;3:e24.
33. Virnig BA, Fisher ES, McBean AM, Kind S. Hospice use in Medicare managed care and fee-for-service systems. Am J Manag Care. 2001;7(8):777–86.
34. Byock IR. End-of-life care: a public health crisis and an opportunity for managed care. Am J Manag Care. 2001;7(12):1123–32.
35. Brumley RD. Future of end-of-life care: the managed care organization perspective. J Palliat Med. 2002;5(2):263–70.
36. Brumley RD, Enguidanos S, Cherin DA. Effectiveness of a home-based palliative care program for end-of-life. J Palliat Med. 2003;6(5):715–24.
37. Brumley R, Enguidanos S, Jamison P, Seitz R, Morgenstern N, Saito S, McIlwane J, Hillary K, Gonzalez J. Increased satisfaction with care and lower costs: results of a randomized trial of in-home palliative care. J Am Geriatr Soc. 2007;55(7):993–1000.
38. Emanuel L, Alexander C, Arnold RM, Bernstein R, Dart R, Dellasantina C, Dykstra L, Tulsky J, Palliative Care Guidelines Group of the American Hospice Foundation. Integrating palliative care into disease management guidelines. J Palliat Med. 2004;7(6):774–83.
39. Nidetz A, Fishman E, Jacobs M, Daniels C, Tamang S. Palliative care management services in a Medicare Social HMO. J Pain Symptom Manage. 2005;29(1):109–11.
40. Aiken LS, Butner J, Lockhart CA, Volk-Craft BE, Hamilton G, Williams FG. Outcome evaluation of a randomized trial of the PhoenixCare intervention: program of case management and coordinated care for the seriously chronically ill. J Palliat Med. 2006;9(1):111–26.
41. Della Penna R, Martel H, Neuwirth EB, Rice J, Filipski MI, Green J, Bellows J. Rapid spread of complex change: a case study in inpatient palliative care. BMC Health Serv Res. 2009;9:245.
42. Enguidanos S, Vesper E, Lorenz K. 30-day readmissions among seriously ill older adults. J Palliat Med. 2012;15(12):1356–61.
43. Edens PS, Harvey CD, Gilden KM. Developing and financing a palliative care program. Am J Hosp Palliat Care. 2008;25(5):379–84.
44. Head BA, LaJoie S, Augustine-Smith L, Cantrell M, Hofmann D, Keeney C, Pfeifer M. Palliative care case management: increasing access to community-based palliative care for Medicaid recipients. Prof Case Manag. 2010;15(4):206–17.
45. Elliott MN, Haviland AM, Cleary PD, et al. Care experiences of managed care medicare enrollees near the end of life. J Am Geriatr Soc. 2013. doi:10.1111/jgs 12121. Epub ahead of print.
46. Byock I, Twohig JS, Merriman M, Collins K. Promoting excellence in end-of-life care: a report on innovative models of palliative care. J Palliat Med. 2006;9(1):137–51.
47. Personal communication from the Circle of Life Children Center of New Jersey. http://www.circleoflifenj.org/index.php?lang=en
48. Oleske JM, Czarniecki L. Continuum of palliative care: lessons from caring for children infected with HIV-1. Lancet. 1999;354:1287–90.
49. Master R, Dreyfus T, Connors S, Tobias C, Zhou Z, Kronick R. The Community Medical Alliance: an integrated system of care in Greater Boston for people with severe disability and AIDS. Manag Care Q. 1996;4(2):26–37.
50. Personal communication from the chapter's authors regarding VNSNY CHOICE SelectHealth in New York; February 2013.
51. Bodenheimer T, Berry-Millett R. Care management of patients with complex health care needs. Robert Wood Johnson Foundation Research Synthesis report no. 19;2009. ISSN 2155-3718.
52. http://www.commonwealthfund.org/Publications/Case-Studies/2013/Jan/VNSNYs-Choice-Program.aspx. Accessed 23 Feb 2013.

Part IV
Platforms for Improvement

Chapter 11
Models of Care Delivery and Coordination: Palliative Care Integration Within Accountable Care Organizations

Dorothy Deremo, Monique Reese, Susan D. Block, Vicki A. Jackson, Thomas H. Lee, Lori Bishop, and Robert Sawicki

The "Missing Piece"

The At Home Support™ Program

The System (Maturity of Both ACO and PC)

Our journey in creating At Home Support™ began over 10 years ago as part of Hospice of Michigan (HOM)'s mission, vision, and strategic plan. Rich in experience with coordinating care under a capitated shared risk model for Medicare and

---

D. Deremo, R.N., M.S.N., M.H.S.A., F.A.C.H.E.
Hospice of Michigan, Detroit, MI, USA

M. Reese, D.N.P., A.R.N.P., F.N.P.-C., A.C.H.P.N.
UnityPoint Health, Urbandale, IA, USA

S.D. Block, M.D.
Department of Psychosocial Oncology and Palliative Care, Dana-Farber Cancer Institute and Brigham and Women's Hospital, Boston, MA, USA

V.A. Jackson, M.D., M.P.H.
Palliative Care Division, Massachusetts General Hospital, Boston, MA, USA

Harvard Medical School, Boston, MA, USA

T.H. Lee, M.D.
Chief Medical Officer, Press Ganey,
Boston, MA, USA

L. Bishop, R.N., C.H.P.N.
UnityPoint Health/UnityPoint at Home, Urbandale, IA, USA

R. Sawicki, M.D. (✉)
Division of Supportive Care, OSF HealthCare,
800 N.E. Glen Oak Avenue, Peoria, IL 61603, USA
e-mail: Robert.sawicki@osfhealthcare.org

Medicaid beneficiaries, the organization began to expand services and test a new model of care based on core strengths: providing community based, family centered care for vulnerable populations. A collaborative research initiative lead by HOM's research, innovation, and education Institute, the Maggie Allesee Center for Innovation (MAC) provided the foundations for the outcomes-based At Home Support™ program. In the midst of healthcare reform and a concerted effort in creating coordinated patient centered care under the Accountable Care Organization (ACO) model, a synergistic partnership and natural "fit" was created between At Home Support™ and the Detroit Medical Center (DMC) Michigan Pioneer ACO.

At Home Support™ was implemented in 2007 in collaboration with two large Health Maintenance Organizations (HMOs). Quality and cost outcomes were primary drivers and were defined at the beginning of each relationship providing the strategy for measuring success. Both HMOs were interested in improving access to supportive care and in improving cost outcomes for patients in the last year of life. Two different payment structures were tested: a per diem and fee for service model. The MAC developed and proposed eligibility criteria based on end of life criteria for four disease categories: Stage IV lung cancer, Stage III–IV heart failure, Stage IV lung conditions, and a debility category. The debility category included criteria for advanced stage neurological, renal, and multisystem organ failure disease conditions. All aspects of the program were measured including types and numbers of services, cost associated with delivering the service, and patient/caregiver related health outcomes (e.g., pain, dyspnea and functional status, caregiver relationship to patient, advance directives). In 2010, the MAC, in collaboration with Wayne State University, secured a grant to rigorously measure cost outcomes. In late 2011, the preliminary results supported a 30 % decrease in total costs net of At Home Support™ costs for patients receiving At Home Support™ services [1]. The data findings provided the foundation for discussions with the newly formed DMC Michigan Pioneer ACO.

At Home Support™ is unique in design and is not by definition a traditional home care model, a chronic disease model, or a hospice model. The At Home Support™ model incorporates a community-based approach that "supplements", versus replacing, existing healthcare services. An interdisciplinary team of specialty trained nurses, social workers, and patient family assistants provide advanced illness strategies. The staff complete a training program created by the MAC to meet defined program outcomes. Advance illness management (AIM) strategies include a focus on surrogate decision making, creating a safety net for remaining independent at home, and teaching skills to effectively navigate the healthcare system. The use of goals of care discussion to assist in family centered care transitions between aggressive and supportive care is a key strategy. The model of care described as the "Care Giver Model" focuses on the role of the caregiver in the shared decision making process. Evidence-based disease management protocols for disease management (e.g., GOLD standards for the management of lung conditions) are combined with psychosocial approaches (e.g., addressing the burdens of illness) to incorporate social cognitive theory, public health principles of prevention, and caregiver engagement. The integration of palliative care principles and practices is a vital element of the model. The delivery of care is primarily in the home, but patients can be followed and supported in various settings.

Table 11.1 Key misperceptions of the At Home Support™ Program

The program is "hospice in disguise," or "hospice lite"
The program is designed to assume management of the patient, severing long-term relationships between physician and patient
The program is a competing home care service, or "home care on steroids"
The program is a case management model created to observe, manage, and dictate physician practices
Concern for losing funds to vendor as part of the shared savings plan
"We already do this"
"We can do this"

Care plans and visit frequency are established with the patient and family and in accordance with identified needs, illness severity (functional status), and goals of care. Critical to the model delivery system is access to care via a 24/7 AIM At Home Telesupport Center. Strategies include routine and as needed home visits and individualized treatment plans designed to keep patients in their own homes and providing an alternative to unwanted emergency room and acute care utilization.

Process of Negotiating Inclusion

Creating synergy and a collaborative partnership in the newly formed ACO required addressing misperceptions and issues related to AIM (see Table 11.1), specifically, (1) the perception that "we already do this," (2) the perception "we can probably do this ourselves," and (3) the perception that the system was able to effectively identify high risk and resource intensive members. As the new ACO was creating community relationships, leadership from HOM presented "The Missing Piece" highlighting the importance for the ACO of establishing a strategic plan to address caring for their most vulnerable population: those with serious and complex illnesses.

HOM leadership challenged the perception that the current system was designed to manage patients with serious and complex illness, and the notion that the skill set of AIM could easily be replicated. Data and program experience demonstrated how standard chronic disease models, focused primarily on medication compliance and physician access, become ineffective as a patient progresses to advanced stages of chronic disease, often with multiple chronic conditions and functional dependency. Addressing the needs of those with progressive illness and their caregivers was emphasized as a specialized skill set (skills that would take the ACO months to years to build). At Home Support™ offered a proven, experienced, turnkey solution.

In addition to challenging key misperceptions, the next task was to engage the ACO in their ability to identify the sickest most complex tier three patients. Tier three patients are defined as the 10 % of the ACO population that account for 64 % of total costs [1]. Our research identified a significant subset of the Tier 3 cohort, we have named Tier 3A. The Tier 3A cohort is 5 % of the seriously ill patients with Stage IV chronic disease in a Medicare network that accounts for 50 % of the total healthcare costs—the Pareto principle on steroids. At Home Support™ offered a turnkey solution in the form of a predictive model to identify

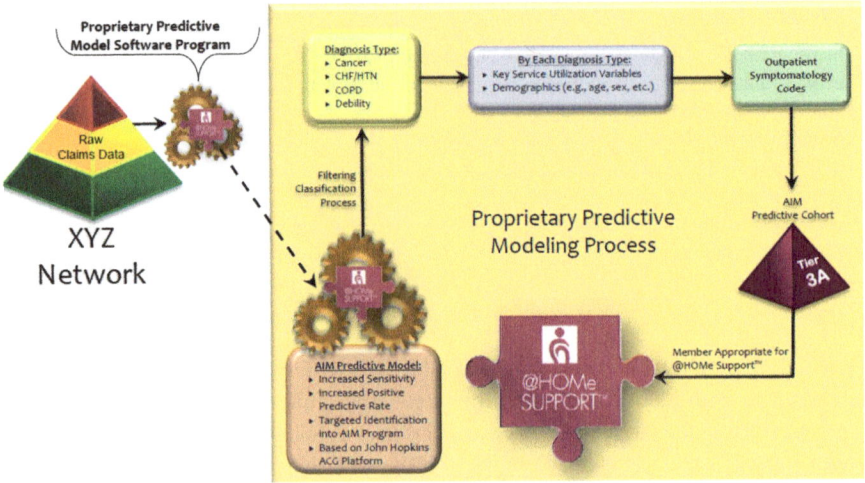

Fig. 11.1 AIM predictive model for member identification

the Tier 3A target population that would benefit most from AIM. Unlike traditional models that require physicians to recognize limited prognosis and then make referrals, the predictive model approach allows for efficient member identification and the ability to offer immediate intervention (See Fig. 11.1).

Challenges, Opportunities, and Lessons Learned

System navigation has created both challenges and opportunities for a successful partnership between HOM and the Michigan ACO. Our previous partnership experiences provided us with a proactive plan to address the known challenges of working within highly complicated and relatively closed systems. Physician engagement, reliability of member contact information, and the availability of "real time" data remained common challenges that complicate integration of AIM services within a conventional system. As the ACO was being formed, HOM emphasized the importance of contacting individual ACO physicians to describe and communicate the focus and intent of the AIM program. Because AIM is different than hospice, home care, or other community-based programming, clarifying the outcomes, the target population, and method of member identification was essential in the initial planning phases. Equally important to physician engagement is the relationship-building, support, and advocacy of the ACO physician leadership team to guide and ensure effective integration of this innovative program structure.

The data exchange and data sharing process is essential to effectively and efficiently identify members that would most benefit from AIM. Although fundamental to model design, this process does come with limitations. A data exchange process is only as reliable as the information that is entered in the system. Challenges due to the inaccuracy of demographic data (including contact information for members), paucity of "real time" data, and accessibility to medical records/clinical markers continue to be areas for improvement.

Favorable preliminary outcomes continue to support our previous findings. Outcomes of the program under scrutiny include comparison of total costs by patient (baseline to actual), ER diversions, hospitalization, and patient/caregiver satisfaction. Preliminary indications showed a decrease in total costs attributed to both ER and hospitalization avoidance. Initial patient/caregiver satisfaction scores are also high with the program. Finally, initial indications also show a significant increase in Family Evaluation of Hospice Care scores, an NQF–endorsed measure of patient/family experience with hospice, for patients transitioned to hospice from At Home Support™ versus those that enroll in hospice directly.

Input from ACO leader, Dr. Gregory Berger, Executive Medical Director of the Michigan Pioneer ACO

The goals of the Michigan Pioneer ACO include 33 quality metrics that comprise an eight item CAHPS survey for member satisfaction and 25 quality measures. Specific to the collaborative, there are five key quality indicators: emergency room utilization, hospital readmissions, hospital days, physician visits within 7 days post discharge, and a Caregiver Satisfaction Survey.

The leadership of the DMC Michigan Pioneer ACO recognized that 80 % of Medicare expense occurs in the last 2 years of life and that innovative approaches are needed to address an aging baby boomer population. An important goal for the ACO is to provide effective solutions by integrating models that focus on relief of symptoms and improving quality of life for patients and families and interventions to address advance care planning on all levels. Some of the unique benefits of the Personalized Home Care Program (the private label branding the DMC Pioneer chose to use instead of At Home Support™) are that members have a choice and options. Barriers to needed services such as the hospice requirement for physician certification and prognosticating time until death have been eliminated.

Integrating an innovative model such as Personalized Home Care Program within an ACO does come with challenges. Creating awareness among providers, the need for data sharing among differing electronic systems as well as developing network relationship within the hospital systems, emergency room, skilled nursing facilities and palliative care initiatives are a few examples. Some of the efforts to address these challenges include creating effective tools from both the clinical and cost perspectives for providing the "right care at the right time." One of the key elements for success has been creating a collaborative team approach by holding regular meetings of providers across all settings and organizations to develop strategies specific to the population being served and institutions involved. Dr. Berger says that real change will come by "changing physician and provider behavior." We recognize that this is pioneer work at this time and the care models for the future are being developed and tested. Dr. Berger believes that other institutions working within the ACO continue to be creative and hopeful in an era of change.

Partners Health System

Partners Health System (PHS), encompassing Brigham and Women's Hospital (BWH), Massachusetts General Hospital (MGH), and affiliated community hospitals, has had a Palliative Care Committee providing system-wide leadership and serving as a system-integrating focus, for more than 12 years. Our academic health centers and BWH-affiliated Dana-Farber Cancer Institute (DFCI) have had palliative care services since 1996 (MGH) and 2001 (BWH/DFCI); our community-based hospitals (North Shore Medical Center, Newton Wellesley Hospital, Brigham and Women's Faulkner Hospital), have subsequently developed palliative care programs. In efforts to develop a complete system of palliative care, in 2006, PHS bought a local hospice, and subsequently transferred its ownership to Hospice of the North Shore and Greater Boston, which is now the preferred provider organization for PHS. Rehabilitation and long-term and home care services are integrated into the care system. DFCI, in collaboration with Boston Children's Hospital, has a large pediatric palliative care program, and MGH a smaller one. MGH and DFCI/BWH have a joint fellowship training program; additional educational activities are supported through the Harvard Medical School (HMS) Center for Palliative Care.

PHS palliative care efforts have focused on a number of key initiatives:

- Creating a system of palliative care that allows us to provide integrated, coordinated care across the continuum, meeting patients' needs in all settings of care, from hospital, to clinic, to rehabilitation, home care, and hospice settings.
- Developing uniform standards for palliative care across the system (e.g., all PHS hospitals must have an inpatient palliative care program).
- Learning from and disseminating best practices.
- System-wide initiatives such as the development of a major EMR enhancement to provide a "single source of truth" about advance care planning throughout our system, developing a PHS-wide survey of family perceptions of quality of care of all patients dying in our system, triggers for palliative care consultation, and outpatient palliative care models.
- Pay for Performance initiatives to expand palliative care access, advance care planning, and Medical Orders for Life-Sustaining Treatment (MOLST) implementation.
- A system-spanning End-of-Life Care Value Dashboard, providing a snapshot of institutional performance on key palliative care quality indicators.
- Financial support for faculty development through the Harvard Medical School Center for Palliative Care Program in Palliative Care Education and Practice and other efforts.

These initiatives, many of which began before Accountable Care arose on the horizon, have provided us with a robust platform that has accelerated and supported our response to the ACO environment.

PHS leadership, including that of the hospitals, has long had a commitment to palliative care "because it is the right thing to do." In preparation for the new ACO environment, leaders recognized the contribution palliative care can make to healthcare "value," especially in the care of our sickest (and most expensive) patients, and invested in enhancing and enlarging our hospital-based programs and provided new resources to expand the reach of palliative care within the hospital, and, most importantly, in the outpatient setting. One of the turning points in our palliative care efforts, a PHS-sponsored leadership retreat, took place 2 years before we became an ACO. At the retreat, a family member of a patient who died was interviewed and her story, illustrating major opportunities for improvement in our system, catalyzed hospital- and system-wide momentum for improvement.

Partners became a Pioneer ACO in 2011, leading to even more emphasis on "system-ness" and the role of palliative care in improving the care of our sickest patients. System leadership has articulated that the goal of healthcare reform initiatives, such as the ACO, is to improve quality and reduce costs, thus enhancing value [2]. The focus on palliative care integration has centered on improving quality by matching the care provided to the patient with the patient's individual goals and values. Although this approach has been shown to be cost-effective, system leaders emphasize that cost should not be the driver of palliative care integration, as that approach has the potential to erode patients', families', and referring clinicians' trust in our system. Measuring outcomes that are important to patients and working consistently to improve them is a pathway to creating and enhancing the value of care.

The palliative care growth strategy at PHS has recognized that, because of the workforce shortage in palliative care and the large volume of patients who could benefit from palliative care services, we must work to improve generalist palliative care delivered by clinicians in other fields. By investing in the training of non-palliative care clinicians, the standard of practice across the system is elevated. For example, by developing a Serious Illness Communication Checklist, with clinician training, triggers, and a structured format for goals of care discussions and documentation, effective communication practices developed in palliative care can be disseminated to other clinicians. Our work on triggers for palliative care consultation grew out of a recognition that palliative care could add value to many patients who are not currently being seen. Measurement is also playing a key role in driving change in our system. Recognizing that we do not have a system to learn about the experiences of patients who are dying in our system and their families, we developed and are implementing a survey of all family members about their perceptions of the care received by loved ones at the end of life to help us identify both best practices and opportunities for improvement. Our end-of-life care dashboard will allow us to continue to track key outcomes in these domains and to measure our progress. Future initiatives include integrating palliative care into our medical homes, developing an outpatient palliative care case management program for complex patients with advanced illness to help patients remain at home, and improving our hospice care.

We are fortunate to be able to leverage the HMS Center for Palliative Care to support educational initiatives across the system, including faculty development, which has contributed to training many of the palliative care leaders in our system and the PHS-wide palliative care community. The PHS Palliative Care Committee reports to the Chief Quality and Safety Officer at PHS, providing a strong linkage with other clinical programs focused on quality and safety.

We have confronted remarkably few barriers in the integration of palliative care into our ACO. One of the most significant continues to be the paucity of well-trained palliative care clinicians, which limits our capacity to expand. Other issues include: developing consistent and efficient measurement approaches across the system, information technology to provide timely support for new initiatives, and addressing the complexities of culture change in our high-tech hospital environments.

UnityPoint Health

Palliative Care as a Key Strategy in an Accountable Care Organization (ACO) Model

The System

UnityPoint Health (formerly Iowa Health System) is one of the nation's largest integrated health systems. Through affiliations with 27 hospitals in metropolitan and rural communities, more than 280 physician clinics, and the full array of home health services, UnityPoint serves communities across Iowa and Illinois and is dedicated to providing innovative care that achieves its vision of Best Outcome for Every Patient Every Time.

Integrating Palliative Care

Since 2005, UnityPoint Health and UnityPoint at Home (formerly Iowa Health Home Care) have been investing in palliative care services. Initially, work began in two of the system's nine geographic regions, Cedar Rapids and Des Moines. By 2009, both regions had attended the Center to Advance Palliative Care Leadership Centers and had expanded their programs to include the acute setting and the patient's home.

As the health system began developing initiatives in response to healthcare reform focused on achieving the objectives of the Triple Aim (better care for individuals, better health for populations, better value for all), it identified palliative care as a key strategy for the seriously ill population based on the outcomes its regional palliative care programs had already achieved: decreased utilization of acute services, improved symptom management, and better patient/family satisfaction.

This led to the creation of a charter to advance system-wide integration of palliative care in 2010. The original charter included two key components: (1) identify physicians in each region to achieve board certification in palliative medicine by October 2012 and (2) create palliative care metrics to identify and disseminate best practices and support program improvement/development. The health system assigned executive sponsors and provided an IT analyst, clinical innovations advisor, and project manager. This team created a system-wide model for palliative care.

Pioneer ACO

In December of 2011, UnityPoint Health—Fort Dodge and UnityPoint Clinic were selected to participate in the Pioneer ACO model. Two other entities—the Berryhill Center for Mental Health and UnityPoint at Home—helped form what is considered to be the "anchor" for the ACO. UnityPoint Health now has four additional regions participating in a Medicare Shared Saving Program in addition to an accountable care contract with a private insurance provider.

Development of a system-wide palliative care program continued to evolve during this time to ensure our ability to respond to the needs of the seriously ill patient population. All regions came together to share the current state of palliative care and create a common vision for the future. Participation included all members of the interdisciplinary team, including physicians, nurse practitioners, registered nurses, social workers, chaplains, and administration.

Strategic analysis of the strengths, weakness, opportunities, and threats for palliative care, both regionally and system-wide, led to identification of common themes and specific areas for opportunity. This process set the stage for cross-region collaboration and mutual accountability. The group developed a standardized definition of palliative care, program standards (which included the adoption of the *Clinical Practice Guidelines for Quality Palliative Care, second Edition*), and a set of metrics. Data collection, storage, and analysis were standardized and centralized at the system level so that all regions were collecting and reporting data consistently. Committees were created to lead and support specific initiatives and to ensure sustainability. The Palliative Care Provider Steering Committee meets quarterly; the Palliative Care Affinity Group, made up of clinical administrators, meets monthly; and the Metric Committee meets weekly. Some key individuals participate in all groups to assist with transfer of information and standardization. The Clinical Innovations Advisor, Project Manager, and IT Analyst participate in all work groups. By 2012, seven regions had successfully implemented Palliative Care programs. Palliative Care programs vary across regions and may encompass one or several sites of care, including hospital inpatient consult services, outpatient clinic, home-based, and/or nursing home services (Fig. 11.2).

Challenges and Outcomes

Physician Certification and Workforce Shortages

Palliative care program development was one of many system-wide innovation projects occurring at this time and was competing for the time and attention of our providers against other equally important initiatives. For this reason, only half of the

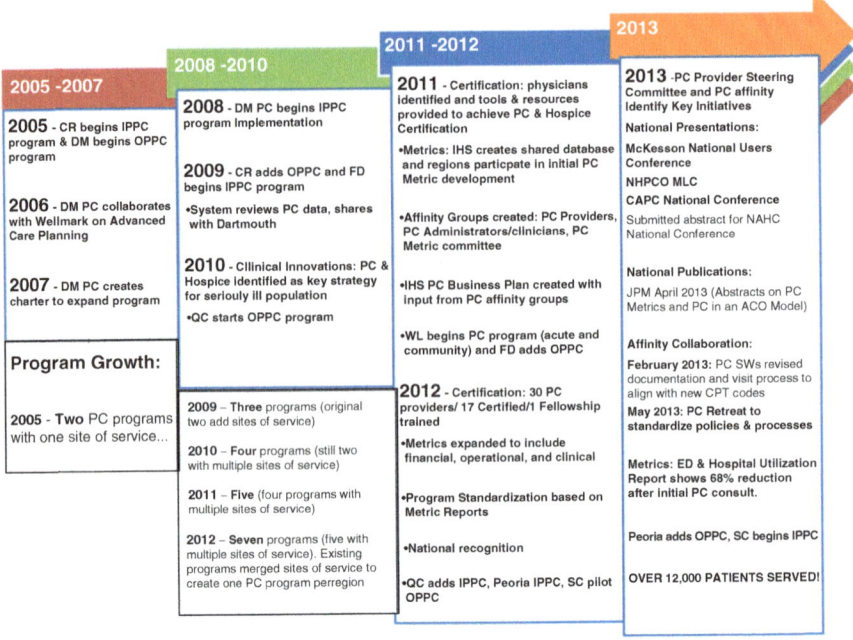

Fig. 11.2 20 Mile march

physicians identified to pursue palliative care board certification actually were certified. Nurse practitioners are recognized as a valued provider on the palliative care team, and UnityPoint Health continues to actively recruit more for the program. Currently 17 of our 30 providers (physicians and nurse practitioners) are palliative care board certified. UnityPoint is working with its palliative care providers to create a productivity model in order to identify the point in time when volume has grown sufficiently to justify recruitment of additional providers.

Metric Participation

Building relationships across regions was a critical first step before data could be shared and analyzed collectively. The palliative care committees and groups promote transparency and trust. All regions participate in the Metrics Committee and network to replicate best practices identified through the quarterly Palliative Care Metric Report.

Metric Evolution

All regions participate in identifying metrics and creating standard definitions and specifications (e.g., data source, inclusions, exclusions, etc.). The IT analyst owns the metric report, definitions, processes (e.g., data collection and entry), and

Table 11.2 Palliative care metric table of contents

Sites of service
Inpatient: Acute & Emergency Department
Outpatient: Community (home, assisted living, and long-term care) & Clinic
1. Operational
(a) Number of consults (Inpatient & Clinic)
(b) Number of admissions (Community)
(c) Rate of consults per hospital admissions (Acute)
(d) Length of stay for admissions pre & post consults—average and median (Acute, Community, and Hospice)
(e) Rate of provider visits per consults (Acute and Community)
(f) Reasons for discharge (Inpatient and Community)
(g) Readmissions to acute care (Outpatient)
2. Financial
(a) Cost savings on impact days (Acute)
(b) Medical group charges and revenue (Inpatient and Outpatient)
3. Clinical
(a) Pain scores (Inpatient and Outpatient)
(b) Dyspnea scores (Inpatient and Outpatient)
(c) Advanced Care Planning (Inpatient and Outpatient)
4. Patient satisfaction/experience
(a) Press Ganey (Acute and Clinic)
(b) SHP (Strategic Healthcare Programs)

database to ensure that all get updated as metrics are refined. UnityPoint Health has over 2 years' worth of data on operational, financial, and clinical metrics. We are utilizing existing customer satisfaction surveys (Press Ganey and SHP) to flag patients that have received palliative care for the satisfaction metric. As we are just now implementing a standardized electronic health record across the hospital care settings, we are still manually collecting and entering inpatient data; however, in the community site of service, we are able to pull data directly from the electronic record (McKesson). We plan to map data elements in Epic by end of 2014 to eliminate manual entry (Table 11.2).

Program Development

Metrics have positively influenced palliative care program development. Regions with the best outcomes had implemented a dyad leadership model including both a physician and nonphysician administrator and had integrated inpatient and outpatient palliative care across all sites of service. This successful model was then recommended for all regions. High performers on Consultation Rate metric in the acute setting utilized palliative care physicians, leading to a system-wide recommendation for palliative care physician staffing in all in-patient facilities. Poor results in the community setting on Advanced Care Planning metric led to expanding clinician support in the EHR through creation of an advanced directive dictionary in the electronic record software. All sites of service report 40–50% reductions in pain and dyspnea scores, supporting the added value of palliative care consultation to our primary care and specialty providers. As our programs expand into the emergency room, clinic, and pediatric settings, we are simultaneously expanding our metrics. We plan to use the same metric definitions as much as possible across all sites of service (Fig. 11.3).

Financial Constraints

The financial metrics (billable revenue, cost savings, and cost avoidance) have helped regions identify the value of investing in team members who can bill under Medicare and other payors: physicians, nurse practitioners, and licensed social workers. Rising income, in turn, has helped regional and system CEOs and CFOs appreciate the return on investment and recognize the need for program growth as additional referral opportunities are identified through analysis of claims data and through embedding palliative care triggers within the electronic health record (Table 11.3).

Lessons Learned

Investment in data-driven decision making to identify and replicate best practices promoted transparency and enhanced trust allowed us to overcome initial barriers to system-wide collaboration.

System-wide support for resources (IT analyst, project manager, clinical innovation advisor) needed to launch standardized metric development escalated palliative care program growth and unification.

All sites of service share in program investment. We were able to unify our programs in each region based on data; however, sharing staff and program costs between hospitals and home care settings represented a new way of thinking for each region. As Phyllis Stadtlander, president and CEO of UnityPoint at Home, puts it, "The Palliative Care program is owned by the patient and family, rather than owned by a hospital or the home care team."

Collaboration breeds success. Thanks to the foundation created by scheduling collaborations through the Steering Committee, Affinity Group, and Metric Evolution Committee, regions work together on a regular basis to discuss best practices and overcome barriers. Regions routinely host site visits with other regions across the system and share expertise to provide education within their region. PC Metrics include discharge disposition, so we can track patients referred to home health care, hospice, etc. Hospice tracks and compares the average length of stay and median length of stay of hospice patients referred from palliative care to its total patient population. This identifies opportunities to get patients to the right service at the right time and place. We are also collaborating with other ACO clinical programs, services, and innovations to ensure smooth transitions for the seriously ill patient population.

Engage stakeholders on an ongoing basis. Our executive sponsors continue to support palliative care by keeping it in the forefront of system level initiatives and

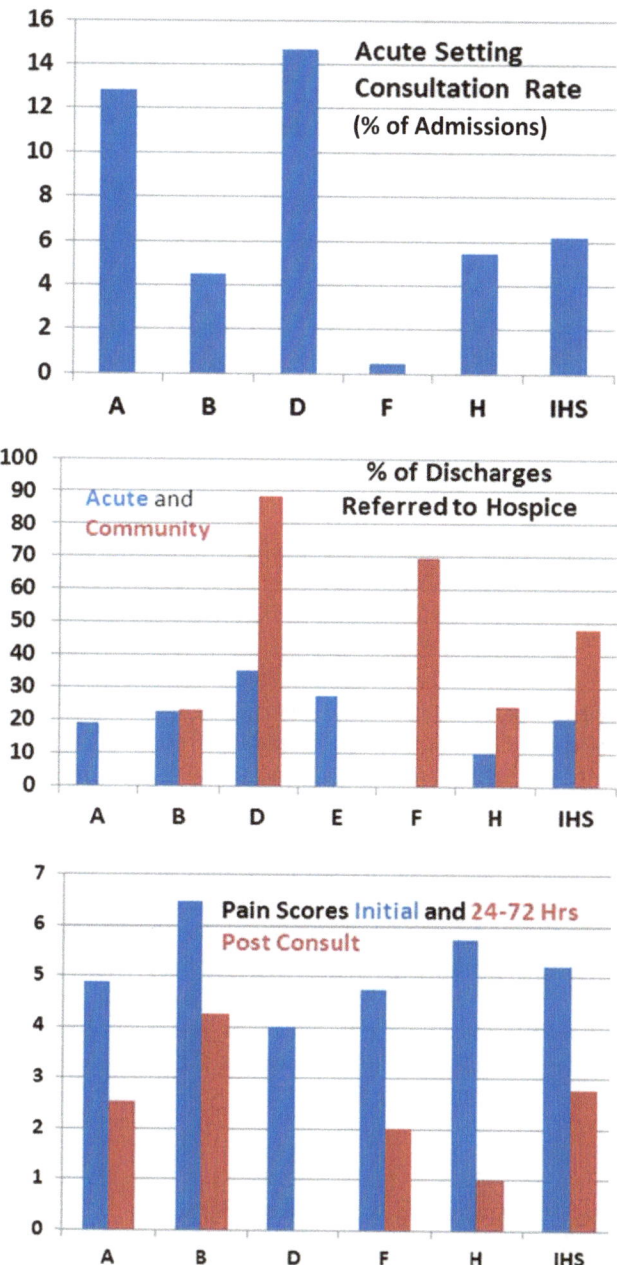

Fig. 11.3 Examples of palliative care metrics. Each letter represents palliative care programs per region within UnityPoint Health. IHS represents the system average. Data are reported quarterly but report always represents a rolling 12 months. Old reports are archived so they can be accessed as needed. Acute is the hospital inpatient setting and community is home and nursing home setting. Clinical metrics reflect pain scores on initial consult and then 24–72 h post-initial consult

Table 11.3 Return on investment report

2012	Revenue	Cost savings on impact days	Cost avoidance	Total	Operational cost	ROI
Return on investment in palliative care						
A	$106,980	$981,564	$238,954	$1,327,498	$839,920	*$487,578*
B	$145,687	$1,481,259	$1,328,256	$2,955,202	$811,759	*$2,143,443*
C						
D	$61,746	$233,372	$297,711	$592,829	$314,002	*$278,827*
E[a]	$57,322	$678,015	$192,634	$927,971	$175,240	*$752,731*
F[a]	$19,981	NA	$242,813	$262,794	$101,185	*$161,609*
G[a]	$750	NA	$127,555	$128,305	$11,871	*$116,434*
H	$670	$130,075	$458,817	$589,562	$223,255	*$366,307*
Total	$393,136	$3,504,285	$2,886,740	$6,784,161	$2,477,232	**$4,306,929**

Each letter represents a palliative care program within UnityPoint Health Revenue based on actual reimbursement received
[a]Indicates program with one site of service

dashboards. Metric reports are sent to leaders at the system, regional, and program level on a quarterly basis. We provide system and regional presentations to keep leadership and other clinicians apprised of our outcomes and value. When the IT analyst, project manager, and clinical advisor see outliers within our PC Metric and/or Cost Reports, we work with that program to ensure data integrity (quality assurance) and identify performance improvement opportunities.

Accountability and transparency are essential to sustainability. As we operate in a time between two methods of reimbursement—today's fee-for-service environment versus the future's focus on achieving the Triple Aim—we need to effectively function in both worlds. We have recently enhanced our cost avoidance by comparing our palliative care population to itself as a historical control. We have looked at the utilization patterns of this group 90 and 180 days pre- and post-initial palliative care consultation, regardless of where the initial consult occurred. The group was broken down into 12 separate populations based upon the month of the initial palliative care consult. We can analyze this data by payer, diagnosis, program, deaths, and demonstrate a significant decrease in utilization (emergency room and hospital) post-palliative care consult. Coupled with our positive clinical outcomes, these data support the value of palliative care (Fig. 11.4).

Input from System and Regional Leaders

Bill Leaver

President and Chief Executive Officer, UnityPoint Health
"UnityPoint Health has a fundamental commitment to coordinated care. We consider the patient first as a person and aim to provide the care and support necessary to

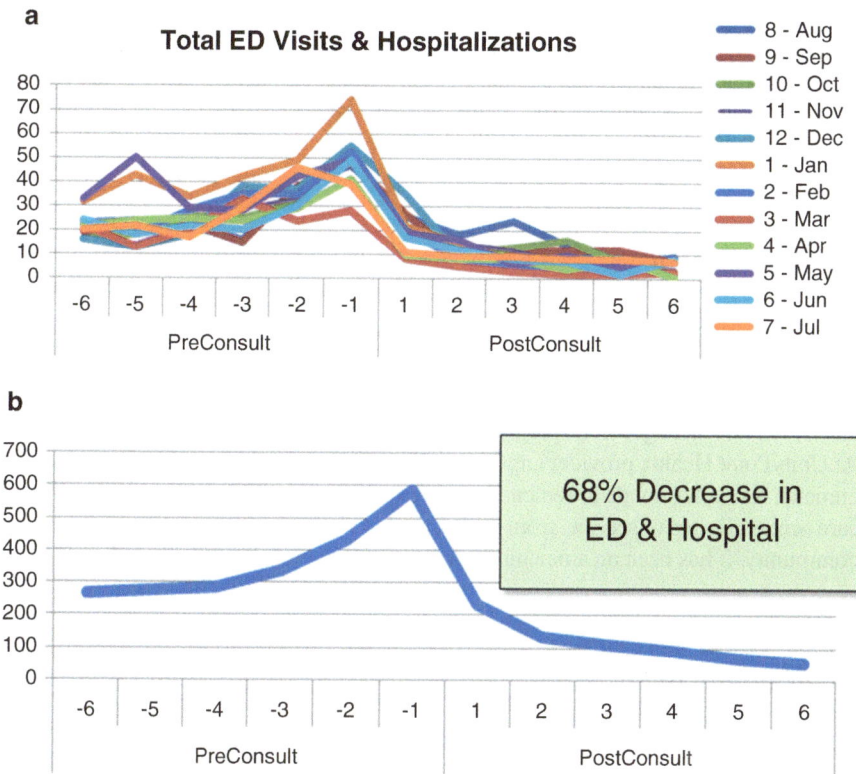

Fig. 11.4 Cost Report graphs: Vertical axes represent episodes of ED visits and hospitalizations. Horizontal axes represent months with negative numbers as pre-consult and positive numbers as post-consult. The line between −1 and 1 marks the initial consult. (**a**) 12 separate and distinct patient populations are represented. (**b**) Total population. Note: patients discharged due to death are not included

achieve each patient's unique goals and optimize their wellness. This core principle enables our innovative palliative care to surround the patient with a team of professionals who are truly led by a physician. By integrating acute, community, and clinic palliative care into a single, system-wide clinical program, we improve outcomes and the patient experience."

Kevin Vermeer

Executive Vice President/Chief Strategy Officer and ACO Chief Executive Officer, UnityPoint Health

"Through the collection and analysis of data, UnityPoint Health demonstrates how palliative care drives high quality patient outcomes while reducing the overall cost of care. We must identify and deploy care strategies capable of achieving the Triple Aim. Our ability to develop metrics specific to palliative care gives us important tools to develop an integrated, standardized clinical program across our entire region. Because we are becoming a true 'point of unity' with our data, we can generate the types of results that are in demand—both by the patients and payers."

Dr. Alan Kaplan

President and Chief Executive Officer, UnityPoint Clinic
Senior Vice President and Chief Clinical Officer, UnityPoint Health

"As providers nationwide begin to develop clinical strategies specifically for population health management, programs like palliative care will elevate in status. At UnityPoint Health, provider engagement both at the physician and advance practice clinician levels has made a tremendous difference in our ability to integrate palliative care across all sites of service, from the hospital to clinics and in the patient's home and community. It has been an amazing team effort and the results are outstanding."

Dr. Monique Reese

Vice President and Chief Clinical Officer, UnityPoint at Home

"We are committed to providing patient-centered, high quality, cost-efficient care to improve the quality of life of the patients and families we serve. UnityPoint Health Palliative Care teams have been successful in delivering our vision of Best Outcome for Every Patient Every Time."

The OSF (Order of St. Francis) Healthcare Experience

The System

OSF Health Care is an integrated healthcare delivery system, with clinical facilities that include eight acute care hospitals, a multi-specialty physician medical group, Home Care and Hospice, and a Nursing Home. There are over 14,000 employees, including over 600 employed physicians. For several years, OSF has been actively working to streamline care and integrate programs, with the intention of both improving care and preparing for new models of healthcare delivery.

Supportive (or palliative) Care issues became high priority for senior leaders' due in part to concerns raised by front-line staff relating to moral distress and ethical questions, as well the desire to improve care quality and efficiency for the highest risk

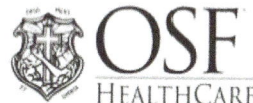

Fig. 11.5 OSF supportive care model

ACO patients. Supportive Care, a system-wide initiative (Fig. 11.5), was charged with developing inpatient palliative care services and a system-wide model of advance care planning. Senior level administrators from across the system sit on a Governance Council, which provides direction to a system-wide Operations Council with representation from all facilities. Regional Committees serve to remove barriers and monitor quality measures, and a Division of Supportive Care at the Corporate Office oversees these activities for palliative care. Hospice services are programmatically integrated. OSF is beginning to expand palliative care to the outpatient environment. Outpatient palliative care services are currently focused on Home Health patients with palliative needs. This model is expanding to include homebound patients who are not currently receiving Home Health services. Going forward, we aim to reach patients in other settings, who are at high risk of hospitalization, including the heart failure clinic and cancer center, and focus on facilitating advance care planning.

Pioneer ACO

OSF is a Pioneer ACO, beginning in 2011. From the outset, the Supportive Care Division was heavily involved with planning the Pioneer ACO application. The ACO team, comprised of senior leaders from across the system, recognized that management of persons with complex and serious illness would be important. Our medical group developed a Primary Care Medical Home model, including Care Managers who help to manage the care of complex patients. Eligible patients were identified both through direct referrals from physicians and staff for those patients felt to be at high risk due to chronic or complex needs, and by use of risk stratification data derived from CMS claims data. We are planning a Pilot project to improve patient risk stratification, navigation, and coordination of care, aligned with the work of Accountable Care and the Medical Home. The challenge for OSF is how to afford the models of care necessary for the future while living in a hybrid state where the great majority of reimbursement is still based on fee for service payment for volume of procedures instead of pay for performance or outcome.

Care Managers

Care Managers contact identified high-risk patients directly and define gaps in care, such as medication reconciliation and compliance, costs, transportation, keeping, appointments, diet, and others. Care Managers assume overall care plan coordination and oversight, and assess for the presence of palliative needs, including conduct of goal setting and advance care planning, with a goal that 100 % of Care Managed patients have a documented discussion and advance directive.

Advance Care Planning

Our advance care planning model, OSF Care Decisions, focuses on high risk patients within the ACO population, but any patient can have a Care Decisions discussion. During a Care Decisions discussion, a trained facilitator meets with a patient and her family, discusses their values and goals, and then relates those to potential future medical decisions. The outcome of that discussion is an advance directive, preferably a Power of Attorney for Healthcare, as well as a documented record of the discussion to serve as a reference in the future.

Prior to training, the facilitators, primarily nurses and social workers, but also a few chaplains, are identified in the Medical Group offices, Home Care services, and Hospital departments. When identified, their managers are asked to verify that they will include this advance care planning duty as part of their routine work, and be given time and resources to do it. Facilitator training includes a full day session of didactic and interactive sessions, followed by role-playing skills validation. Audits are done to ensure quality, and yearly refreshers/updates are held.

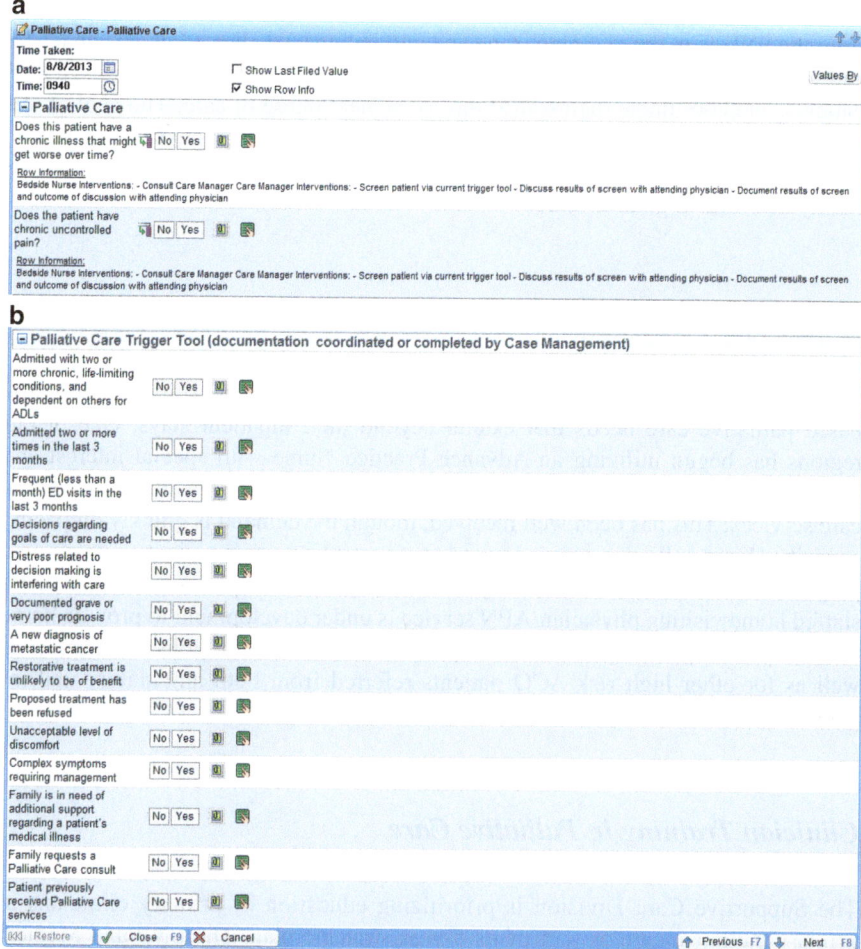

Fig. 11.6 Transitions of care navigator section regarding palliative care. (**a**) Screening items for every patient admitted. (**b**) Additional items completed if screen is positive

Transition Management

Like other systems, OSF has long suffered from fragmentation of facilities and services, and beginning the process of integration is no small challenge. Care Transitions Projects currently focus on discharge from the acute care setting to the post-acute setting, whether that be home with or without home care services, or to a skilled nursing facility. The Transitions of Care projects include modified tools (Fig. 11.6) to assess risk for hospital readmission (including unmet palliative needs), robust medication reconciliation, staff-to-patient callbacks, standardized discharge processes/instructions/forms, and provider handoffs.

Skilled Nursing Facility (SNF) transitional care model, for patients going home from the SNF, is in the planning stage and will include a dedicated physician leader and several APNs Advance Practice Nurses (APNs), who will actively manage SNF patients, and coordinate their transitions to the next phase of care. The goal of this service is to bridge the gaps in information between SNFs and other settings, reduce burdensome transitions, and improve quality by matching care plans to person and family determined goals of care.

Home Palliative Care

Patients who have been seen by palliative care teams in the hospitals have home-based palliative care needs that extend beyond their inpatient stays. One of our regions has begun utilizing an Advance Practice Nurse with special interest and training in palliative care to augment the usual Certified Home Health Agency home care services. This has been well received, though the demand is quickly outpacing capacity. Home palliative care is limited to existing home care patients with chronic progressive diseases, who are likely to someday need hospice services. A better staffed home visiting physician/APN service is under development to provide home follow-up for inpatient palliative care patients who are not eligible for hospice, as well as for other high risk ACO patients referred from both ambulatory and in-patient settings.

Clinician Training in Palliative Care

The Supportive Care Division is prioritizing education of primary clinicians in primary palliative care as part of its 5-year strategic plan. The SNF and Medical Home clinicians will be the primary audience for training in primary palliative care skills. Generalist palliative care training is necessary because need for these services outstrips specialty palliative care staff capacity.

Perspective of ACO Leadership

Our ACO team identified four major themes for system-wide accountable care in OSF: patient engagement, care management, care of SNF patients, and Advance Care Planning. Surprisingly, overall costs for patients who died rose significantly in the first half of 2012. It is unclear why the costs for this group increased over the year, but it has raised the interest of ACO leadership in assuring timely access to quality palliative care. Palliative care improves quality measures (symptoms, occurrence of advance care planning, readmissions, hospital mortality) and is seen as a tool to help bend the cost curve, critical to the success of an ACO. We have shown a significant improvement in the number of ICU patients who have their Code Status identified and symptom scores show a steady improvement for palliative care patients. Average daily costs in the hospital are significantly lower after a palliative care consult than before.

The challenges we currently face include continued staff fatigue with the relentless pace of change and resource limitations. Leadership is necessary to change the fee for service culture of care. Resources will continue to be scarce and emphasizing advance care planning and primary palliative education is paramount. Palliative Care is a strategic measure on the system-wide executive scorecard (metrics linked to payment for executives), keeping it at the forefront of the executives' thinking. The current scorecard includes a measure of the number of designated high risk ACO patients who have a full OSF Care Decisions advance care planning session completed, and a measure of the percentage of inpatient palliative care consults that receive the full complement of palliative services, including physician or mid-level provider, social services, and pastoral care.

Box 11.1

Motivators for ACO-palliative care integration

- Reducing hospitalization rate
- Reducing emergency department visits
- Reducing in-hospital mortality
- Reducing 30-day readmissions
- Increasing patient satisfaction
- Desire to address caregiver burden
- Desire to fill the care gap for patients ineligible for hospice
- Institutional mission focus & alignment
- Population health management

Key misconceptions

- Specialized services are not needed
- Clinicians already provide comprehensive care to this population
- Advance Directives alone are adequate
- Palliative care only appropriate for those at "end of life"
- Claims/utilization data adequate to identify high risk target population

Challenges

- Primary Care Providers may be initially reluctant to share care of their patients with others

(continued)

(continued)
- Patient contact (e.g., phone numbers) data can be missing or poor
- Poor quality of clinical data inputs for predictive modeling
- Lack of real-time claims/utilization data for predictive modeling
- Avoiding duplication of services: coordinating with existing home care and other services
- Overstretched Resources/Program Investment

Utilization metrics/CEO dashboard

- Number of Hospital Admissions per patient, proportion with >1 admission
- Hospital and Intensive Care Unit Lengths of stay
- Number of ED Visits per patient
- Hospital Direct Costs
- 30-day readmission
- Hospital days in last 6 months of life
- Proportion having surgery in last 30 days of life
- Proportion having chemotherapy in last 14 days of life
- In-Hospital Death (number and proportion)
- Penetration of palliative care services to at risk/eligible population
- Home Health Care Referral
- Hospice Referral & mean Hospice Length of Stay
- Cost saving estimates (through reduced ER/hospital utilization)
- Attrition due to Drop Out or Change in Managed Care Plan Coverage

Clinical metrics

- Pain score documented, proportion with severe pain >2 consecutive assessments
- Dyspnea
- Patient satisfaction
- Caregiver satisfaction
- Rate of advance care planning in high risk patients (healthcare proxy, medical/physician orders for life sustaining treatments, DNR/DNI orders)
- Proportion of care concordant with patient/family preferences

Table 11.4 Models and characteristics of palliative care integration within ACOs

	Michigan Pioneer ACO & Hospice of Michigan	Partners Health System	Order of St. Francis (OSF) Health Care Pioneer ACO	UnityPoint Health (one Pioneer ACO) & four regions in MSSP/PI ACO
Service characteristics:				
Telesupport 24/7/365	Yes	Yes	Pending	Yes
Coaches in hospitals & ER	Yes	No	No	Yes
Transitional Care Planning	Yes	Yes	Yes	Yes
Healthcare Navigation	Yes	Yes	Yes	Yes
Facilitated Advance Care Planning	Yes	Yes	Yes	Yes
Home visits	Yes	Yes	Yes	Yes
Family Assessment & Support	Yes	Yes	Yes	Yes
Social Needs Assessment & Support (e.g., poverty, substance abuse, neglect)	Yes	Yes	No	Yes
Setting of services				
Home	Yes	Yes	Yes	Yes
Outpatient Clinic	No	Yes	Pending	Yes*(not all yet)
Long-Term Care	Yes	Yes	Yes	Yes
Inpatient	Yes	Yes	Yes	Yes
Model of care				
Consultative	Yes	Yes	Yes	Yes
Co-management	Yes	Yes	Yes	Yes
Care Coordination	Yes	Yes	Yes	Yes
Blended model	Yes	Yes	Yes	Yes
Team composition[a]				
MDs/DOs	1 FTE	28 (approx)	1.5 FTEs	(Pioneer/MSSP)
NPs/PAs	1 FTE	19	2.0 FTEs	MD: 1/PT
RNs	13 FTEs	4	1.0 FTEs	NP: 1/1
SWs	4 FTEs	7	0	RN: 1/1
Aides	13 FTEs	0	0	SW:PT/PT-1
Volunteers	14 part-time	?	0	Aides: 0
Chaplains	0.1 FTE	3	0	Volunteers: PRN

(continued)

Table 11.4 (continued)

	Michigan Pioneer ACO & Hospice of Michigan	Partners Health System	Order of St. Francis (OSF) Health Care Pioneer ACO	UnityPoint Health (one Pioneer ACO) & four regions in MSSP/PI ACO
Other	2 Enrollment specialists		2.0 Support FTEs at system level; 300+ ACP Facilitators (integrated in to usual duties)	Chaplain: PRN
				Clinical Pharm: PRN
Community Partnerships & Coordination	SW coordination with community partners	ELNEC training; collaboration with mental health providers	High Quality SNF's with specific agreements ACP education with other systems in communities we serve Parish Nursing	Supporting community-wide IPOST implementation; Parish nurses; ELNEC training for NH partners; collaboration with mental health & public health

[a]Not including hospital-based services

References

1. Conwell, L. C. (2005). Characteristics of people with high medical expenses in the US civilian non-institutionalized population, 2002. (Statistical Brief #73).
2. Lee TH. Care redesign—a path forward for providers. N Engl J Med. 2012;367:466–72.

Chapter 12
Implementing a Care Planning System: How to Fix the Most Pervasive Errors in Health Care

Bernard J. Hammes, Linda A. Briggs, William Silvester, Kent S. Wilson, Sue Schettle, John R. Maycroft, Julie Sandoval, Ann E. Orders, and Melissa Stern

Introduction

In the course of a single lifetime, medical science has made unprecedented strides in managing serious illness. But as good as the US healthcare system is, in 2000, the Institute of Medicine estimated that as many as 268 patients died needlessly each day due to preventable hospital errors [1]. Progress has been made to address most errors.

B.J. Hammes, Ph.D. (✉)
Gundersen Health System,
1900 South Avenue, La Crosse, WI 54601, USA
e-mail: bjhammes@gundluth.org

L.A. Briggs, M.A., M.S., R.N.
Gundersen Health System, La Crosse, WI, USA

W. Silvester, M.D.
International Society of Advance Care Planning and End of Life Care,
Melbourne, VIC, Australia

K.S. Wilson, M.D.
Honoring Choices Minnesota, Minneapolis, MN, USA

S. Schettle
Twin Cities Medical Society, Minneapolis, MN, USA

J.R. Maycroft, M.P.P.
Wisconsin Medical Society, Madison, WI, USA

J. Sandoval, M.D.
The Permanente Medical Group, Oakland, CA, USA

A.E. Orders, M.H.A.
Continuum of Care and Health Care Reform, Kaiser Permanente, Pasadena, CA, USA

M. Stern, M.B.A.
Life Care Planning, Kaiser Permanente, Pasadena, CA, USA

For example, the use of bar codes in hospitals reduces medication errors [2–4]. Surgical treatment to the wrong body part and hospital-acquired pneumonia rates have declined, thanks to work redesign and procedural checklists [5].

That said, a significant medical "error" remains in shadow. Today's medical complexity often leads to fragmentation and depersonalization of care, with the focus of such care often on the science of treating a disease or injury, rather than on a thorough understanding of the individual who is sick [6]. When people are healthy, fragmentation of care is not a major problem because receiving care episodically actually fits our needs. But when patients develop serious, progressive illnesses, they need more personalized, coordinated care over months and years. It is at this point that our current healthcare arrangements can truly fail patients. We know from research and personal experience that many of the sickest patients suffer needlessly because they receive treatments that offer little benefit but great burden—treatments not aligned with patients' values and goals [7]. To withhold a desired treatment, or to start a treatment that is inconsistent with a patient's goals, values, and beliefs, is perhaps the most serious error a healthcare provider can make.

Just as other types of medical errors can be prevented by redesigning systems, so, too, can these errors. Previous efforts to correct these errors have failed. For example, we have learned that merely having patients sign advance directives (ADs), such as living wills or powers of attorney for health care, does not improve the care we provide [8]. Some writers have declared not only that ADs do not work [9], but that they *cannot* work [10]. Legislation, regulation, and court decisions have clarified the right of adults to refuse medical care, but they have not structured a healthcare system where patients with serious illnesses have a voice in their care that is routinely sought, heard, and followed [11].

Redesigning the Health System

The healthcare system must be redesigned to ensure that patients have their values and preferences clearly expressed, documented, and honored by incorporating them into healthcare decisions. Even the most ardent critics of statutory living wills realize that such a system is needed to achieve success [9].

Redesign will require clear and specific design principles:

1. Care planning must be built into routine patient care. Healthcare professionals need to know how and when to initiate planning conversations. This planning service must be organized and its members trained to act as a team. Strategies must be developed to engage and motivate patients to participate. Prompts must be developed to ensure that care planning discussions occur when needed, initiating discussions at regular and critical points of care and revisiting them whenever major changes in a patient's health occur.
2. The focus of care planning is on conversations, skillfully facilitated by trained and competent healthcare professionals. The investment in skilled facilitation results in an effective and unique type of planning. Such conversations engage

patients by helping them understand their own preferences, values, and goals, and by encouraging them to reflect on how future choices might be made in light of these beliefs. Such unique planning discussions include the individuals who are closest to the patient—whomever they consider "family." Skillfully facilitated conversations shift the focus of planning away from the completion of a legal document (although this might be one feature of planning).
3. The outcome of these conversations needs to be a plan that reflects the patient's realized values and preferences and is clinically specific enough for the patient's health condition. The plan needs to be clear to the patient who is planning, to those close to the patient, and to any health professional providing care. Importantly, such plans must communicate the authentic goals of the person and specify when certain outcomes would be considered too burdensome relative to the benefits.
4. Plans must be available whenever and wherever the patient receives care, including in nursing homes and the community. Immediate availability is less important when patients are relatively healthy (we can assume they want all possible life-prolonging efforts to be made in the early stages of an emergency) but is vital when patients have advanced illness and are likely to be unable to speak for themselves.
5. Plans must be interpreted with thoughtful professional judgment when serious medical decisions are faced and the patient is incapable of communicating. Plans must be revisited regularly to determine whether a change in either the assessment of illness or the patient's values necessitate a revision to the plan. By reflectively using care plans, it is possible to integrate the advantages of both care planning and just-in-time decision-making [12].
6. The healthcare system must be able to deliver a range of services in multiple settings, including one's home or nursing home, that enable the patient's care plan to be honored. For example, if a long-term care facility resident wants some interventions that may prolong life and improve comfort but does not want to return to the emergency department or hospital, such a plan matters only if the long-term facility can provide the desired care.

When these principles are implemented, the potential exists for important improvements in the care of patients with serious illness:

- Person- and Family-Centered and Determined Care: When a patient's values, beliefs, and preferences are reliably known, communicated, and honored, care will be focused on treating the person rather than the disease.
- Shared Decision-Making: When the process of planning is undertaken in the way described, the goals and preferences of the patient, the perspectives of the family, and the recommendations of the patient's physicians can be carefully considered in making plans for future care.
- Reduced Fragmentation: When medical records and other communication processes are designed to communicate care plans, care becomes more personalized and coordinated in all settings at any time.
- Concurrent Care: Management of disease and palliative services are no longer an either/or choice; rather, patients can receive both desired palliative and disease-specific care in the "dose" that fits their medical condition and informed preferences.

Evidence of Success in Redesigning the Healthcare Delivery System: The Story of Respecting Choices®

Can these design principles be implemented? Clearly, the answer is "Yes." Perhaps the first, surprising realization is that these principles can be implemented in most healthcare systems without significant regulatory or statutory changes.

Development and implementation of the six principles began in La Crosse, Wisconsin in 1991, when its four major healthcare providers agreed to collaboratively create a new approach to advance care planning (ACP). A program, now called Respecting Choices® (RC), was developed and implemented between 1991 and 1993. After the program had been fully implemented for 2 years, a study of 540 consecutive deaths of adult residents in all La Crosse County health organizations over an 11-month period—the first La Crosse Advance Directive Study [13] (LADS I)—found that:

- The prevalence of written ADs, mainly statutory powers of attorney for health care, was 85 %.
- These plans were in the medical record where the patient received end-of-life care 95 % of the time.
- Preferences to *forgo* treatment were consistent with treatments provided 98 % of the time.

LADS I was replicated in 2007–2008 for the same population over a 7-month period (LADS II) [14]. LADS II investigated 400 consecutive deaths in all healthcare organizations in La Crosse County and found:

- The prevalence of written ADs was 90 % (90 % of which were the La Crosse Region Power of Attorney for Healthcare, available at http://www.gundluth.org/upload/docs/Services/POAHCVersionAEE81.pdf).
- 99 % of the time the written AD was in the medical record where the patient received end-of-life care.
- 99 % of the time preferences either to *have* or to *forgo* treatment were consistent with treatment provided.

LADS II also determined that (1) 67 % of decedents also had a Physician Orders for Life-Sustaining Treatment (POLST) form; (2) these forms were found at the organization providing end-of-life care 98 % of the time; and (3) treatment provided was consistent with these medical orders in all except two cases [15]. Of the 400 decedents, only 16 did not have some type of care plan (written AD or POLST), 8 of whom had been approached but declined to participate in planning.

These results demonstrate that care planning is now part of routine care, that healthcare professionals are trained to facilitate high-quality discussions, that procedures for documentation, storage, and retrieval of plans make them accessible, and that evidence exists that patients' preferences are incorporated into decision-making and medical orders. Additionally, this community effectively shifted its care model so that patients could more reliably get the care they needed and wanted in places other than the hospital or emergency department.

To achieve this success, RC required the integration of four key and interconnected elements [16]:

- Systems Redesign: To help busy professionals deliver the ACP service in a consistent and reliable way, key systems were redesigned, including ACP workflows, team roles, and tools [16].
- Competency Training: Competency-based training was developed for health professionals and others to facilitate planning discussions at three distinct stages of planning (First Steps®, Next Steps, and Last Steps® ACP). The new role of "ACP facilitator" was endorsed as a key member of the ACP team [17].
- Community Engagement: To deliver consistent messages to the community at large, social marketing strategies are needed to engage individuals in the value of ACP and incorporate it into the fabric of group and social norms.
- Quality Improvement: Continuous performance improvement is necessary to achieve and sustain the quality of an ACP program, to achieve desired outcomes, and to make critical changes efficiently.

To achieve truly person-centered care, each element is essential and designed to work in tandem with the others. The program is most effective when all health organizations in a community or region work collaboratively to implement all four elements.

Scaling Respecting Choices to Help Reform the US Health System

The successful redesign in La Crosse provides a possible model for creation of a more person- and family-centered health system, but there are reasons to be skeptical about expanded use of this approach. The La Crosse region has a modest population (560,000) and is racially homogeneous, with 98 % being White. Health care is delivered by two competing, integrated systems in which all of the practicing physicians are employed by one system or the other. Not only is this delivery system not typical, but the level of collaboration between La Crosse's two competing health systems is also unusual.

Although other locations could encounter barriers to ACP implementation peculiar to their social, demographic, economic, and political circumstances, efforts to spread the program have identified that the biggest barriers to successful replication of the RC model are:

1. Creating strong and sustained administrative and clinical leadership that support this work.
2. Securing and sustaining the needed financial support.
3. Identifying and addressing community fears related to this newly designed system to promote informed decision-making.
4. Developing a reliable road map so the redesign can be undertaken with predictable timeframes, costs, and outcomes so that leaders can invest in such changes with confidence.

Despite the differences between La Crosse and other places and these real barriers, the RC approach to ACP has been transferred effectively to other countries, metropolitan communities, statewide efforts, and large healthcare systems. Although these places are very different from La Crosse, the key to success was addressing the four barriers listed above.

Australia: Respecting Patient Choices® [18]

The first documented transfer of this model occurred in 2002 in the Austin Hospital in Melbourne, Australia. This transfer began with an engagement of the RC team in La Crosse and a careful attention to both the four essential elements and barriers. After a successful demonstration in their own facility, these leaders obtained financial support (which has been sustained) from their state and federal departments of health to license the RC program and to adopt it for dissemination in Australia. They rebranded the program as "Respecting Patient Choices" (RPC) (www.RespectingPatientChoices.org.au). They have successfully tested RPC in "aged care" (long-term care) facilities [19] and proven the success of the model in a randomized, controlled clinical trial of ACP in elderly people admitted to the hospital [20]. They now have the materials, the resources, and the approach to disseminate across their country. In Australia there has been a growing awareness of the need to discourage futile care [21] and the need for quality ACP in aged care homes [22, 23]. RPC has been implemented in at least 30 major health services and hundreds of aged care facilities in Australia, and continues to be adopted in new communities each year. Australia was successful at spreading this program because they required any healthcare organization that wanted to implement RPC to use standardized ACP practices and materials, to train RPC consultants (facilitators), and to monitor outcomes using well-established performance improvement methods. They have also developed a training package [24] to teach doctors and other health professionals how to discuss ACP.

Honoring Choices® Minnesota: The Twin Cities Medical Society Initiative [25]

While documented successful transfers of RC in the United States occurred earlier [26–28], the first implementation in a large metropolitan area began in 2008. The Twin Cities Medical Society (TCMS), through its foundation, took the lead to improve ACP outcomes in the metropolitan Twin Cities (St. Paul and Minneapolis) and, eventually, statewide. TCMS contracted with RC for services to design an effective rollout of the La Crosse model for the Twin Cities metro area. This rollout used the four design elements to effectively address the four major barriers previously described.

The project began by first engaging clinical leadership from the metro area to test the support for such a project. High-level meetings with senior administrative healthcare leaders produced agreement that the seven major health systems would collaborate on developing standardized First Steps ACP practices and materials using the RC model, and would devote resources to the overall effort. With the strong commitment of both clinical and administrative healthcare leaders, TCMS first undertook the task of raising needed funds. Contributions were received from healthcare organizations and health insurance companies, as well as other businesses and private foundations. With funding secured, TCMS and the faculty at RC engaged the major health systems. During this period, TCMS created an overarching advisory committee that decided on a project name, "Honoring Choices Minnesota," and helped design a more readable, easier to use, standardized healthcare directive document and patient education materials that are now available in five languages. The materials are available at www.metrodoctors.com. When the pilots had been designed and the written materials developed, RC faculty trained facilitators to provide competent ACP services in the pilot projects. Several pilot projects were undertaken to redesign work flows in order to initiate planning conversations and to make referrals to trained ACP facilitators, as well as to improve medical records processes so that advance care plans could be reliably stored, retrieved, and transferred as needed. Pilots were conducted for 6 months to test the reliability of the workflows, the medical records systems, the materials, and the ACP facilitators. (Reports from these "pilots" can be found at: http://www.metrodoctors.com/index.php?option=com_content&view=article&id=135:2012-sharing-the-experience-conference&catid=145:sharing-the-experience-conference&Itemid=506.) One month after the pilots were completed, a "Sharing the Experience" conference was held, where the outcomes, lessons learned, and plans for sustainability and expansion of the scope of the work were reported for each pilot. This work was then continued with a second, third, and fourth round of pilots.

As the ACP clinical capacity expanded, TCMS began to engage other leaders in the community. They found interested and resourceful partners in Twin Cities Public Television (TPT) and the Citizens League. The broader community engagement provided an opportunity to gain wider understanding and support of the work and to appeal for broader financial support. Together, these groups developed a sophisticated community engagement strategy that included conducting facilitated focus group discussions with Minnesotans from various social and cultural groups. These interactions were taped and housed on a sophisticated Website, www.honoringchoices.org. TCMS continues to provide presentations and has developed public service announcements and full-length television documentary programs. Their broad-based community engagement strategy focuses on interdenominational faith communities, multicultural groups, employers, identity groups, associations, and health and human service organizations. They have also developed a strong volunteer Ambassador program with over 60 individuals trained and motivated to carry forward the Honoring Choices Minnesota message into their communities.

Honoring Choices Wisconsin: The Wisconsin Medical Society Project

The Wisconsin Medical Society has taken note of the Twin Cities model and aims to expand it as a statewide project following a similar pattern to address the major barriers. Similar to Honoring Choices Minnesota (and with generous assistance and advice from TCMS), the new "Honoring Choices Wisconsin" is beginning with pilot projects in seven southeastern and south-central Wisconsin organizations with the guidance of the RC faculty. These organizations, which include hospitals, a health maintenance organization that serves elderly and disabled patients, and a Veterans' Affairs site, trained together under the RC First Steps program. They agreed to collaborate and not compete, to a shared language and common patient education materials, to share lessons throughout the pilot process, and to contribute financially to the project. The pilots launched in March of 2013. With success, Honoring Choices Wisconsin hopes to expand into additional regions of the state and to make ACP a routine part of care. The Wisconsin Medical Society is also beginning outreach to community groups and stakeholders across the state to generate conversation at the community level, and plans to develop an advance directive readable at a fifth-grade level. The healthcare community has been grateful to see physicians take the lead in this ambitious effort.

Kaiser Permanente of Northern California

Kaiser Permanente of Northern California (KPNC) serves over 3.3 million members, making it the largest health system in the United States to implement the RC model. The system has more than 6,000 physicians, 21 hospitals, and 40 ambulatory clinics across northern California, from Fresno to Santa Rosa. The region comprises a wide range of cultural, ethnic, and socioeconomic backgrounds. While the implementation is young, an organization of this size is in a unique position to demonstrate ways to scale the RC model and bring the service to a highly diverse population. Early lessons show the value of achieving a high degree of leadership alignment as the cornerstone of such an implementation.

The path to this implementation began in late 2011, when a core group of clinical, operational, and health plan leaders met to explore how best to support adult members in planning for their future healthcare needs. After a comprehensive scan of the ACP environment, the leadership group identified RC as the approach upon which to build their services.

KPNC began engaging with RC over a series of telephone calls and meetings that soon led to a decision to adopt the model. Building leadership alignment was the goal of a 2-day summit organized for over 250 leaders across the organization with diverse but relevant functions and focus. KPNC invited RC leaders to its headquarters in Oakland, California, and the summit came to serve two purposes: (1) to provide education about and to consider plans for rolling out the model in order to establish engagement early on in the implementation process and (2) to begin to demonstrate how the RC model was different from what existed in the organization at the time.

KPNC completed the contracting process with RC and began planning pilots to test the service, which KPNC has named "Life Care Planning." Consistent with the organization's vision to implement a service for all adult members at every stage of life, leaders set out to pilot all aspects of the RC model: First Steps, Next Steps, and Last Steps. The initial investment in leadership engagement proved useful, as evidenced by leaders in each of KPNC's medical centers eagerly volunteering to develop pilots. Pilots are taking place across the care continuum—from ambulatory clinics to the hospital, from home to skilled nursing facilities. The pilots will be followed by a comprehensive assessment and evaluation to determine the best way to spread the program throughout northern California.

Significant resources were devoted to ongoing communication with stakeholders across all levels of the organization and to the development of systems and structure. Four full-time staff were hired to provide project oversight and to serve as RC content experts (or Faculty) for the region. Communication proved critical, requiring execution of a detailed communication plan that included development of a Life Care Planning brand, presentations to key stakeholder groups, and the publication of the "Life Care Planning Newsletter" to target the organization at large. Local medical centers identified project managers to help oversee pilots and ensure local performance improvement. Finally, to ensure that the appropriate structure was in place, three workgroups formed to focus on key areas: local leadership, patient and provider education, and documentation, storage, and retrieval of care plans in the electronic medical record. Local managers and clinicians participated in the workgroups to provide advice and refine the design and deployment of key systems and tools into operations.

How Respecting Choices Fits with Other, Larger Efforts to Improve Care: Lessons Learned

More time is needed to assess whether these large-scale implementations of RC can achieve a high prevalence of planning. It is expected that they will be successful in substantially increasing the percentage of their population who have care plans at the time of death. It is also expected that plans will be available to health providers involved in decision-making and that those plans will be honored across a large region. The progress of these implementations demonstrates that the technical guidance developed by the RC team provides a reliable pathway for large-scale implementations so that the process, timeframes, and cost can be reliably predicted.

So if RC can be implemented on a large scale, does it really improve quality? Can the RC approach redesign the medical "glide path" identified by Joanne Lynn in SUPPORT [29] so that care of those with serious illness is guided by what matters most to patients rather than by medical protocol and habit?

The evidence for improved care is promising. The retrospective evidence (LADS I and II) reveals a high prevalence of planning and access to these plans by health professionals at the bedside. The evidence also shows that the treatment provided at the end of life is almost always consistent with these plans. Medicare beneficiaries in La Crosse spend far less time in the hospital during the last 2 years of life than is typical in the United States (13.5 vs. 23.5 days) [30]. Furthermore, the mean age of death in La Crosse County increased over the 20 years of use (75.83 years in 2011 vs. 74.87 years in 1991) [31], ages similar to those of other counties in Wisconsin that do not use RC. Thus, evidence suggests that implementation of RC can lead to a high prevalence of knowing and honoring patient preferences, reduced use of hospital services, and no change in mean length of life.

Evidence also demonstrates that this approach to planning is satisfying to patients and families. In randomized controlled trials of the RC Next Steps intervention, patients and their families rate the quality of communication high, and family members have an improved understanding of patient preferences [32, 33].

Finally, in a prospective clinical trial conducted in Australia using the Respecting Choices approach, it was determined that the elderly patients who participated in the planning intervention were significantly more satisfied with all elements of their hospital care, were less likely to receive intensive care at the end of life, were significantly more likely to have their wishes known and honored, had a length of life similar to that of those who did not plan, and had family members who suffered significantly less depression, anxiety, or distress after their death [20].

So to date it appears that it is possible to scale this ACP approach to large populations, including large health systems, metropolitan areas, regions, states, and entire countries. The evidence also suggests that the RC approach, when properly implemented in a community or large health system, can improve patient care.

All four of these large implementations had clear, strong, and sustained administrative and clinical leadership. All had sufficient and sustained funding. In Australia, funding came from state and federal sources. In the Twin Cities and Wisconsin, funding came from a mix of sources, including participating health systems, payers, and private foundations. KPNC funds its own program. Finally, each of these projects have sufficiently engaged both their community leaders as well as the larger community to address the potential, unfounded fears of individuals that ACP is about the denial of wanted and needed treatment.

Although these large ACP projects were not motivated by new policies or regulations, changes in reimbursement policy that would incentivize healthcare organizations to improve quality, including providing more patient-centered care, would increase interest in such programs. In a payment system that paid for better care of patients rather than for each service or procedure provided, not only would this approach to ACP become the norm, but health organizations would be disadvantaged if they failed to implement it. It is important to recognize that reimbursing for RC ACP would be different from reimbursing physicians for having an advance directive discussion (which may or may not improve care of the patient). A policy approach that would reward a health system for both knowing and honoring patient preferences would help drive quality improvement.

Finally, in a world where most of us will die after a prolonged, progressive illness, a well-designed ACP system would provide a unique type of coordinated care—one not driven by protocols like disease management or by personnel like nurse navigators. While these other types of coordination are important, care coordinated through an effective ACP system develops relationship-based care that begins with the patient's story, leads to informed decisions that reflect personal goals, values, and beliefs, and leads to treatment decisions that align with patient preferences. This type of care coordination creates a system that can organize care across settings and over time, helping to eliminate the fragmentation so common in the US health system. And perhaps equally important, such a system demands that a larger group of health professionals be equipped to provide what may honestly be called primary palliative care. When all health professionals in all settings have a responsibility to know and honor patient preference, then the person-centered and person-determined care that is the hallmark of palliative care becomes everyone's work.

Conclusion

This RC redesign of health care developed and tested in La Crosse, Wisconsin, and successfully being implemented in numerous places in the United States and beyond, is a response to the radical shift witnessed in our healthcare system over the last 40 years. We no longer are cared for by a single doctor, nor are the healthcare decisions we make simple. These realities have often resulted in a depersonalized healthcare delivery system—one that is less sensitive to the individuality of each patient and each family.

But it does not need to be this way [34]. Just as we have redesigned healthcare processes to reduce medical errors, we can redesign the healthcare system to be more person-centered and to produce care plans that evolve from shared decision-making so that we deliver the care that is important to people.

Implementing RC systems alone, of course, cannot correct or address all the challenges we face in health care. In this regard it is important to appreciate that this RC approach is complementary and synergistic with several other efforts to improve care. In particular, the RC approach assists strategies such as accountable care organizations (ACOs) [35] and medical homes [36], as well as new approaches to care, such as advanced illness management [37, 38]. For example, the RC approach helps ACOs provide higher quality care in a coordinated fashion across a community or region, it helps a medical home provide more person-centered care for the sickest patients, and it provides an organized way to create and update sophisticated care plans needed to care for patients who have advanced, serious illness.

While RC is no silver bullet, it can be a central tool in the complex tool kit needed for improvement of our health system and the care of patients with serious illness. What is helpful is that its implementation is effective, and implementation need not wait for the passage of new policy or regulation. RC is an improvement that can start now, and there is a clear implementation strategy to make it work anywhere in the United States.

References

1. Kohn LT, Corrigan J, Donaldson MS. To err is human: building a safer health system. Washington, DC: National Academy Press; 2000. http://www.nap.edu/books/0309068371/html/. Accessed 16 May 2013.
2. Poon EG, Cina JL, Churchill W, et al. Medication dispensing errors and potential adverse drug events before and after implementing bar code technology in the pharmacy. Ann Intern Med. 2006;145(6):426–34.
3. Poon EG, Keohane CA, Yoon CS, et al. Effect of bar-code technology on the safety of medication administration. N Engl J Med. 2010;362(18):1698–707.
4. Henneman PL, Marquard JL, Fisher DL, et al. Bar-code verification: reducing but not eliminating medication errors. J Nurs Adm. 2012;42(12):562–6.
5. Gawande A. The checklist manifesto: how to get things right. New York: Metropolitan Books; 2010. p. 209.
6. Stuart B. Advanced care: choice, comfort, and control for the seriously ill. In: Hammes BJ, editor. Having your own say: getting the right care when it matters most. Washington, DC: CHT Press; 2012. p. 99–121.
7. A controlled trial to improve care for seriously ill hospitalized patients. The study to understand prognoses and preferences for outcomes and risks of treatments (SUPPORT). The SUPPORT principal investigators. JAMA. 1995;274(20):1591–8.
8. Castillo LS, Williams BA, Hooper SM, Sabatino CP, Weithorn LA, Sudore RL. Lost in translation: the unintended consequences of advance directive law on clinical care. Ann Intern Med. 2011;154(2):121–8.
9. Fagerlin A, Schneider CE. Enough. The failure of the living will. Hastings Cent Rep. 2004;34(2):30–42.
10. Perkins HS. Controlling death: the false promise of advance directives. Ann Intern Med. 2007;147(1):51–7.
11. Wenger N, Shugarman LR, Wilkinson A. Advance directives and advance care planning: report to Congress. US Department of Health & Human Services Web site. http://aspe.hhs.gov/daltcp/reports/2008/ADCongRpt.htm. Updated 2008. Accessed 8 March 2013.
12. Sudore RL, Fried TR. Redefining the "planning" in advance care planning: preparing for end-of-life decision making. Ann Intern Med. 2010;153(4):256–61.
13. Hammes BJ, Rooney BL. Death and end-of-life planning in one midwestern community. Arch Intern Med. 1998;158(4):383–90.
14. Hammes BJ, Rooney BL, Gundrum JD. A comparative, retrospective, observational study of the prevalence, availability, and specificity of advance care plans in a county that implemented an advance care planning microsystem. J Am Geriatr Soc. 2010;58(7):1249–55.
15. Hammes BJ, Rooney BL, Gundrum JD, Hickman SE, Hager N. The POLST program: a retrospective review of the demographics of use and outcomes in one community where advance directives are prevalent. J Palliat Med. 2012;15(1):77–85.
16. Hammes BJ, Briggs LA. Respecting choices: building a systems approach to advance care planning. La Crosse, WI: Gundersen Lutheran Medical Foundation; 2012.
17. Briggs LA. Helping individuals make informed healthcare decisions: the role of the advance care planning facilitator. In: Hammes BJ, editor. Having your own say: getting the right care when it matters most. Washington, DC: CHT Press; 2012. p. 23–40.
18. Silvester W. Respecting patient choices: scaling care planning to a whole country. In: Hammes BJ, editor. Having your own say: getting the right care when it matters most. Washington, DC: CHT Press; 2012. p. 57–66.
19. Austin Health. Respecting patient choices: final evaluation of the community implementation of the respecting patient choices program. 2006. http://www.health.gov.au/internet/nhhrc/publishing.nsf/Content/018-wilsiletal/$FILE/018%20William%20Silvester%20et%20al%20Submission%20B.pdf. Accessed 16 May 2013.

20. Detering KM, Hancock AD, Reade MC, Silvester W. The impact of advance care planning on end of life care in elderly patients: randomised controlled trial. BMJ. 2010;340:c1345.
21. Silvester W, Detering K. Advance care planning and end-of-life care. Med J Aust. 2011;195(8):435–6.
22. Silvester W, Fullam RS, Parslow RA, et al. Quality of advance care planning policy and practice in residential aged care facilities in Australia [published online ahead of print November 14, 2012]. BMJ Support Palliat Care. doi:10.1136/bmjspcare-2012-000262.
23. Silvester W, Parslow RA, Lewis VJ, et al. Development and evaluation of an aged care specific advance care plan. BMJ Support Palliat Care. 2013;3(2):188–95.
24. Respecting Patient Choices. Respecting patient choices course. Respecting Patient Choices Web site. http://www.rpctraining.com.au/. Accessed 19 March 2013.
25. Wilson KS, Schettle SA. Honoring Choices Minnesota: a metropolitan program underway. In: Hammes BJ, editor. Having your own say: getting the right care when it matters most. Washington, DC: CHT Press; 2012. p. 41–56.
26. Schellinger S, Sidebottom AC, Briggs LA. Disease-specific advance care planning: conversations emphasize patient preferences and provide clarity. Oncology Nurse Advisor. 2010. http://www.oncologynurseadvisor.com/disease-specific-advance-care-planning-conversations-emphasize-patient-preferences-and-provide-clarity/article/178063/ Accessed 18 March 2013.
27. Schellinger S, Sidebottom AC, Briggs LA. Disease-specific advance care planning for heart failure patients: implementation in a large health system. J Palliat Med. 2011;14(11):1224–30.
28. Patient Autonomy State Advisory Council. The report of the Iowa Patient Autonomy in Health Care Decisions Project. 2012. http://www.idph.state.ia.us/hcr_committees/common/pdf/patient_autonomy_pilot/pilot_report_2012.pdf. Accessed 21 March 2013.
29. Lynn J, Arkes HR, Stevens M, et al. Rethinking fundamental assumptions: SUPPORT's implications for future reform. Study to understand prognoses and preferences and risks of treatment. J Am Geriatr Soc. 2000;48(5 Suppl):S214–21.
30. The Dartmouth atlas of health care. http://www.dartmouthatlas.org/. Accessed 9 Sept 2011.
31. Wisconsin Interactive Statistics on Health (WISH), mortality module. Wisconsin Department of Health Services Web site. http://www.dhs.wisconsin.gov/wish/. Updated 2011. Accessed 19 March 2013.
32. Kirchhoff KT, Hammes BJ, Kehl KA, Briggs LA, Brown RL. Effect of a disease-specific planning intervention on surrogate understanding of patient goals for future medical treatment. J Am Geriatr Soc. 2010;58(7):1233–40.
33. Lyon ME, Garvie PA, McCarter R, Briggs L, He J, D'Angelo LJ. Who will speak for me? Improving end-of-life decision-making for adolescents with HIV and their families. Pediatrics. 2009;123(2):e199–206.
34. Hammes BJ. Having your own say: getting the right care when it matters most. Washington, DC: CHT Press; 2012.
35. Song Z, Lee TH. The era of delivery system reform begins. JAMA. 2013;309(1):35–6.
36. Bitton A, Schwartz GR, Stewart EE, et al. Off the hamster wheel? Qualitative evaluation of a payment-linked patient-centered medical home (PCMH) pilot. Milbank Q. 2012;90(3):484–515.
37. American Hospital Association. 2012 Committee on Performance Improvement, James A. Diegel, chair. Advanced illness management strategies. Chicago, IL: American Hospital Association; 2012. http://www.aha.org/content/12/aims_strategies.pdf. Accessed 19 March 2013.
38. American Hospital Association. 2012 Committee on Performance Improvement, James A. Diegel, FACHE, chair. Advanced illness management strategies: engaging the community and a ready, willing and able workforce part 2. Chicago, IL: American Hospital Association; 2012. http://www.aha.org/content/12/aims_strategies_part2.pdf. Accessed 19 March 2013.

Chapter 13
Igniting Action to Integrate Palliative Care in Our US Health System: The Role of Disease-Specific Advocacy Groups—A Cancer Advocacy Case Study

Rebecca Kirch and Andy Miller

Palliative care is hitting its stride as one of the nation's fastest growing healthcare trends, with a robust and growing evidence base, associated quality practice standards and measures, and increasing health professional and consumer understanding and interest. Public policy is the next necessary frontier for action to make further meaningful system-level gains that truly integrate palliative care in mainstream medicine. Partnering with the Center to Advance Palliative Care (CAPC), the National Palliative Care Research Center (NPCRC), and multiple stakeholders, the cancer community has taken extensive concerted action through research support, program delivery, and legislative advocacy to propel palliative care's prominence as a fundamental aspect of delivering high quality person-centered and determined and family-focused care.

Promoting quality of life and preventing suffering alongside disease-directed treatment from diagnosis onward are essential aspects of quality healthcare delivery for people facing serious illness like cancer. This chapter highlights key strategic steps and collaborative activities involved in building a new "Quality of Life" public policy priority agenda featuring palliative care, including details about the development and launch of a national legislative campaign addressing research, workforce, and access barriers.

Helping People Make Good Plans

Person-centered care is more than just a buzzword for patients and families. The momentum building behind the concept reflects the importance that people place on personal choice and control as priorities, and cuts to the very core of what

R. Kirch (✉)
American Cancer Society, Inc., 555 11th Street NW, Suite 300, Washington, DC 20004, USA
e-mail: rkirch@cancer.org

A. Miller, M.H.S.E., M.C.H.E.S.
MillerStephens & Associates, Austin, TX, USA

constitutes good medicine and the essential elements of delivering high quality healthcare services.

All people want to live healthy and disease-free lives for as long as possible, and parents of course want this for their children. When serious illness like cancer does strike, in addition to achieving cure or keeping cancer's progression in check, patients and families also place a premium on maintaining good quality of life and functioning for as long as possible so they can continue to pursue their life goals and enjoy what matters most to them. They want clear communication and quality time with their healthcare team to help them understand treatment options, the implications of those treatments in terms of their survival, functioning, and quality of life, and so they can make informed decisions during and after treatment that align with their personal preferences and goals.

But our acute sick care system has not yet adapted to meaningfully address cancer prevention and early detection for all populations to help preserve their good health and find cancers at an early stage when treatments may be most effective. Nor is it set up to adequately assess and address pain, symptoms, and distress as equal priorities of care alongside disease-directed treatment and continuing across what can be a long trajectory of complex chronic illness. The result is a health system that is technology and disease driven, but shortchanges quality of life considerations for nearly everyone—especially our sickest adults and children.

Our National Institutes of Health research agenda has similarly been largely disease centric in its organization and focus. Though the National Institute of Nursing Research (NINR) was designated as the lead institute for end-of-life research in 1997, it was not until 2009 that an office focused on this important area was established [1]. Further, the annual research budget of NINR is only about $111 million (funding 300 awards in FY2012)—strikingly lower when compared with the research budgets of disease-specific institutes such as the $3.1 billion of the National Cancer Institute (funding 6,115 awards) or $2.3 billion of National Heart Lung Blood Institute (funding 4,673 awards) [2]. Moreover, no NIH institute or center has yet specifically designated a clear home for "quality of life" research addressing the complex array of symptoms, side effects, or late effects that often and increasingly present as chronic conditions and concerns for people undergoing active treatment or in long-term remission. As a result, palliative care has been positioned as the stepchild of all and favorite of none, with comparatively scarce funding resources for palliative care and symptom management research made available among only a small handful of NIH institutes and centers [3]. Similarly, NIH peer review would benefit from more consistently populating its study sections with palliative care research specialized methodological expertise.

In addition, the national public policy agenda has historically been a patchy landscape, divided by disease, body part, or professional discipline with little coordination or connection. Over the past decade, pain medication and prescribing policies have been one of the most active hotbeds of federal and state legislative and regulatory activity in the realm of palliative care-related policy. Most other proposals have focused solely on advance care planning and advance directives, physician or medical orders for life-sustaining treatment (POLST, MOLST, and others), the Medicare hospice benefit, and other aspects of caring for people at the end of life.

As a consequence of the disjointed research, practice and policy, many patients, survivors, and families are left suffering from symptoms, side effects, and late effects across their entire illness trajectory. They endure fragmented care across multiple specialist encounters with little or no care coordination, poor communication with their doctors, and enormous strains on family caregivers.

A series of Institute of Medicine reports and other scholarly consensus initiatives over the past decade addressing quality cancer care [4], palliative care [5], psychosocial care [6], survivorship care [7], and pain care [8] have documented these system shortfalls. These reports have offered consistent and discrete recommendations for needed emphasis of our national research agenda as well as health system and delivery reform across the cancer continuum and quality of life spectrum [9, 10].

Now is the time to dismantle these silos and bring together the diseases and disciplines in promoting a new public policy paradigm that emphasizes personal choice about what is most important, how patients want to be living, is respectful of the practical and social realities of their daily lives, and makes their quality of life a priority on par with delivering disease-targeted therapy.

Quality of Life Is Not a Backburner Matter

Children with pediatric cancer and their families are particularly vulnerable to the severe toxicities associated with aggressive treatment and our single-minded focus on cure that often minimizes QOL concerns [11]. Cure is so often the primary goal, with toxicities, quality of life, growth and development often taking a back seat in treatment and survivorship care planning and delivery [12]. Among adults and seniors as well, the literature has similarly shown that substantial treatment toxicities remain a very real price paid for our many therapeutic advances in cancer [13]. For long-term cancer survivors, significant psychosocial symptoms also often continue or arise and build as one of many potential late effects after active cancer treatment concludes [14, 15].

Yet health information absorbed by the public through media coverage and other outlets often emphasizes the promise of therapeutic breakthroughs and cures while downplaying or failing to describe at all the significant adverse effects and long-term consequences of these treatments [16]. Studies have also shown how important clear clinical communication about prognosis, quality of life, and goals of care is to avoid therapeutic misconception, or other misunderstanding about what cancer treatment can and cannot do in terms of achieving cure or remission [17, 18]. Taken together, these factors can contribute to inflated or unrealistic expectations about what today's treatments can achieve or the quality of life implications that may result.

Treating the person—not only the disease but also the physical and psychological sequelae of the disease and its treatment—is the key to both extending life and enhancing the quality of the time gained. But patients and families do not know what they do not know. Because the clinical focus is so often disease-directed treatment, quality of life and comfort are typically relegated to the back bench. Patients and their families need practical assistance to help them ask questions and articulate their concerns, needs, and wishes. They also require understandable and balanced information and skilled professional communication to help them understand their diagnosis and prognosis as well as participate meaningfully in making good, personalized care plans that are right for them—including making informed decisions about their treatment course and long-term follow-up across what is increasingly becoming a long-term disease trajectory.

Cancer Assumes a Key Supporting Role

A growing body of research findings suggest that concurrent palliative care provided with oncology care improves quality of life and can also increase survival [19, 20]. Even before this pivotal work was published, many of the nation's cancer center leaders were already united in agreement that stronger integration of palliative care services into oncology practice would benefit patients at their institutions [21]. More recently, this evidence has been boosted by findings of additional studies supported through an innovative palliative care research partnership between the American Cancer Society and NPCRC initiated in 2007 that provides dedicated extramural grant support and mentoring for palliative care and symptom management research to build the community of palliative care researchers and collaborative projects among them [22].

In addition to addressing complex symptoms, palliative care improves care coordination, reduces ICU lengths of stay, and helps align treatment with patient and family goals. These care efficiencies delivered by palliative care teams drive better quality care at significantly reduced cost [23, 24] and signal important opportunities to bend the cost curve in cancer care [25].

Adding to this landscape, critical consensus work across the palliative care community led by the CAPC has delivered an essential suite of recommendations for preferred palliative care practices, metrics, technical assistance, and practical tools to help guide palliative care's integration and operationalization in hospital settings [26]. Applying the wisdom and lessons learned from those initiatives will accelerate our opportunities and timeline for the next wave of concerted action bringing palliative care to outpatient and other community care settings so all patients and families have access to high quality palliative care integrated with disease-focused services. This is particularly important in oncology because most cancer and survivorship care (85 %) is ambulatory and happens in community cancer center settings.

In the wake of these events, several cancer collaborative efforts have since issued new measures, standards, and initiatives for integrating palliative care with oncology. In 2011, a consensus initiative convened by LIVESTRONG Foundation identified "symptom management and palliative care" as a top tier essential element of cancer survivorship care; the American Society for Clinical Oncology issued guidance for integrating palliative care with oncology in all cancer cases with high symptom burden or metastatic disease; the American College of Surgeon's Commission on Cancer released its new palliative care standard among a suite of

Table 13.1 Cancer organization activities highlights in palliative care

Cancer organization	Palliative care activities	Website
American Cancer Society	Extramural research grant partnership with National Palliative Care Research Center	http://cancer.org/research/index and http://npcrc.org/
American Cancer Society Cancer Action Network	Quality of life and palliative care legislative initiative	http://acscan.org/qualityoflife
American Society of Clinical Oncology	Provisional clinical opinion: the integration of palliative care into standard oncology care	http://jco.ascopubs.org/
C-Change	Assuring values in cancer care initiative	http://c-changetogether.org/values
Commission on Cancer	Patient-centered care standards for accreditation	http://facs.org/cancer/coc/programstandards2012.pdf
LIVESTRONG Foundation	LIVESTRONG Community Impact Project: Advancing Joint Commission Palliative Care Certification in Cancer Centers	http://www.livestrong.org/What-We-Do/Our-Actions/Programs-Partnerships/Community-Engagement
National Cancer Institute	National Community Cancer Center Partnership	http://ncccp.cancer.gov/about/index.htm

patient-centered care accreditation standards for cancer centers; and C-Change released its consensus objectives for assuring value in cancer care to significantly increase use of palliative care services and increase length of stay for patients enrolled in hospice (see Table 13.1).

During this time, the Joint Commission also launched its advanced certification in palliative care program for the nation's hospitals and the National Quality Forum endorsed several new palliative care and hospice care quality measures. In its first program year, 20 hospitals seeking the new Joint Commission palliative care advanced certification benefitted from an innovative competitive community grant program funded by LIVESTRONG Foundation to subsidize certification costs and provide technical assistance from CAPC.

With palliative care already poised as one of the fastest growing healthcare trends, this series of events also inspired development of a new quality of life-focused public policy agenda for federal and state strategic action.

Emphasizing Personal Choice About Living

For patients and their families, personalized medicine has little to do with molecular profiles. Instead, personalized medicine is all about what is important to a particular person and his or her loved ones—the aspects of life that give them joy and make their lives worth living.

Personal choice based on individual needs and preferences is a key element that all people facing serious illness hold dear and consider fundamental to delivering person-centered and family-focused care. Personal choice is also a cornerstone of palliative care and the communication that is its foundation. Yet in today's environment, these patient and family quality of life priorities are rarely identified or discussed early enough in the course of disease to ensure they are respected, and they are rarely documented in patient medical records across cancer clinical settings to help guide the course of patient care. In a June 2010 national poll among more than 1,000 adult cancer patients, survivors, and caregivers conducted by the American Cancer Society's advocacy affiliate, the American Cancer Society Cancer Action Network (ACSCAN), *fewer than one-third* said that anyone on their healthcare team ever asked what was important to them in terms of quality of life between the time of diagnosis and when cancer treatment began [27].

Today, if personal preferences are addressed at all in clinical settings, the conversations tend to focus solely on advanced care planning in the context of terminal illness and the end of life, relying on completing advanced directives, DNR orders, and other such tools. Those are important strategies, but may actually impede determining what is necessary to deliver truly person-centered and family-focused care and its benefits from the onset. To meet quality of life needs, particularly now when our health system faces unprecedented and rising numbers of people living longer lives with complex chronic conditions, our system must develop standards and protocols for earlier and continuous attention on promoting personal choice about *how patients want to be living*. Clinical triggers for these conversations should identify and document what is important to patients and what are they hoping for before, during, and after active treatment, and continuously as part of care transitions throughout long-term survivorship and at the end of life [28, 29].

Simply stated, it is difficult for people and professionals to plan for or discuss their dying—particularly when they are still very much alive and living. Nor should our health system or public policies require a predictably poor prognosis as the only gateway to getting palliative care or hospice services and the benefits they offer. Research studies, clinical communication emphasis, and associated tools need to transition their focus upstream from an end of life or terminal prognosis to be helpful in addressing personalized quality of life priorities at the onset throughout the often multiyear course of serious illness. Innovative newer patient and family-centered tools like the online offering, PREPARE [30], will help equip patients and families to have these conversations comfortably and personally about identifying what is important to them. This upstream focus enables and empowers patients to articulate their own quality of living formula during treatment and in the weeks, years, or decades they have ahead. Those documented and accessible quality of life goals can then guide informed treatment decisions, long-term survivorship care planning, and advanced care planning preferences as people approach the end of life.

Messaging Matters

The main impediment to achieving this quality of life policy shift and health system integration is really a matter of messaging. While palliative care embodies the very epicenter of what people mean when they talk about wanting person-centered and family-focused care—they do not have the words to ask for the care they want. A 2011 national poll commissioned by CAPC and the American Cancer Society revealed that a large majority of the American public is not at all knowledgeable about palliative care. At the same time, most health professionals, particularly among disease specialties like oncology, associate palliative care with terminal prognosis and believe it only becomes applicable near the very end of life.

Despite this dual identity challenge, the good news is that evidence shows people can understand and want palliative care if we use their own words to describe it. An overwhelming majority of people (92 %) in that poll confirmed that the public would be likely to consider palliative care for themselves or their families and believe patients should have access to palliative care in our nation's hospitals when it was explained as follows:

> Palliative care is specialized medical care for people with serious illnesses. It focuses on providing patients with relief from the symptoms, pain, and stress of a serious illness—whatever the diagnosis. The goal is to improve quality of life for both the patient and the family. Palliative care is provided by a team of doctors, nurses and other specialists who work together with a patient's other doctors to provide an extra layer of support. It is appropriate at any age and at any stage in a serious illness and can be provided along with curative treatment [31].

If patient advocacy organizations, healthcare practitioners, researchers, and others use this terminology consistently to talk about palliative care, great gains can be achieved in raising palliative care awareness among the public, professionals, and policymakers—an important initial strategy for advancing a new quality of life public policy agenda.

Building a Quality of Life National Movement

Evidence consistently demonstrating its benefits over the past decade has positioned palliative care as an essential medical innovation and vital opportunity for cohesive strategic advocacy action to move our system forward with the next generation of delivery reform. Palliative care hits all the high notes required to meet the triple aim trifecta for effective health policy attention and action—better health, better care, and lower cost. Recognizing this as palliative care's decisive moment, the cancer community has taken a leading role together with CAPC, NPCRC, and other national palliative care and hospice organizations in mobilizing collaborative forces to build a national quality of life movement.

The initiative is focused on achieving three objectives: (1) increase palliative care awareness, education, and research emphasis; (2) boost workforce capacity, clinical communication skills, and palliative care training support; and (3) pursue integration of palliative care services and quality standards in all care settings and associated payment reform promoting interdisciplinary care.

Federal Legislative Efforts

To initiate this national campaign in 2013, two federal bills were introduced in the U.S. Congress:

- The "Palliative Care and Hospice Education and Training Act"(PCHETA) (HR1339/ S641) addresses the deficit in palliative care training offered in the nation's medical schools by creating new incentives for the training and development of interdisciplinary health professionals in palliative care. The bill would create up to 24 Palliative Care Education Centers at medical schools across the country to expand interdisciplinary training, as well as establish fellowships that would provide faculty in medical schools and other health profession schools short-term intensive courses focused on generalist-level palliative care. Faculty would be able to use the fellowships to upgrade their knowledge for the care of individuals with serious illnesses, and enhance their interdisciplinary teaching skills.
- The "Patient Centered Quality Care for Life Act" (HR1666) puts in place the building blocks of a national effort to improve the fragmented care that people with cancer and other serious diseases often receive by drawing more national attention to palliative care. First, the bill would require the director of the National Institutes of Health to expand and intensify research on palliative care. This would build upon the already strong scientific rationale for palliative care that demonstrates its ability to improve both quality and length of life at lower cost. Second, the bill expands on the PCHETA legislation by supporting palliative care training for nurses, psychologists, social workers, and other allied health professionals. Finally, the legislation convenes health professionals, patients, public and private payers, and state and federal health officials to develop solutions, tools, and model best practices for providing palliative care to individuals with chronic disease.

Accompanying introduction of these bills, ACS CAN also launched a major new advertising campaign in Capitol Hill publications to educate lawmakers and their staff about the importance of palliative care. The ad, which ran in print and online, emphasizes that palliative care restores patients' quality of life by treating the person as well as their disease (Figs. 13.1 and 13.2).

Model State Legislation

Complementing these federal bills, model state legislation has also been developed urging legislators to partner with the cancer community and other key stakeholders in enacting policies that will increase the availability of palliative care information

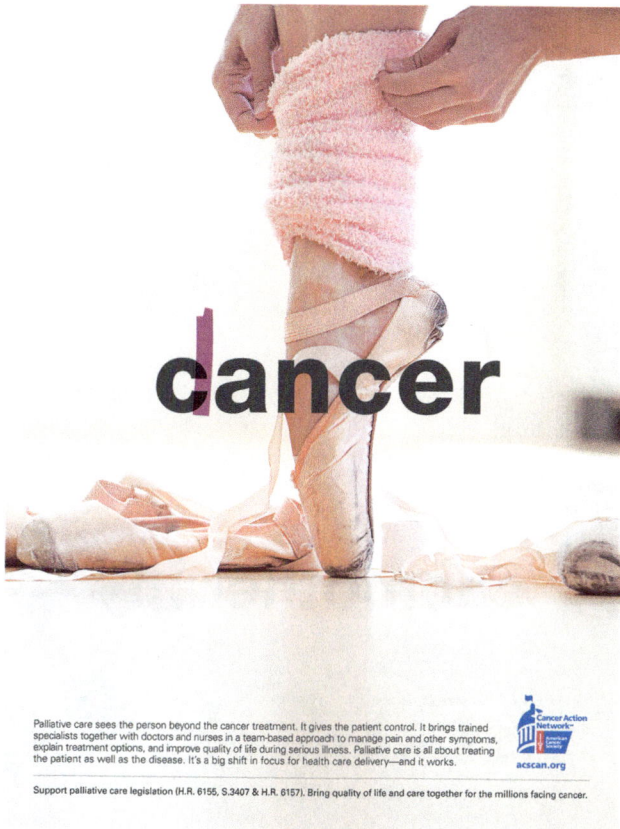

Fig. 13.1 ACSCAN palliative care ad—dancer

and services for all adults and children. Coupled with the federal suite, these state proposals will help build consistent messaging and call for action to integrate palliative care and quality of life in the fabric of care delivery across the country.

The state legislation includes provisions for using interdisciplinary advisory expertise in partnership with State Health Departments and others to educate the public and professionals about palliative care and its benefits as a first order of business. In addition, provisions will be developed to help frame palliative care as a key measure of quality and a core component of available services in all healthcare settings serving the seriously ill, encouraging hospitals, ambulatory care settings, nursing homes, assisted living facilities, home care agencies, and other settings to routinely screen patients for palliative care needs such as poorly controlled pain, depression or other symptoms, lack of clarity about medically achievable goals for care, what to expect in the future and how to plan for it, and family caregiver exhaustion and stress. Requiring identification of these needs would trigger care protocols and associated payment models that reward person- and family-centered, interdisciplinary care, and address current care gaps.

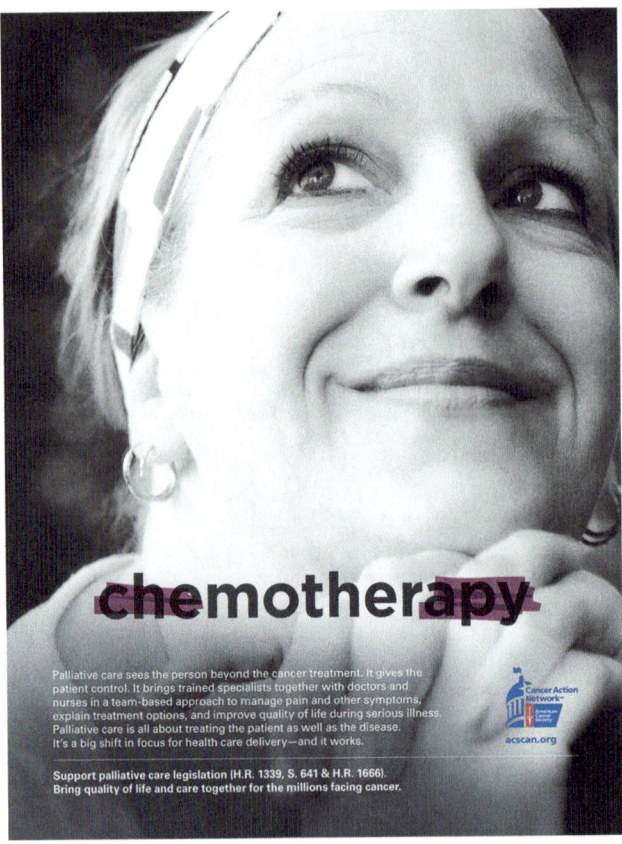

Fig. 13.2 ACSCAN palliative care ad—mother

State-level workforce policy proposals will also be developed to boost mid-career training opportunities in fundamental palliative care clinical skills among health professionals and students of medicine, nursing, social work, and other professions to align educational requirements and professional practices with delivery of core palliative care principles and practices for all who care for the seriously ill. These strategies will accompany ongoing state pain policy advocacy, such as implementing balanced prescription monitoring programs and other policy initiatives that preserve access to pain medications for seriously or chronically ill people with pain and enhance workforce training in pain assessment, management, and responsible prescribing.

With nearly 14 million cancer survivors now living in the USA and two-thirds of newly diagnosed patients expected to be alive in 5 years, increasing survival time alone is no longer enough. Our system must also be equipped to deliver care addressing quality of life needs so these survivors can thrive, both during and after treatment. This is the time for all disease-specific advocates and professional disciplines to take collective action as stakeholder partners in the quality of life movement that will support the needs and hopes of all seriously ill persons and their families.

References

1. Spotlight on End-of-Life Research. https://www.ninr.nih.gov/researchandfunding/spotlight-on-end-of-life-research. Accessed 15 Jan 2013.
2. NIH budget and spending. http://report.nih.gov/budget_and_spending/index.aspx. Accessed 21 May 2013.
3. Gelfman LP, Morrison RS. Research funding for palliative medicine. J Palliat Med. 2008;11(1):36–43.
4. Hewitt M, Simone JV, editors. Ensuring quality cancer care. Washington, DC: The National Academies Press; 1999.
5. Foley KM, Gelband H, editors. Improving palliative care for cancer. Washington, DC: The National Academies Press; 2001.
6. Adler NE, Page AEK, editors. Cancer care for the whole patient: meeting psychosocial health needs. Washington, DC: The National Academies Press; 2008.
7. Hewitt M, Ganz PA, editors. From cancer patient to cancer survivor—lost in transition: an American Society of Clinical Oncology and Institute of Medicine symposium. Washington, DC: The National Academies Press; 2006.
8. Institute of Medicine, editor. Relieving pain in America: a blueprint for transforming prevention, care, education, and research. Washington, DC: The National Academies Press; 2011.
9. National Cancer Legislation Advisory Committee Records, 1998–2001; 2001.
10. National Action Plan for Cancer Survivorship. http://www.livestrong.org/What-We-Do/Our-Approach/Platforms-Priorities/National-Action-Plan. Accessed 15 Jan 2013.
11. Oeffinger KC, Mertens AC, Sklar CA, Kawashima T, Hudson MM, Meadows AT, et al. Chronic health conditions in adult survivors of childhood cancer. N Engl J Med. 2006;355(15):1572–82.
12. Wolfe J, Grier HE, Klar N, Levin SB, Ellenbogen JM, Salem-Schatz S, et al. Symptoms and suffering at the end of life in children with cancer. N Engl J Med. 2000;342(5):326–33.
13. Niraula S, Seruga B, Ocana A, Shao T, Goldstein R, Tannock IF, et al. The price we pay for progress: a meta-analysis of harms of newly approved anticancer drugs. J Clin Oncol. 2012;30(24):3012–9.
14. Gao W, Bennett MI, Stark D, Murray S, Higginson IJ. Psychological distress in cancer from survivorship to end of life care: prevalence, associated factors and clinical implications. Eur J Cancer. 2010;46(11):2036–44.
15. Stanton AL, Ganz PA, Rowland JH, Meyerowitz BE, Krupnick JL, Sears SR. Promoting adjustment after treatment for cancer. Cancer. 2005;104(11 Suppl):2608–13.
16. Fishman J, Ten Have T, Casarett D. Cancer and the media: how does the news report on treatment and outcomes? Arch Intern Med. 2010;170(6):515–8.
17. Weeks JC, Catalano PJ, Cronin A, Finkelman MD, Mack JW, Keating NL, et al. Patients' expectations about effects of chemotherapy for advanced cancer. N Engl J Med. 2012;367(17):1616–25.
18. Mack JW, Smith TJ. Reasons why physicians do not have discussions about poor prognosis, why it matters, and what can be improved. J Clin Oncol. 2012;30(22):2715–7.
19. Temel JS, Greer JA, Muzikansky A, Gallagher ER, Admane S, Jackson VA, et al. Early palliative care for patients with metastatic non-small-cell lung cancer. N Engl J Med. 2010;363(8):733–42.
20. Smith TJ, Temin S, Alesi ER, Abernethy AP, Balboni TA, Basch EM, et al. American Society of Clinical Oncology provisional clinical opinion: the integration of palliative care into standard oncology care. J Clin Oncol. 2012;30(8):880–7.
21. Hui D, Elsayem A, De la Cruz M, Berger A, Zhukovsky DS, Palla S, et al. Availability and integration of palliative care at US cancer centers. JAMA. 2010;303(11):1054–61.
22. National Palliative Care Research Center. http://www.npcrc.org/. Accessed 15 Jan 2013.
23. Morrison RS, Dietrich J, Ladwig S, Quill T, Sacco J, Tangeman J, et al. Palliative care consultation teams cut hospital costs for Medicaid beneficiaries. Health Aff (Millwood). 2011;30(3):454–63.

24. Morrison RS, Penrod JD, Cassel JB, Caust-Ellenbogen M, Litke A, Spragens L, et al. Cost savings associated with US hospital palliative care consultation programs. Arch Intern Med. 2008;168(16):1783–90.
25. Smith TJ, Hillner BE. Bending the cost curve in cancer care. N Engl J Med. 2011;364(21):2060–5.
26. Palliative care tools, training & technical assistance. http://www.capc.org/. Accessed 15 Jan 2013.
27. National poll: facing cancer in the health care system. http://www.acscan.org/healthcare/cancerpoll. Accessed 15 Jan 2013.
28. Berman A. Living life in my own way—and dying that way as well. Health Aff (Millwood). 2012;31(4):871–4.
29. Kirch R. Palliative care and quality of life: patient-centered care case study. Arch Intern Med. 2012;172(15):1170–2.
30. Prepare. https://www.prepareforyourcare.org/. Accessed 15 Jan 2013.
31. Public opinion research on palliative care. 2011. http://www.capc.org/tools-for-palliative-care-programs/marketing/public-opinion-research/2011-public-opinion-research-on-palliative-care.pdf. Accessed 13 Jan 2013.

Chapter 14
What Do You Mean You Don't Also Offer Palliative Care? Effective Public Engagement to Harness Demand to Improve Care for Serious Illness

Sharyn M. Sutton and Marian S. Grant

Drivers of Potential Change

Healthcare Reform

It is increasingly evident that there are problems with the current way we care for those with serious illness in this country. Previous chapters of this book have detailed those issues and we may have reached a critical tipping point in the realization that continuing the current system will continue to result in poor outcomes on all levels for patients, their families, and the country. This is part of what is driving healthcare reform. Many of the outcomes that will be more closely measured and rewarded in future health care, such as improved quality of life, symptom management, patient and family satisfaction, and reducing unnecessary and burdensome hospital readmissions and interventions, can be achieved through the addition of early, concurrent palliative care [1–5].

The Aging Population

The aging of the baby boomer generation (the oldest of some 78 million boomers will turn 68 in 2014) is projected to have a tremendous impact on health care in the USA. The system will face not only a burgeoning older population but also patients whose views on health and aging are very different from those of past generations.

S.M. Sutton, Ph.D., **Masters of Arts in Communication** (✉)
The John Hopkins University, Washington, DC, USA
e-mail: sharyn.sutton@gmail.com

M.S. Grant, D.N.P., C.R.N.P., R.N.
University of Maryland School of Nursing, Baltimore, MD, USA

Age does not seem to be a relevant frame of reference for many boomers. They are less likely to define their lives by age, life stages, or events than as a continuum to build upon. They focus not on their potential decline but on the future, on what's next and what else needs to be done [6]. They are now seeing the deficits with the current healthcare system as they try to navigate it on behalf of their parents. In doing so, they have made the following unpleasant discoveries.

First, there is not much choice in the care for serious illness. The system makes the blanket assumption that everyone wants "everything" done and funnels patients into the hospital and technological life-extending, or death-prolonging, treatments. There is little focus on patients' individual values or wishes and no system to identify or honor them. Palliative care, with its focus on identifying patient goals of care, is one solution to this problem but boomers are discovering that, unfortunately, access to palliative care resources are currently limited. Next, accessing what resources are available is also difficult. Patients and families face substantial information gaps. They are unclear as to what help is needed and available, unaware of whom to ask, lack knowledge of care services available in their communities and which are covered by Medicare or insurance. Research shows, for instance, that most people are unaware of home health and hospice services, what they provide, how to access these services and how they are financed [7, 8]. People tend to overestimate how much private insurance or Medicare will help them and are unlikely to plan or save adequately for the costs of a serious illness. Patients and families are shocked when they learn that many needs they consider "health and medical," such as personal care for bedridden patients, are not classified as **legitimate medical needs** and are therefore not covered by Medicare. They are also worried about the cost of long-term care and are largely unaware of their options or that Medicare does not cover long-term care [9].

The good news is that boomers are awakening to these problems and starting to demand changes. And the numbers of boomers will transform health care, just as they have redefined every other marketplace. Hospitals in the 1970s and 1980s competed to offer services like birthing suites for boomers who insisted on making birth a less medical and more personal experience. Now healthcare systems will be faced with a growing demand for a similar approach to serious illness. The winners will be those that learn to respond positively to that demand.

Growing Evidence to Support the Use of Early Palliative Care

The evidence that concurrent palliative care delivered at the same time as disease-modifying treatment continues to demonstrate improvement in quality of care, increased longevity and reductions in costs [10–12]. With "evidence-based practice" driving medical guidelines and protocols, it will become increasingly difficult to ignore such findings. Palliative care will need to become an integrated part of standard care for most serious illnesses, especially if patient-centered care is to become a reality.

Healthcare Provider Educational Requirements

Research has shown that effective communication among providers, patients, and their families can improve medical outcomes, increase patient and family satisfaction, and reduce burden on the healthcare system [1–5]. Fortunately, improving communication is already occurring as the topic "communicating bad news," along with "improving pain control," is one of the most requested areas for physician training programs on serious illness/end-of-life care [13]. In addition, providers need specific strategies and training to bridge the gulf between the culture of medicine and the patient and family's cultural and individual experiences of illness [14].

There are now clinical practice guidelines for communicating prognosis and engaging seriously ill persons and their families about what matters most to them in the context of a serious illness. These guidelines contain practical strategies for health professionals, with examples of helpful words and phrases that can be used [15]. Internal medicine residency training now includes "Interpersonal and Communication Skills" as a key competency. Providers will be trained and assessed on their ability "to communicate effectively with patients, families, and the public, as appropriate, across a broad range of socioeconomic and cultural backgrounds [16]." However, the resources to implement training and assessment of healthcare provider competencies in this crucial skill are sorely lacking.

Public Engagement Challenges

Shifting the Focus Away from Advance Directives/Advance Care Planning

Historically, experts believed a population that planned in advance or became more accepting of death as a natural part of life could better deal with the process of dying. As a result, major investments were made in public engagement campaigns to promote Advanced Care Planning (ACP) and/or to "change America's death-defying culture." These were unsuccessful and will continue to be unsuccessful for several reasons. First, research has found little evidence in support of the use of Advance Directives (AD) ADs and instead confirms public resistance to the concept of planning ahead for serious illness and death. People can't imagine themselves as seriously ill or dying nor can they predict ahead of time their wants and needs which change as the situation changes [17, 18].

Even if people have ADs, they are not that helpful in the earlier stages of serious illness as they only address very limited, specific situations concerning life-prolonging technology at the end of life. As a result, preparing ADs and general conversations prior to serious illness can be ineffective as they often have little effect on treatment decisions that occur during the long and unpredictable course of the illness or even after the person has lost the ability to make their own decisions, including decisions to resuscitate [19, 20].

One program where ADs/ACP have been shown to help people make decisions throughout the course of a serious illness is Respecting Choices®. This 3-stage model has been successful in widely implementing ADs but did so within an integrated health system in a small, homogeneous community [21]. Implementing this model on a broader scale would require full system redesign and community-wide outreach, neither of which is currently structurally or financially feasible.

Finally, ADs/ACP are typically linked to decisions necessary at the end of a serious illness and so are neither personally relevant nor practically or strategically aligned with addressing issues earlier and throughout an illness. While the transition to end of life is a critical and important aspect of serious illness, the realities of death mean that the use of ADs and preparing ahead of time for end-of-life decisions (ACP) provides only limited benefits for few people—and in some cases can be detrimental [22].

Stopping the Focus on Death and Dying

The research base documenting people's resistance and lack of interest in planning ahead of time for terminal illness continues to grow [9, 23–26]. Public engagement on end of life cannot compete with more powerful messages offering personal benefits for dealing with daily life today [9, 23, 24].

For example, Robert Wood Johnson funded a national communication campaign (1995–2005) that involved over 1,000 health and public groups. The campaign's primary goals were: (1) to improve medical communication and decision making for patients; (2) to change the culture of care for the dying in healthcare institutions; and (3) to change American culture and attitudes about death and dying. An evaluation found that the campaign attracted little public interest and actually appeared to benefit primarily the coalition partners, rather than its intended audience, the public [27].

Most seriously ill patients have great difficulty in **making care decisions as illness progresses** let alone advance planning for care prior to illness. Patients either do not have strongly formed preferences or do not adequately understand the effects of different treatment options near the end of life [28].

Another major reason for refocusing communication resources away from death and dying and on care earlier in the disease process is that the majority of patients with serious illness are **either not dying or do not know if they are actually nearing the end of their life**. More than 75 % of those dying are people over age 65 suffering from multiple chronic conditions (e.g., congestive heart failure, emphysema, and diabetes) [29]. The decline of these patients is a multiyear and unpredictable process, and marked by sudden severe episodes of illness requiring hospitalization, from which they recover. This familiar pattern can repeat itself for years until the final time when the patient fails to recover. There is a second group of elderly patients suffering from frailty of old age, stroke, or dementia who also follow an unpredictable trajectory of dying. Only 22 % **of elderly patients are dying of advanced solid tumor malignancies** that tend to follow an expected or somewhat predictable course of dying [23].

So it is medically difficult to know when, for instance in the case of heart failure, a person has moved into the end-stage. And patients with serious chronic illnesses are rarely told that their condition is terminal and are therefore often left unaware that they are dying until the very end [30, 31]. While patients and families are often accused of being "in denial of death," a strong case has been made that they are responding rationally to a complex and emotional situation with very little support or guidance from the medical system [32]. Therefore messages on death and dying lack the personal relevance that is needed for effective communication for most seriously ill people.

Finally, most people who need palliative care are NOT dying but LIVING (for a long time) with serious and complex illness. Public engagement must frame messages in the context of ongoing serious illness to which patients and families can relate and include calls to action that increase the likelihood of good care decisions during the prolonged and unpredictable course of disease.

Shifting the Focus from Palliative Care's Financial Savings to Quality of Care and Choice

Numerous studies show cost savings from the inclusion of palliative care for serious illness. However, it would be both a substantive and a strategic mistake to sell early palliative care primarily on its potential to save money. First, cost savings occur as a side effect—or epiphenomenon—of better quality of care. The patient whose pain is well managed at home does not require repeated 911 calls, ED visits, and hospitalizations to manage symptom crises. Second, linking any medical care to cost savings raises questions of motive. Quality of care and cost of that care are seen as positively correlated which don't fit with the unintended cost savings resulting from quality palliative care. Palliative care "adds" services and personal attention. How can adding care cost less?

Without understanding the complex reasons why palliative care reduces system costs, it raises public fears about rationing and "death panel" rhetoric. Professionals understand that palliative care's focus on patient goals and choices, linked to expert management of symptoms and ongoing caregiver support for family needs, often avoids the automatic diagnostic testing, burdensome medical treatments of no benefit, and repeated symptom distress crises that have become routine experiences for most serious illnesses. Despite the central focus of palliative care on understanding and honoring patient and family priorities, some have misinterpreted this focus, sometimes for political purposes, to mean that palliative care is against testing, treatment, and patient choice. Cost messages are also confusing because cost is highly dependent on the reimbursement or payment system, a system that is in flux as part of healthcare reform. Therefore, it would be both more accurate and more honest to focus instead on the truth that palliative care improves quality of care, quality of life, survival, the degree to which care is aligned with what matters most to patients and their families—personal choice—and maximizes individual control over their own lives and medical care. Focusing on improved quality of care and personal choice and control is not only an accurate description of the purposes and benefits of palliative care, but it will always be more motivating to the public than cost savings.

Recommendations

Demonstrate That Good Care Is Possible and Focus on Positive, Empowering Situations/Stories

Most successful marketing focuses on experiences that are appealing as opposed to ones that are negative. This is true for serious illness where people want information to be presented in positive ways [33]. They do not want to hear horror stories and tend to be more interested in how they can remain as healthy and independent as possible. However, this will require a shift in perspective on the part of healthcare advocates driving public engagement.

The first shift is to focus on what people want, as opposed to what experts think they need. From product marketing to political campaigns significant resources are invested in research to understand the consumer's reality—how they see and understand the world. This audience research drives the way services and messages are designed and promoted. However, this is rarely the case for expert-driven sectors like health care where little is invested in effective message development. Instead the focus of communication is on "educating the public" to understand and communicate using expert terminology, and based on the expert's needs and expectations.

Research that begins with the patient's own frame of reference is more likely to provide unbiased responses about his/her values, attitudes and decision making, based on his/her life experience. Some groups are starting to conduct studies that are more patient oriented. The methodology of the SCAN Foundation, the Center to Advance Palliative Care, the American Cancer Society, AARP Services Inc., and the National Journal are designed so that the patient provides the starting point [34].

The second shift is to use palliative care success stories where the patient survives and thrives, as opposed to stories about good deaths. There are stories about how people with serious illness, some of which were curable, were able to better tolerate curative treatment with the help of palliative care and either lived a long, better quality of life, or were indeed cured. The public will be more interested and motivated by such stories than they will about ones describing "a good death," which are not relevant or meaningful to people who are not actually dying. One example of how changing the focus from death to living increases consumer appeal is the Make-A-Wish Foundation that used to market itself as granting wishes for dying children. Parents did not want their children to have a wish since this meant they were dying. This changed when the Foundation altered its positioning to granting wishes of children with life-threatening medical conditions to enrich human experience with hope, strength, and joy [35]. In fact, stories about "a good death" are not relevant, as noted previously, because they bring up death and most people who need palliative care are not dying but *living*.

It is critical for public engagement strategies to promote concurrent palliative care through stories that demonstrate how it benefits patients and families facing serious illness. Given its timely, personal relevance this message is particularly important to share with today's baby boomers as they care for their aging parents.

The stories that show the benefits and share hope will be much more effective than those that are frightening, address dying, or show the hopeless incompetence of the current healthcare system.

Provide Clear Direction to People about Palliative Care

First people must be made aware that it is possible to receive the type of care that palliative care offers. Currently over 78 % of adults in the USA do not know what palliative care is [36]. At the same time, palliative care has a negative image among the minority of patients who have knowledge of it as it is often linked to hospice and hospice's mandate to stop curative and life-prolonging treatment. Pubic engagement efforts need to correct this misunderstanding as palliative care is an option at any stage of an illness and should be provided concurrent with curative treatment for serious illness.

Once appropriately described, the desire for concurrent curative and palliative care is very high across gender, race/ethnicity, educational level, and cancer diagnosis [36]. In fact, were it a new consumer product, its appeal would forecast a blockbuster. Additional selling points are that palliative care also helps patients align treatments with their goals. Recent research confirms that people want care that enhances their independence [37] and their quality of life [38]. Most say they would choose a shorter, higher-quality life over a longer, lower-quality life. They also want to avoid being a burden to their family and to have adequate information about treatment for serious illness [38]. For chronic and late-stage illness, the majority says [39] they prefer to stay in their homes, rather than in other settings, with the support of their families, who are their most trusted caregivers [40]. Most seriously ill patients want [38, 41, 42]:

- To spend quality time with family and friends
- To have their pain managed
- To have their spiritual wishes and needs respected
- To be assured that loved ones are not emotionally and financially devastated

Palliative care identifies and seeks to meet such goals and public engagement efforts on its behalf need to make that very clear.

Help People Demand Early Palliative Care Despite Provider Resistance

While public efforts need to distinguish "palliative care" from "end-of-life" and "hospice care," the same effort needs to be aimed at healthcare providers since many still mistakenly believe that palliative care *is* end-of-life care, and offer it only when curative attempts are no longer viable. As a result, despite data suggesting better quality of life and survival outcomes from simultaneous palliative care and disease-directed treatment [43], some providers are unwilling to refer a patient still undergoing curative or disease-modifying treatment to a palliative care team.

A study of board-certified physicians found that 96 % believe improving quality of life for seriously ill patients is more important than extending life as long as possible—and that the health system should put a higher priority on palliative care for patients who need and want it. Despite these near unanimous opinions on palliative care, 42 % were concerned that palliative care could interfere with doing whatever it takes to extend patients' lives as long as possible. Two-thirds of the surveyed physicians said their patients are not well informed about their palliative care options, and almost 25 % were reluctant to recommend palliative care for fear that their patients may believe they're not doing everything possible to extend their lives. In addition to these issues, limitations in resources and services are perceived by clinicians to be significant barriers to providing palliative care [44].

Physician attitudes are important since, for the majority (76 %) of people, physicians and other health providers appear to remain the most trusted source for information on care options for serious illness [38]. Therefore, public engagement appeals need to prepare "early adopters" in the public to come to the healthcare system fully informed and empowered to demand the best care.

Provide Clear Calls to Action That Support Market and System Change

Once people are in need of palliative care and understand that it is possible to have their needs met, messaging needs to clarify where and how they can access it. At present, palliative care is available in over 85 % of all large hospitals and 54 % of all hospitals, although fewer than half of the public, for-profit, and small community hospitals report presence of a palliative care team [45]. However, even in the hospitals where such services exist, only a fraction of those patients in need actually receive palliative care. Research is needed on what actions patients and their families can take to ensure access to these services.

Given hospitals house most non-hospice palliative care, it is likely that the first time patients and families encounter palliative care will be during a hospitalization. This needs to change as most serious illness is initially diagnosed and managed in the outpatient arena. Therefore, another opportunity for advocating palliative care is to increase the outpatient and community resources to provide and promote it there.

There are a number of system changes that need to be put in place to support early palliative care for serious illness. Current CMS regulations do not always pay for palliative care delivered in skilled nursing facilities. The Medicare Hospice Benefit does not pay for concurrent curative and hospice care for adults. This forces people to make difficult choices, which can delay their use of palliative care or hospice. As more people experience the suffering of serious illness, then learn about the benefits concurrent palliative care makes possible, but find that it is not available to them because of policy and reimbursement issues, public demand for change will grow. Advocates must be ready to leverage the public will for change into meaningful policy demands.

Conclusion

With the right emphasis, public engagement could result in more and more patients and families insisting on concurrent curative and palliative care. This would force hospitals, health systems, and community providers to meet those needs in an increasingly competitive marketplace. This demand would support increased funding for more palliative care generalist and specialty level provider training. It would prompt policy makers to change legislation that currently impedes palliative care for serious illness. The end result would be improved care for those with serious illness and better use of increasingly limited healthcare resources. A win–win for all.

References

1. Gerteis M, Edgman-Levitan S, Daley J, Delbanco TL, editors. Through the patient's eyes: understanding and promoting patient-centered care. San Francisco: Jossey-Bass; 1993.
2. Lilly CM, De Meo DL, Sonna LA, et al. An intensive communication intervention for the critically ill. Am J Med. 2000;109:469–75.
3. Lautrette A, Darmon M, Megarbane B, et al. A communication strategy and brochure for relatives of patients dying in the ICU. N Engl J Med. 2007;356:469–78.
4. Curtis JR, Treece PD, Nielsen EL, et al. Integrating palliative and critical care: evaluation of a quality-improvement intervention. Am J Respir Crit Care Med. 2008;178:269–75.
5. Mosenthal AC, Murphy PA, Barker LK, et al. Changing the culture around end-of-life care in the trauma intensive care unit. J Trauma. 2008;64:1587–93.
6. AARP, unpublished, proprietary data on aging Americans; 2005.
7. Long-term care study conducted by Lake Research Partners, 18–23 Dec 2010. The SCAN Foundation.
8. Sofaer S, Hopper SS, Firminger K, Naierman N, Nelson M. Addressing the need for public reporting of comparative hospice quality: a focus group study. Jt Comm J Qual Patient Saf. 2009;35(8):422–9.
9. Survey of California voters 40 and older conducted by Lake Research Partners and American Viewpoint. The SCAN Foundation and UCLA Center for Health Policy Research, 16 Aug 2011.
10. Bakitas M, Doyle Lyons K, Hegel M, Balan S, Brokaw F, Seville J, Hull J, Li Z, Tosteson T, Byock I, Ahles T. Effects of a palliative care intervention on clinical outcomes in patients with advanced cancer. JAMA. 2009;302(7):741–9.
11. Morrison RS, Penrod JD, Cassell JB, Causel-Ellenbogen M, Litke A, Spragens L, Meier DE. Cost savings associated with U.S. hospital palliative care consultation programs. Arch Intern Med. 2008;168(16):1783–90.
12. Morrison RS, Dietrich J, Ladwig S, Quill T, Sacco J, Tangeman J, et al. Palliative care consultation teams cut hospital costs for Medicaid beneficiaries. Health Aff. 2011;30(3):454–63.
13. Robinson K, Sutton S, Von Gunten CF, et al. Assessment of the education for physicians on end-of-life care (EPEC™) project. J Palliat Med. 2004;7(5):637–45.

14. Delbanco T, Gerteis M. A patient-centered view of the clinician–patient relationship. 2014 [Updated 14 Oct 2013]. http://www.uptodate.com.proxy1.library.jhu.edu
15. Clayton JM, Hancock KM, Butow PN, Tattersall MHN, Currow DC. Clinical practice guidelines for communicating prognosis and end-of-life issues with adults in the advanced stages of a life-limiting illness, and their caregivers. Med J Aust. 2007;186(12):77.
16. Green ML, Aagaard EM, Caverzagie KJ, Chick DA, Holmboe E, Kane G, Smith CD, Iobst W. Charting the road to competence: developmental milestones for internal medicine residency training. J Grad Med Educ. 2009;1(1):5–20.
17. Almack K, Cox K, Moghaddam N, Pollock K, Seymour J. After you: conversations between patients and healthcare professionals in planning for end of life care. BMC Palliative Care. 2012;11:15. doi:10.1186/1472-684X-11-15.
18. Parker SM, Clayton JM, Hancock K, et al. A systematic review of prognostic/end-of-life communication with adults in the advanced stages of a life-limiting illness: patient/caregiver preferences for the content, style, and timing of information. J Pain Symptom Manage. 2007;34(1):81–93.
19. U.S. Department of Health and Human Services, Assistant Secretary for Planning and Evaluation, Office of Disability, Aging and Long-Term Care Policy, Advance Directives and Advance Care Planning: Report To Congress, Aug 2008.
20. Fagerlin A, Schneider C. Enough: the failure of the living will. Hastings Cent Rep. 2004;34:30–42.
21. Hammes BJ, Rooney BL. Death and end-of-life planning in one Midwestern community. Arch Intern Med. 1998;158:383–90.
22. Shapiro S. Advance directives: the elusive goal of having the last word. NAELA J. 2012;VIII(2):205–32.
23. Advance Care Planning: preferences for care at the end-of-life. Agency for Healthcare Research and Quality. Research in Action, Issue # 12, Mar 2003.
24. Pew Research Center. Growing old in America: expectations vs. reality. Washington, DC: Pew Research Center; 2009.
25. AARP Planning for long-term care: a survey of midlife and older women, Oct 2010.
26. For more on the use of non-medical advance planning models, see: Fried TR, Redding, CA, Robbins ML, Paiva A, O'Leary JR, Iannone, L. Stages of change for the component behaviors of advance care planning. J Am Geriatr Soc. 2010;58(12):2329–36. doi:10.1111/j.1532-5415.2010.03184.x.
27. Balch Associates. Assessment of last acts program provides recommendations for future direction. http://www.rwjf.org/reports/grr/038049.htm. Accessed 22 Mar 2007.
28. Halpern SD, Loewenstein G, Volpp KG, Cooney E, Vranas K, Quill CM, McKenzie MS, et al. Default options in advance directives influence how patients set goals for end-of-life care. Health Aff (Millwood). 2013;32(2):408–17. doi:10.1377/hlthaff.2012.0895.
29. Hogan C, Lynn J, Gabel J, et al. Medicare beneficiaries' costs and use of care in the last year of life. Final report to MedPAC. Washington (DC); 2000.
30. Lynn J. Serving patients who may die soon and their families. JAMA. 2001;285(7):925–32.
31. Lynn J, Schall MW, Milne C, et al. Quality improvements in end of life care: insights from two collaboratives. Jt Comm J Qual Improve. 2000;26(5):254–67.
32. Bennett A. Summary report of national summit on advanced illness, coalition to transform advance care.
33. 2011 Public opinion research on palliative care. Center to Advance Palliative Care and American Cancer Society Action Network. Long-term care study conducted Lake Research Partners, 18–23 Dec 2010. The SCAN Foundation.
34. UHG-AARP Services Advance Care Planning Roundtable in DC, Apr 2010. 2011 Public opinion research on palliative care. Center to Advance Palliative Care and American Cancer Society Action Network. Long-term care study conducted by Lake Research Partners, 18–23 Dec 2010. The SCAN Foundation.
35. Arnold R. Half-full or half-empty: making the message of palliative care palatable. J Palliat Med. 2005;8(3):474–6.
36. 2011 Public opinion research on palliative care. Center to Advance Palliative Care and American Cancer Society Action Network.

37. Fried TR, Bradley EH, Towle VR, Allore H. Understanding the treatment preferences of seriously ill patients. N Engl J Med. 2002;346:1061–6. doi:10.1056/NEJMsa012528.
38. Living well at the end of life: a national conversation. National Journal and the Regence Foundation, Mar 2011.
39. Majority of Americans agree "There's No Place Like Home" for care of elderly family members. Harris Interactive Poll conducted for Amedisys; 2010.
40. Whitlatch CJ, Feinberg LF. Family care and decision making. In: Cox C, editor. Dementia and social work practice: research and interventions. New York: Springer; 2007.
41. Final chapter: Californians attitudes and experiences with death and dying. California Healthcare Foundation, Feb 2012.
42. Allshouse KD. Treating patients as individuals. In: Gerteis M, Edgman-Levitan S, Daley J, Delbanco TL, editors. Through the patient's eyes: understanding and promoting patient-centered care. San Francisco: Jossey-Bass; 1993.
43. Temel JS, Greer JA, Muzikansky A, Gallagher ER, Admane S, Jackson VA, Dahlin CM, Blinderman CD, Jacobsen J, Pirl WF, Billings JA, Lynch TJ. Early palliative care for patients with metastatic non-small-cell lung cancer. N Engl J Med. 2010;363(8):733–42. doi:10.1056/NEJMoa1000678.
44. Living well at the end of life: a national conversation. National Journal and the Regence Foundation, Nov 2011.
45. Center to Advance Palliative Care. http://www.capc.org/reportcard/.

Chapter 15
Research Priorities in Palliative Care for Older Adults

R. Sean Morrison

Society is facing one of the largest public health challenges in its history—the growth of the population of older adults. Improvements in public health, the discovery of antibiotics, and advances in modern medicine have resulted in unprecedented gains in human longevity. For most Americans, the years after age 65 are a time of good health, independence, and integration of a life's work and experience. Eventually, however, most adults will develop one or more chronic illnesses with which they may live for many years before they die. Over three-quarters of deaths in the USA are due to chronic diseases of the heart, lungs, brain, and other vital organs [1]. Even cancer, which accounts for nearly a quarter of US deaths, has become a chronic, multi-year illness for many. For a minority of patients with serious illness (e.g., metastatic colon cancer), the time following diagnosis is characterized by a stable period of relatively good functional and cognitive performance followed by a predictable and short period of functional and clinical decline [2]. However, for most patients with serious illness (e.g., heart or lung disease, Parkinson's disease, dementia, stroke, neuro-muscular degenerative diseases, and many cancers), the time following diagnosis is characterized by months to years of physical and psychological symptom distress; progressive functional dependence and frailty; considerable family support needs; and high healthcare resource use [2–5]. Indeed, currently and over the next decades most physicians will be caring for seriously ill elders with multiple comorbidities, lengthy duration of illness, and intermittent acute exacerbations interspersed with periods of relative stability [1]. Abundant evidence suggests that the advanced stages of disease for most are characterized by inadequately treated physical distress; fragmented care systems; poor communication between doctors, patients, and families; and enormous strains on family caregiver and support systems [6].

R.S. Morrison, M.D. (✉)
Brookdale Department of Geriatrics and Palliative Medicine,
Icahn School of Medicine at Mount Sinai, One Gustave L. Levy Place,
New York, NY 10029, USA
e-mail: sean.morrison@mssm.edu

Palliative Care for Older Adults

Palliative care for elders differs from what is usually appropriate in younger adults because of the nature and duration of chronic illness during old age. The prototypical example of a palliative care patient is that of a 55-year-old mother of two with advanced ovarian cancer. Care for this patient would include chemotherapy until it no longer meets the patient's goals of care, treating her symptoms (e.g., nausea, pain, fatigue), addressing her psychological and spiritual concerns, supporting her partner, and helping to arrange for care of her children after her death. The majority of this patient's care occurs at home (with or without hospice) or in the hospital, and the period of functional debility is brief (months). In reality, an 88-year-old widowed woman with advanced heart failure, diabetes mellitus, osteoarthritis, mild cognitive impairment, and frailty typifies the most common example of a patient requiring palliative care. Palliative care for this patient involves treating the primary disease process (advanced heart failure), managing her multiple chronic medical conditions and comorbidities (diabetes mellitus, arthritis) and geriatric syndromes (cognitive impairment, frailty), assessing and treating the physical and psychological symptom distress associated with all of these medical issues, and establishing goals of care and treatment plans in the setting of an unpredictable prognosis. Additionally, the needs of her caregiver(s) are also different from those of the caregiver of the younger patient. Individuals caring for geriatric patients are often adult children with their own family, work responsibilities, and medical conditions, and these roles must be balanced with the months to years of personal care that they must provide to their aging parent. Finally, because older adults often make multiple transitions across care settings (home, hospital, rehabilitation, long-term care), especially in the last months of life, palliative care programs for older adults must assure that care plans and patient goals are maintained from one setting to another. Thus, palliative care for the elderly is centered on the identification and amelioration of functional and cognitive impairment; the development of frailty leading to dependence on caregivers; symptom, emotional, and spiritual distress; and bereavement needs of adult children and elderly partners. The overlap between the traditional fields of geriatrics and palliative care is shown in Fig. 15.1.

The Knowledge Base of Palliative Care for Older Adults

Although serious illness occurs far more commonly in the elderly than in any age group, the evidence base for palliative care in older adults is sparse [7]. For example, the majority of symptom prevalence studies have focused on patients with cancer and AIDS, have not included the oldest old, have excluded patients with associated comorbidities, or have focused almost exclusively on pain. Indeed, the incidence and prevalence of pain in older populations is not even known. Studies have suggested that the prevalence of significant pain in community-dwelling older adults

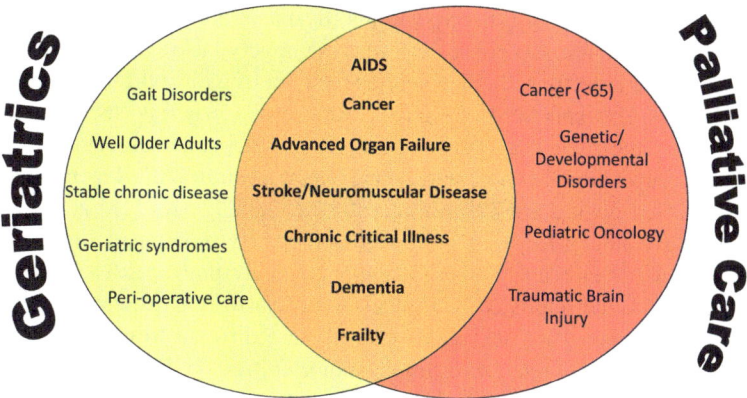

Fig. 15.1 The intersection between geriatrics and palliative care

may be as high as 56 % [8] and that almost one-fifth of older adults take analgesic medications on a regular basis [9]. Similarly, it has been suggested that 45–80 % of nursing home residents have substantial pain and that many of these patients have multiple pain complaints and multiple potential sources of pain [10]. Available data also point to a high prevalence of non-pain symptoms in older adults with serious illness. In retrospective interviews with family members of patients who died of non-cancer illnesses in the UK, 67 % of patients experienced moderate to severe pain, 49 % had trouble breathing, 27 % reported nausea, 36 % reported depression, and 36 % reported sleep disturbances [11]. In an analyses of patients with heart failure, end-stage liver disease, lung cancer, and COPD from the SUPPORT trial over 20 % of patients consistently experienced severe dyspnea during the 6 months prior to death [12–14]. A companion study to SUPPORT reported almost identical pain findings for a cohort of hospitalized patients 80 years and older [15] and also noted a high prevalence of anxiety and depression in the last 6 months of life [16].

Preliminary studies suggest pain and other symptoms are underassessed, undertreated, and are associated with a number of negative outcomes in older adults [17]. Pain is perhaps the best studied symptom and data from several studies suggest that untreated pain is associated with depression, decreased socialization, sleep disturbance, impaired ambulation, and increased healthcare utilization in older adults [18]. These studies are limited by small sample sizes, have included relatively healthy subjects with defined conditions (e.g., osteoarthritis), focused on postoperative surgical patients, or been confined to one disease state (e.g., cancer). Additionally, these studies have not included frail older adults nor adults with multiple comorbidities and have not examined the association of pain with outcomes such as gait disturbances, rehabilitation and functional recovery, frailty, and functional dependence [18]. Studies in older adults that have included these outcomes (functional recovery, frailty, falls, and function) have typically not included pain and other symptoms as independent variables [19–21]. Studies on the prevalence, assessment, and impact of other symptoms (dyspnea, anxiety, nausea, fatigue) on quality of life, function, and other outcomes are largely lacking.

The evidence base for the effective management of pain and other symptoms in older adults is also sparse. Although the American Geriatrics Society published guidelines for the treatment of acute and persistent pain, these guidelines were largely based upon small cohort studies and expert opinion [22]. Recommendations for age-adjusted dosing are not available for most analgesics [18] and almost all analgesics have side effect profiles that are particularly problematic in older adults [22]. Interventions directed at other symptoms (e.g., dyspnea, nausea, anxiety) have rarely included older adults or have focused on relatively narrow conditions (e.g., chemotherapy induced nausea) and the results are difficult to generalize to older adults with advanced illness and multiple comorbidities [7]. Finally, even studies in younger adults have rarely linked the treatment of pain to outcomes other than symptom relief. Although symptom relief is critically important, and whereas many have argued that patient comfort should be sufficient stimulus to alter pain management practices [1, 23, 24], the documented difficulties in shifting clinician priorities and behaviors [25] over the past several decades suggest that empirical data regarding the adverse effects of pain and other symptoms on specific clinical outcomes are required in order to change practice patterns and improve patient care.

The burdens of serious illness extend to patients' families and friends [4, 5, 26]. More than 50 million individuals serve as informal caregivers to the seriously ill [27]. Due to recent efforts to reduce hospitalization rates and lengths of stay, there is increased reliance on informal caregivers to provide care for family members or friends with serious illness. The majority of these caregivers are older adults who endure stress and burden related to both caring for the individual in the setting of serious illness and in coping with their death. An increasing body of research demonstrates adverse financial, physical, and psychological effects on caregivers of patients with serious chronic illness. For example, a study of 893 caregivers of patients with terminal illness, reported that over one third of caregivers had substantial stress and 86 % stated that they needed more help with transportation (62 %), homemaking (55 %), nursing (28 %), or personal care (26 %) than they were currently receiving or could afford [5]. Caregivers with care needs were significantly more likely to consider suicide, have depressive symptoms, and to report that caring for patients interfered with their lives and reduced their independence [4]. Caregiving has also been shown to be an independent risk factor for death, major depression, and associated comorbidities [28].

Research Funding for Palliative Care

Federal funding through the National Institutes of Health, the Veteran's Administration, and the Agency for Healthcare Research and Quality is low and inadequate. A recent study reported that from 2006 to 2010 grants related to palliative care research comprised 0.2 % of total grants awarded by NIH [29]. Furthermore, three agencies—the National Cancer Institute (0.4 % of all NCI awarded grants), the National Institute for Nursing Research (7.6 % of all NINR awarded grants), and the National Institute on Aging (0.8 % of all NIA awarded grants) funded 82 % of all palliative care research awards [29]. Indeed, the same study found of the 1,253 original research papers published in palliative care from 2006 to 2010, only one-fifth were supported by federal research dollars [29]. There are several possible reasons to account for these findings. The absence of a federal agency specifically charged with a focus on palliative care and on persons with serious illness may be a contributing factor to low levels of research support for care of people with serious and complex illnesses. With few exceptions, the NIH institutes are disease-specific and thus palliative care, with its applicability to all serious illnesses, does not fit well within a particular institute's scope. Although NINR has focused on palliative and end-of-life care, its relatively small budget compared to other Institutes considerably limits the amount of palliative care research that can be realistically funded. Recent budget cuts have further hampered the NIH Institutes' abilities to fund new research or new investigators that might be perceived as outside their core missions. Finally, neither an Institute-specific nor a Center for Scientific Review Study Section that specifically focuses on palliative care has been established. Existing study sections have, at most, one or two reviewers with expertise in palliative care research. Thus, peers with appropriate content and methodological expertise in palliative care rarely review palliative care grant submissions.

Research Gaps

An adequate evidence base for palliative care for older adults will require new knowledge including the development and testing of innovative models of care delivery, the development of new research instruments, designs, and analytic techniques; application of established instruments, designs, and techniques from other fields to palliative care and aging research; and changes in federal funding priorities and review processes. Recommendations resulting from a recent conference sponsored by the National Institute on Aging, the National Palliative Care Research Center, and the Mount Sinai Older Adults Independence Center to identify priorities in geriatric palliative care research are detailed below.

Knowledge Gaps: Gaps in knowledge relate to several key areas. First, a clear research definition of serious illness that goes beyond the traditional disease-specific ("advanced cancer," "NY class IV CHF") or prognosis specific ("last year of life") definitions is needed. Such a definition will likely incorporate symptom burden, functional status, cognition, treatment burden, social morbidity, and diagnosis. Second, the longitudinal nature and needs of older adults with serious illness and their caregivers have yet to be well described. If new models of care are truly going to meet the needs of an aging society, longitudinal studies on non-dementia and non-cancer populations and that include caregivers are required. Third, the impact of suffering on the caregiving experience and effect of palliative care on caregiver outcomes needs to be elucidated. Fourth, additional research is needed on decision making and advance care planning—both for cognitively intact and cognitively impaired individuals and their families. Fifth, despite the millions of dollars dedicated to research in Alzheimer disease by the National Institute on Aging, few if any clinical trials have been funded or performed to examine ways to alleviate symptoms, improve care planning, or reduce burdensome transitions and complications for persons with end-stage dementia. Sixth, evaluation of symptom interventions beyond disease-specific models is needed. Finally, the development and evaluation of appropriate new models of delivering palliative care outside of hospital and hospices needs to be undertaken and such models should include both formal and informal caregiving strategies and interventions and comparative and cost-effectiveness analyses.

Gaps in Research Design and Methods: Traditionally, research in pain and other symptoms has relied upon patient self-report as the gold standard of assessment [30]. For patients with cognitive impairment, such assessment may be impractical or simply impossible and reliable means of assessing pain and other symptoms through behavioral observation or through the use of proxies are required. Unfortunately, existing observational scales [31] require considerable skill, experience, and familiarity with the patient to administer and validated scales employing proxy respondents are not available [18]. Researchers also face complexities in studying patients with multiple symptoms that may interact with each other—particularly since it may be difficult to distinguish symptoms caused by the patient's illness from those resulting from treatments. Such patients thus require instruments that assess a wide constellation of symptoms and assess multiple dimensions within each individual symptom. Whereas a few such instruments exist, they are relatively complex, lengthy, and burdensome and have not been validated in older adults [32–35]. Indeed, in a recent population-based study of adults with recently diagnosed rectal cancer, subjects who were older had poor performance status or were receiving active palliative care were significantly more likely to have missing data on physical functioning and global quality of life data than younger and more highly functional patients over the 2-year study [36]. Although some research questions in geriatric palliative care may be addressed using the gold standard of clinical research—the randomized controlled trial, many others may only be feasibly addressed through observational data and quasi-experimental designs. Thus, improvements in care may well require careful and innovative use of non-randomized and sometimes uncontrolled settings [1]. Finally, specific analytic issues unique to palliative care in older adults also require attention. For example, the problem of missing or distorted data is considerable in palliative care research [1]. Data can be missing because patients with advanced disease die during studies or are unable to report directly about their symptoms, concerns, or attitudes because their illness, treatment, or both have left them confused, weak, or unconscious. Sophisticated research methods to deal with nonrandom missing data are required in palliative care research but are not yet widely used. Many studies in palliative care are observational or employ quasi-experimental designs and thus require analytic techniques that strengthen the inferences that can be made from the studies.

Addressing the Knowledge Gap

Policy initiatives to address this knowledge gap are relatively straightforward and could be rapidly integrated within current biomedical research funding structures. First, strong consideration should be given to the development of a Center for Scientific Review (CSR) study section that specifically focuses on serious illness and moves beyond disease and biology-specific topic areas. At a minimum, key review panels that are currently assigned palliative care grants both within CSR (e.g., Health Services Organization and Delivery Study Section, Behavioral Medicine: Interventions and Outcomes, Aging Systems and Geriatrics Study Section) and individual Institutes [Clinical Aging (NIA), Clinical Studies (NCI)], should contain at least 3–4 members with expertise in palliative care. Second, NIH, AHRQ, and Patient-Centered Outcomes Research Institute (PCORI) need to develop specific Program Announcements (PAs) and Requests for Applications (RFAs) targeted to the research priorities detailed above. Studies submitted under these PAs/RFAs should consider sociodemographic/system factors, be required to include the cognitively impaired and frail, and all implementation studies should include a knowledge translation and implementation plan. Third, despite fiscal constraints, increased investment in palliative care research is needed—beyond the current 0.2 %. At a minimum, of 2 % of current Institute budgets should be reallocated to focus on the needs of patients and families with serious illness and developing and evaluating new models of care delivery [37]. Fourth, strong consideration should be given to establishing an Office of Palliative Care Research modeled after the Office of AIDS Research [38] to oversee distribution of research funding. This is particularly important given that the priorities for palliative care research cross multiple diseases and conditions and are not well matched by the current disease-specific silos of NIH. Finally, existing NIH career development award mechanisms need to be better utilized to support junior investigators and mid-career palliative care investigators in order to address the lack of established researchers in this area.

Conclusion

In summary, there is a pressing need to improve the evidence base for palliative care in older adults. The areas of research that need to be addressed include establishing the prevalence of symptoms in patients with chronic disease, evaluating the association between symptom treatment and outcomes, increasing the evidence base for symptom treatment, understanding patients' psychological/spiritual well-being and quality of life and elucidating sources of caregiver burden, reevaluating service delivery, and adapting research methodologies specifically for palliative care. Changes in the review process and funding priorities by the National Institutes of Health, Agency for Healthcare Research and Quality, and the PCORI are also critically needed in order to address the gaps in research and develop the knowledge that clinicians need to appropriately care for older adults with serious illness.

References

1. Field MJ, Cassel CK, editors. Approaching death: improving care at the end of life. Washington, DC: National Academy Press; 1997.
2. Lunney JR, Lynn J, Foley DJ, Lipson S, Guralnik JM. Patterns of functional decline at the end of life. JAMA. 2003;289(18):2387–92.
3. SUPPORT Principal Investigators. A controlled trial to improve care for seriously ill hospitalized patients. The study to understand prognoses and preferences for outcomes and risks of treatments (SUPPORT). JAMA. 1995;274(20):1591–8.
4. Emanuel EJ, Fairclough DL, Slutsman J, Emanuel LL. Understanding economic and other burdens of terminal illness: the experience of patients and their caregivers. Ann Intern Med. 2000;132(6):451–9.
5. Emanuel EJ, Fairclough DL, Slutsman J, Alpert H, Baldwin D, Emanuel LL. Assistance from family members, friends, paid care givers, and volunteers in the care of terminally ill patients. N Engl J Med. 1999;341(13):956–63.
6. Signorielli N. Physical disabilities, impairment and safety, mental illness, and death. In: Mass media images and impact on health. Westport, CT: Greenwood Press; 1993. p. 37–42.
7. Morrison RS, Meier DE, editors. Geriatric palliative care. New York: Oxford University Press; 2003.
8. Helm RD, Gibson SJ. Pain in older people. In: Cronbie IK, Croft R, Linton SJ, Lerexche L, Von Dorff M, editors. Epidemiology of pain. Seattle: IASP Press; 2000. p. 102–12.
9. Cooner E, Amorosi S. The study of pain in older Americans. New York: Louis Harris and Associates; 1997.
10. Ferrell B. Pain evaluation and management in the nursing home. Ann Intern Med. 1995;123:681–7.
11. Seale C, Cartwright A. The year before death. Brookfield, VT: Ashgale; 1994.
12. Claessens MT, Lynn J, Zhong Z, et al. Dying with lung cancer or chronic obstructive pulmonary disease: insights from SUPPORT. Study to understand prognoses and preferences for outcomes and risks of treatments. J Am Geriatr Soc. 2000;48(5 Suppl):S146–53.
13. Roth K, Lynn J, Zhong Z, Borum M, Dawson NV. Dying with end stage liver disease with cirrhosis: insights from SUPPORT. Study to understand prognoses and preferences for outcomes and risks of treatment. J Am Geriatr Soc. 2000;48(5 Suppl):S122–30.
14. Levenson JW, McCarthy EP, Lynn J, Davis RB, Phillips RS. The last six months of life for patients with congestive heart failure. J Am Geriatr Soc. 2000;48(5 Suppl):S101–9.
15. Desbiens NA, Mueller-Rizner N, Connors Jr AF, Hamel MB, Wenger NS. Pain in the oldest-old during hospitalization and up to one year later. HELP Investigators Hospitalized Elderly Longitudinal Project. J Am Geriatr Soc. 1997;45(10):1167–72.
16. Somogyi-Zalud E, Zhong Z, Lynn J, Hamel MB. Elderly persons' last six months of life: findings from the Hospitalized Elderly Longitudinal Project. J Am Geriatr Soc. 2000;48(5 Suppl):S131–9.

17. Reyes-Gibby CC, Aday L, Cleeland C. Impact of pain on self-rated health in the community-dwelling older adults. Pain. 2002;95(1–2):75–82.
18. Ferrell BA, Whiteman JE. Pain. In: Morrison RS, Meier DE, editors. Geriatric palliative care. New York: Oxford University Press; 2003. p. 205–29.
19. Magaziner J, Hawkes W, Hebel JR, et al. Recovery from hip fracture in eight areas of function. J Gerontol A Biol Sci Med Sci. 2000;55(9):M498–507.
20. Fried LP, Tangen CM, Walston J, et al. Frailty in older adults: evidence for a phenotype. J Gerontol A Biol Sci Med Sci. 2001;56(3):M146–56.
21. Tinetti ME, Speechley M, Ginter SF. Risk factors for falls among elderly persons living in the community. N Engl J Med. 1988;319(26):1701–7.
22. American Geriatrics Society. The management of persistent pain in older adults. http://www.americangeriatrics.org. Accessed 15 Nov 2007.
23. Meier DE, Morrison RS, Cassel CK. Improving palliative care. Ann Intern Med. 1997;127(3):225–30.
24. Cassell EJ. The nature of suffering and the goals of medicine. N Engl J Med. 1982;306(11):639–45.
25. Foley KM. Pain relief into practice: rhetoric without reform. J Clin Oncol. 1995;13(9):2149–51.
26. Levine C. The loneliness of the long term caregiver. N Engl J Med. 1999;340:1587–90.
27. National Alliance for Caregiving and AARP. Caregiving in the U.S. National Alliance for Caregiving and AARP; 2004.
28. Schulz R, Beach S. Caregiving as a risk factor for mortality: the Caregiver Health Effects Study. JAMA. 1999;282:2215–9.
29. Gelfman LP, Du Q, Morrison RS. An update: NIH research funding for palliative medicine 2006 to 2010. J Palliat Med. 2013;16(2):125–9.
30. Agency for Health Care Policy and Research. Management of cancer pain: adults. Cancer Pain Guideline Panel. Am Fam Physician. 1994;49(8):1853–68.
31. Hurley A, Volicer B, Hanrahan P, et al. Assessment of discomfort in advanced Alzheimer patients. Res Nurs Health. 1992;15:369–77.
32. Daut RL, Cleeland CS, Flanery RC. Development of the Wisconsin Brief Pain Questionnaire to assess pain in cancer and other diseases. Pain. 1983;17(2):197–210.
33. Portenoy RK, Thaler HT, Kornblith AB, et al. The Memorial Symptom Assessment Scale: an instrument for the evaluation of symptom prevalence, characteristics and distress. Eur J Cancer. 1994;30A(9):1326–36.
34. Dudgeon D, Raubertas RF, Rosenthal SN. The short-form McGill Pain Questionnaire in chronic cancer pain. J Pain Symptom Manage. 1993;8(4):191–5.
35. Dudgeon D. Multidimensional assessment of dyspnea. In: Portenoy RK, Bruera E, editors. Palliative care research. New York: Oxford University Press; 2003.
36. Kopp I, Lorenz W, Rothmund M, Koller M. Relation between severe illness and non-completion of quality-of-life questionnaires by patients with rectal cancer. J R Soc Med. 2003;96(9):442–8.
37. Morrison RS, Meier DE. Pallliative care, access, quality, and costs. In: Yount PL, Olsen LS, editors. The healthcare imperative: lowering costs and improving outcomes: workshop series summary. Washington, DC: National Academies Press; 2010. p. 498–503.
38. NIH Office of AIDS Research (OAR). OAR Home. http://www.oar.nih.gov/. Accessed 12 May 2013.

Chapter 16
Medical and Nursing Education & Training

Charles F. von Gunten and Betty R. Ferrell

Introduction

Physician behavior controls 95 % of the health care spending in the USA. If the needs of older adults with serious illness are to be met in ways that are different from today, then the education and training of physicians and nurses will need to be different. Nurses are also key providers of care and amidst the major demands of an aging society and workforce shortages, nurses are assuming an increasing role as primary care providers. There are two overridingly important features that are important if this change is to be achieved.

First, the fundamental approach to decision-making for the older adult with serious illness needs to change. The palliative care approach as contrasted to the standard approach to serious illness is this: overall goals of care are established for the patient in the context of his or her family, first; the goals take into account what is known about the illness, what is inevitable versus what is modifiable, the prognosis, and patient and family preferences; then, plans to achieve these goals are established. In contrast, the standard approach is to first identify all of the problems through diagnostic testing then set about to solve each of the biological problems. This approach, which has guided American medicine since the 1970s, assumes that a person's health is the sum of the component biological parts. It also assumes that each time the patient presents to the medical system, the patient needs a "workup." This quote, from the medical literature of the 1970s, captures the thrust of this

---

C.F. von Gunten, M.D., Ph.D. (✉)
OhioHealth System, Kobacker House, 800 McConnell Drive, Columbus, OH 43215, USA
e-mail: charles@pallmed.us

B.R. Ferrell, R.N., Ph.D.
Department of Nursing Research and Education, City of Hope, Duarte, CA, USA

approach. "If only patients could leave their damaged physical vessels at the hospital for repair, while taking their social and emotional selves home [1]."

Second, clinicians are developed by apprenticeship; they learn by doing. Consequently, meaningful changes in the behavior of clinicians will not be achieved unless they observe the desired approaches modeled by others that they respect, that they practice under supervision, and that are expected and rewarded when they are in practice. For that to occur, the healthcare system must be structured to enable these trained physicians and nurses to act. No behavior will persist in the face of sustained negative reinforcement. The greatest mistake that is made in medical and nursing education and training is to view it as a cognitive exercise; if the doctor or nurse is told, or persuaded, she will behave differently. In contrast, doctors and nurses will do what they see others do, and are rewarded for doing in terms of praise, recognition, gratitude and that the system makes easy to do. If it is difficult to do the "right thing"; if there is negative social stigma attached to the practice of palliative care in the context of mainstream health care; if there are negative consequences in terms of income or status, the desired changes in physician and nursing behavior will not occur.

To make the case for these two assertions, this chapter will first summarize the background of clinical palliative care in the USA and its impact on palliative care education. Then, we will review the needs assessments that have been used to justify and stimulate contemporary approaches to introduce and improve palliative care education. We will then review some major approaches to meet those needs, including the establishment of training criteria in medical and nursing education, the establishment of the specialty of palliative medicine and nursing and the structure for its practice in American Health Care. Finally, we will describe the policy changes that will ensure the medical workforce is able to meet the needs of older adults with serious illness.

Background

In the USA, as elsewhere in the western world, the care of older adults with serious illness was a routine part of life until the last half of the twentieth century. Before that time, it was expected that older people would become frail and ill, and eventually die; it was "normal." By the second half of the century, the product of the investment in applying the scientific method to human illness was to deconstruct "getting old and dying" into component parts. It was "old fashioned" and "unscientific" to think of older people dying from natural causes. Rather, they were dying of the consequences of atherosclerotic diseases (myocardial infarctions, stroke, congestive heart failure) or lung disease (primarily smoking-induced emphysema) or dementia. The scientific method demonstrated successful cure of such common causes of death as pneumococcal pneumonia and infectious diarrhea. It follows that these other causes of death and disability would similarly fall to the scientific method.

The images and models of health care and the medical profession changed. Doctor's offices and hospitals were explicitly designed to look more like scientific laboratories and less like homes and businesses. Doctors and nurses began to dress as if they worked in a laboratory by wearing laboratory coats. The principal skills expected from physicians and nurses changed from people-oriented communication, interpretation, and advice skills to the ordering, scheduling, obtaining, and interpretation of a variety of diagnostic tests and the prescription of evidence-based treatments. This approach markedly reduced infectious diseases as a cause of death, while chronic degenerative diseases such as cancer, heart failure, and dementia became more common. Inevitably, however, it became apparent that science could not eliminate disease and death and person-centered concerns including function, cognition, and quality of life were marginalized in favor of focusing on those things that were amenable to the new scientific model of American medicine.

Very similar changes have occurred in the nursing profession. Nursing has advanced to provide baccalaureate, masters, and doctoral education with much greater emphasis on evidence-based practice taught by Ph.D. nurses who no longer practice nursing. The roles of nurses have expanded tremendously to accommodate the throughput and volume demands of a burdened healthcare system but often neglecting the primary needs of patients and their families.

The disconnect began being discussed in the 1960s [2]. The scientific method illustrated that patients wanted to talk about their impending death when modern medicine was not able to change the eventual outcome [3]. The publication of *On Death and Dying* by Dr. Elizabeth Kuebler-Ross from the University of Chicago Medical School in 1969 capped this period [4]. A remarkable feature of her work was that she interviewed real patients facing death in teaching sessions with medical students, residents, and other students in a manner similar to that used in teaching other medical subjects. As it relates to the thesis of this chapter, what makes Kuebler-Ross's work striking and effective is she role-modeled the new behavior in front of doctors working with real patients.

Interestingly, teaching hospitals and "standard" medicine didn't change. Rather, a grass-roots "hospice movement" started in North America resulting in the founding of a large number of hospice programs that primarily provide care as support teams in the patient's home, far away from the settings where the attitudes, knowledge and skills of new physicians and nurses were established through apprenticeship in the nation's teaching hospitals [5]. In other words, this innovation in health care happened in a way that was invisible to medical and nursing education and training.

Need for Palliative Care Education

It should be no surprise, then, that the education of medical students, nursing students, and other health professionals about serious advanced illness and palliative care in North America is poor. In response, private and public groups have worked to determine the core competencies that physicians, nurses, and others should possess in order to provide adequate palliative care for patients and their families. This evolution culminated in the determination by the Liaison Committee for Medical Education (LCME), the accrediting body for all 126 medical schools in the USA, that all accredited medical schools must include education in palliative care [6]. Similar standards were established for the 16 Canadian medical schools. Similar commitment has been made by the American Association of Colleges of Nursing (AACN) [7].

Some medical schools have described curricula on death and dying [8–16]. However, descriptions of instruction indicate that the education is provided predominately through scattered didactic courses in death and dying during the preclinical years. Their effectiveness is limited by the absence of immediate clinical application of the material, and therefore, no opportunity to develop the necessary skills to alleviate the suffering of the patient and their loved ones [17–19]. Although most medical schools offer some formal teaching of the subject, there is considerable evidence that current training is inadequate, most strikingly in the clinical years. A 1997 article by Billings and Block characterizes the present as well: "Curricular offerings are not well integrated; the major teaching format is the lecture; formal teaching is predominantly preclinical; clinical experiences are mostly elective; there is little attention to home care, hospice, and nursing home care; role models are few; and students are not encouraged to examine their personal reactions to these clinical experiences [17]."

Although several national organizations have presented curricula and position statements on the importance of this subject, no clear standards or widely adopted curricula have yet emerged for either undergraduate or graduate training in palliative medicine in the USA, or for clinical practice in the hospital, nursing home, or hospice, with the exception of one facet of palliative care—pain management.

Postgraduate training of physicians is little better [20–22]. A survey of oncologists reported their training to be poor and that the greatest source of information about palliative care was "trial and error" [23]. A national study in Internal Medicine found that residents, faculty, and their program directors rated their palliative care training as inadequate [17]. Cancer pain education research has shown that residents lack basic pain assessment skills, knowledge of opioid pharmacology, and skills of pharmacological management [20–26]. Internal Medicine residents have poor skills in conducting advance directive discussions and discussing resuscitation orders, crucial to appropriate planning during serious illness [27–29]. In the SUPPORT trial, neither interns nor their attending faculty were consistently accurate, nor were attending physicians more accurate than interns, in assessing patient treatment preferences [30].

Response to Needs for Palliative Care Education

Recent initiatives have begun to address palliative care education. These efforts include development and dissemination of new educational recommendations, training materials, and educational training requirements at both the medical school and residency levels [31–47]. The American Board of Internal Medicine (ABIM) added the domain of "End-of-Life Care" to its residency training requirements. Family Medicine has since recommended this area to its residency training programs [45].

Efforts to incorporate palliative care education within existing residency programs face daunting obstacles. Some barriers reflect challenges unique to palliative care, including physicians' attitudes and fears about their own mortality, assessing and treating pain, and acknowledging and communicating transitions. Content of a palliative care curriculum responsive to these barriers includes evidence-based symptom assessment and management practices, cultural and spiritual context of medical interventions and the ethical principles and communication skills that relate to interactions between and among professionals, patients, and their families. A major step forward to meet this need was the development and initial dissemination of the Education for Physicians on End-of-Life Care by the American Medical Association [9] that has reached more than 90,000 practicing physicians [48]. This curriculum has been widely adapted to teach medical students, residents, nursing students, social workers, chaplains, and the public. This is due largely to the modular construction, ease of adaptability, and innovative teaching methods such as trigger video tapes that are all provided to the teacher by the project.

The companion national effort for nursing has been the End-of-Life Nursing Education Consortium (ELNEC) Project also initially funded by the Robert Wood Johnson Foundation to develop educational tools for undergraduate nursing faculty to ensure that core skills in palliative care were taught as part of the core nursing curriculum [49]. The ELNEC curriculum has been adapted for nurses in practice as well as in special populations and settings (oncology, pediatrics, critical care, geriatrics advanced practice). Since 2000, the AACN has partnered with the City of Hope to develop and disseminate palliative care education to undergraduate and graduate nursing faculty and students through the ELNEC. In the first 12 years of this project, over 15,000 nurses and other members of the interprofessional healthcare team, from all 50 states, the District of Columbia, Puerto Rico, and 77 countries have attended a national ELNEC train-the-trainer course.

However, as in medicine, a significant shortcoming is that nurses learn best when didactic material is paired with direct clinical encounters under the supervision of expert clinical preceptors. Structured mentoring of nurses new to palliative care is needed.

Barriers to Palliative Care Education

Reform of existing curricula to include palliative care confronts challenges that pervade professional education reform in general. While the changing societal needs, and an aging chronically ill population require that medical and nursing education respond in kind, there is no clear evidence of "what works" in education reform. The written descriptions of the outcome of similar past efforts suggest that we most often reaffirm the difficulty of implementing and sustaining reform [50].

One way to identify a domain of practice for which competence is expected is to include that domain in formal assessment. Yet, the majority of residency programs report that written evaluations by the faculty supervisors on clinical rotations are the only means by which palliative care competence is assessed [43]. Nurses in undergraduate education are evaluated primarily on written exams and in graduate education settings through written papers or feedback from clinical mentors who likely are not well trained in palliative care. Even in ethics, where many programs provide required education, very few provide supervised clinical experiences. This limits the occasions in which palliative care skills can be systematically observed and assessed. Thus, considerable burden is placed on the teaching faculty to assess the constellation of requisite knowledge (e.g., drug therapy for dyspnea), attitudes (e.g., fear of addiction), and clinical skills (e.g., discussing treatment goals), which shape how clinicians provide palliative care. But the premise that programs can simply extend existing resources to take on this burden seems unwarranted, given that programs often reported the absence of faculty skilled in palliative care, and infrequent structured performance based assessments.

Knowledge: Insufficient for Change

Sadly, much of palliative care education in North America hinges on the assumption that knowledge will change practice. Yet, we know that education alone does not change patient and family experience. Or, to be more precise, education targeted to improve knowledge and attitudes does not change behavior [51].

Although the conclusions are discouraging, they shouldn't be surprising. We have learned the same things from education about tobacco, alcohol, sex, diet, hand washing, hypertension, and advance directives. Attitudes and knowledge are necessary, but insufficient, to change behavior.

Formal Recognition of Palliative Medicine and Palliative Nursing

The 1997 report from the US Institute of Medicine (IOM) sets the stage for specialization in the healthcare system's approach to End-of-Life Care by calling for the development of specialty-led professional expertise in palliative medicine in the USA to make this knowledge widely available in US health care [26]. The IOM report recognized the benefits formal recognition of palliative medicine would confer, stating that a formal specialty would:

- focus attention more powerfully on an existing knowledge base that is both insufficiently understood and inadequately applied and that is in need of further growth;

- recognize more explicitly and publicly that palliative care is an appropriate goal of medicine;
- conform to the value and recognition structure of medical professionals—providing credibility with peers (and perhaps patients and others) as a source of knowledge, guidance, and referral;
- attract leaders to the field; and
- nurture the development of the field and its knowledge base.

Palliative medicine was subsequently recognized as a specialty of 11 parent Boards by the American Board of Medical Specialties in 2006. At the same time, The Accreditation Council for Graduate Medical Education recognized the formal training path leading to the new specialty in 2006.

The unprecedented feature of the recognition deserves comment. Eleven specialties recognize hospice and palliative medicine as a subspecialty of their area: (1) internal medicine (which includes all of its subspecialties including cardiology, pulmonology, nephrology, oncology, etc.), (2) family medicine, (3) pediatrics, (4) surgery (including all of its subspecialties like urology, hand surgery, and plastic surgery), (5) radiation oncology (as part of radiology), (6) physical medicine and rehabilitation, (7) neurology, (8) psychiatry, (9) anesthesiology, (10) obstetrics and gynecology, and (11) emergency medicine. Never before in the history of organized medicine have all of these specialties agreed that ONE training pathway after training in the core specialty can lead to ONE certification.

This event underlines the thesis of this chapter—palliative medicine contradicts, and actually overcomes, the hyperspecialization and fragmentation of medicine that characterizes its development since World War II. To accept that there is a subspecialty of palliative medicine means that the generalist features belong in each of the 11 specialties—in other words, in all of medical care.

From the point of view of preparation of the physician workforce, primary or generalist palliative care is the responsibility of all physicians. This includes basic approaches to the relief of suffering and improving quality of life for the whole person and his or her family. It also means the skill of being able to establish overall goals for care for those with serious illness. Overwhelmingly, physicians with primary not specialist-level-palliative care skills will care for the majority of people with serious illness. The same is true for the nursing profession. While nurses are playing key roles in hospices and palliative care programs, nurses across all specialties and all settings of care provide care for the seriously ill and dying.

Secondary palliative care, also called specialist palliative care, is the responsibility of specialists and hospital or community based palliative care or hospice programs. The role of the secondary specialist or program is to provide consultation and assist the managing service. These are the people who will be "board certified" in palliative medicine or nursing. These are not the people to whom patients and their families are "turned over" when there is "nothing more we can do." Rather, they care for the smaller number of patients who require specialist skills that exceed the time or abilities of their primary caregivers.

Tertiary palliative care is the province of academic centers where new knowledge is created through research, and new knowledge is disseminated through education. In addition, tertiary palliative care centers are likely to care for the most challenging cases.

It should be obvious then, that palliative medicine and nursing needs to be integrated throughout the care system [52, 53].

The need for palliative care has been reinforced in concurring opinions from the US Supreme Court that refused to recognize a constitutional right to assisted suicide [54]. The American College of Physicians and the ABIM have both called for general physician competency in the care of persons with terminal illness [55, 56].

The field of palliative nursing has also developed as a specialty with similar demands for both specialization but also integration of palliative care into all areas of nursing. The Hospice and Palliative Nursing Association (HPNA) includes over 10,000 members and the certification of nurses in the specialty is through the National Board for Certification of Hospice and Palliative Nurses. HPNA and NBCHPCN (www.hpna.org) have offered valuable leadership in development of the specialty but nurses in all settings from neonatal intensive care, oncology, ICU, long-term care, emergency departments, and other areas require palliative care skills if they are to effectively care for seriously ill patients and families. There is also a need for palliative care education for Advanced Practice Nursing (APN) as these nurses will assume even greater responsibilities in future healthcare delivery.

Policy Implications

1. Nursing schools, like medical schools, will prepare nurses in palliative care at all levels including undergraduate, graduate (masters), and doctoral including the new Doctorate in Nursing Practice—DNP.
2. Every physician and nurse will need to demonstrate primary palliative care competencies during required clinical training; graduated clinical responsibility during medical school, nursing school, and postgraduate training will be required.
3. Every center training physicians and nurses will have specialist-level palliative care programs that include consultation, dedicated specialist inpatient units, and specialist outpatient and home care services in which all medical and nursing trainees play essential roles in providing the care under supervision of experts.
4. Extensive continuing education in palliative care is required for physicians and nurses already in practice.
5. Nurses will be enabled to assume a much greater role in delivery of palliative care through advanced practice roles in all settings of care.
6. Persistent failure to demonstrate palliative care competencies despite opportunities for remedial training will result in loss of clinical privileges and licensure to practice in the same ways that other failures in standard clinical practice result in sanctions.
7. Failure to demonstrate palliative care competencies are grounds for civil litigation in the same manner as other forms of malpractice.

Road Map for Change

To achieve these policy and behavior changes will require concerted efforts at various levels. We will outline what this might look like.

The Liaison Committee for Accreditation of Medical Schools (LCME) will refine its existing criteria that all medical schools include palliative care education to include more details. Currently, there is no direction about how or when such education should occur. Since preclinical education without clinical education is useless, accreditation should rest on the demonstration that all medical students complete a clinical rotation in hospice and palliative care that includes measurement of basic palliative care competencies in pain and symptom assessment, communication skills to set goals of care in advanced disease, and working with an interdisciplinary team. Since the majority of teaching hospitals now have access to clinical palliative care [57], this should be a straightforward development.

The American Association for the Colleges of Nursing would move beyond supplying its faculty with tools from the ELNEC curriculum to helping its members develop clinical correlates for the didactic curriculum that some, but not all, schools have nursing have adopted.

The Residency Review Committees (RRCs) of the Accreditation Council for Graduate Medical Education (ACGME) will refine accreditation criteria for postgraduate training in each of the specialties from which graduates may be eligible for subspecialty training in hospice and palliative medicine. This strategy builds on the logic that there cannot be a subspecialty without basic training in the specialty. While that basic competency training should exist logically, it does not exist practically for the 11 specialties that cosponsor subspecialty training in hospice and palliative medicine.

This would best be achieved by a federally or privately sponsored initiative to convene working groups of the RRCs, constituents from each of the specialties, and constituents from the subspecialty of hospice and palliative medicine that are drawn from the specialty. For each, a track of training that leads logically from the first postgraduate year of training in surgery, or family medicine, or internal medicine, or radiation oncology, to completion of core specialty training and is then built upon for those who choose to pursue subspecialty training in hospice and palliative medicine, would be defined. Then, the accreditation requirements would match the path.

The AACN would analogously work with its schools that provide masters and doctoral level training to assure that programs develop advanced practice nurses in palliative care with adequate clinical components to the education in affiliated programs.

Since palliative care is interdisciplinary, these approaches of medicine and nursing could be facilitated by extramural funding that incentivizes schemes that train both physicians and nurses together. This could be federal or private foundation funding.

The American Board of Medical Specialties could facilitate the coordination of testing for the co-sponsoring specialties for the field of hospice and palliative medicine to assure that a component of their examinations includes questions tied to the curricular requirements developed by the RRCs. This could be facilitated by a process analogous to that proposed for the RRCs to include the collaboration between test committees in the various disciplines to assure that appropriately written questions written at the appropriate level appear in each of the examinations for certification in each of the 11 disciplines.

Because the federal government continues to provide the majority of funding to medical schools and their associated residency programs for physicians, it could play an important role in a way that is analogous to the role it played when geriatrics was first introduced as a new specialty in the 1970s.

The federal government could provide grants to medical schools and nursing schools who propose to develop well-designed, logically progressive programs that continue from undergraduate to graduate programs of medical education that would fund curriculum development and protected faculty time.

The federal government could provide grants to medical schools and nursing schools to stimulate faculty recruitment and development in hospice and palliative medicine in sufficient numbers to provide clinical, education, and research to further the field.

References

1. Lorber J. Good patients and problem patients: conformity and deviance in a General Hospital. J Health Soc Behav. 1975;16:213–25.
2. Mor V, Greer DS, Kastenbaum R. The hospice experiment: an alternative in terminal care. In: Mor V, Greer D, Kastenbaum R, editors. The hospice experiment. Baltimore: Johns Hopkins University Press; 1988. p. 6.
3. Ptacek JT, Eberhardt TL. Breaking bad news. A review of the literature. JAMA. 1996;276(6): 496–502.
4. Kuebler-Ross E. On death and dying: what the dying have to teach doctors, nurses, clergy and their own families. New York: Macmillan; 1969.
5. Hospice Standards. National Hospice Organization, Arlington, Virginia, USA, 1979. Approaching death: improving care at the end of life. Committee on Care at the End of Life, Division of Health Care Services, Institute of Medicine, National Academy of Sciences; 1997.
6. Accreditation and the Liaison Committee on Medical Education. Standards for Accreditation of Medical Education Program Leading to the M.D. Degree; May 2001.
7. American Association of Colleges of Nursing. http://www.aacn.nche.edu/elnec. Accessed 20 Sept 2012.
8. Grauel RR, Eger R, Finley RC, Hawtin C, et al. Educational program in palliative and hospice care at the University of Maryland School of Medicine. J Cancer Educ. 1996;11:144–7.
9. Ross DD, Keay T, Timmel D, et al. Required training in hospice and palliative care at the University of Maryland School of Medicine. J Cancer Educ. 1999;14:132–6.
10. Ross DD, O'Mara A, Pickens N, Keay T, et al. Hospice and palliative care education in medical school: a module on the role of the physician in end-of-life care. J Cancer Educ. 1997;12:152–6.
11. Bishop M, Heaton J, Jaskar D. Collaborative end-of-life curriculum for fourth year medical students. Presented as module W-11 A collaborative end-of-life care curriculum at the 11th Annual Assembly of the American Academy of Hospice and Palliative Medicine; 23–26 Jun 1999; Snowbird, UT.
12. Policzer JS. Approach to teaching palliative medicine to medical students. Presented as module W-11 A collaborative end-of-life care curriculum at the 11th Annual Assembly of the American Academy of Hospice and Palliative Medicine; 23–26 Jun 1999; Snowbird, UT.

13. Thompson AR, Savage MH, Travis T. Palliative care education—the first year's experience with a mandatory third-year medical student rotation at the University of Arkansas for Medical Sciences. Presented as module W-11 A collaborative end-of-life care curriculum at the 11th Annual Assembly of the American Academy of Hospice and Palliative Medicine; 23–26 Jun 1999; Snowbird, UT.
14. Weissman DE. Palliative medicine education at the Medical College of Wisconsin. Wis Med J. 1995;94:505–8.
15. Burge FL, Latimer EJ. Palliative care in medical education at McMaster University. J Palliative Care. 1989;5:16–20.
16. Steen PD, Miller T, Palmer L, et al. An introductory hospice experience for third-year medical students. J Cancer Educ. 1999;14:140–3.
17. Billings JA, Block S. Palliative care in undergraduate medical education. Status report and future directions. JAMA. 1997;278:733–8.
18. United States General Accounting Office. Suicide Prevention: Efforts to Increase Research and Education in Palliative Care. GAO/HEHS-98, 128.
19. Barzansky B, Veloski J, Miller R, Jonas H. Palliative care and end-of-life education. Acad Med. 1999;74:S102–4.
20. Approaching death: improving care at the end of life. Committee on care at the end of life, Division of Health Care Services, Institute of Medicine, National Academies Press, Washington DC; 1997.
21. Foley KM, Gelband H, editors. Improving palliative care for cancer National Cancer Policy Board, National Research Council. Washington, DC: National Academies Press; 2001.
22. Block SD, Sullivan AM. Attitudes about end-of-life care: a national cross-sectional study. J Palliat Med. 1998;1:347–55.
23. American Society of Clinical Oncology. Cancer care during the last phase of life. J Clin Oncol. 1998;16(5):1986–96.
24. Hill CS, Fields WS, Thorpe DM. A call to action to improve relief of cancer pain. In: Hill CS, Fields WS, editors. Advances in pain research and therapy. New York: Raven; 1989. p. 353–61.
25. Sloan PA, Donnelly MB, Schwartz RW, Sloan DA. Cancer pain assessment and management. Pain. 1996;67:475–81.
26. Von Gunten CF, Weitzman Von Roenn JH. Housestaff training in cancer pain education. J Cancer Educ. 1994;9:230–4.
27. Tulsky JA, Fischer GS, Rose MR, Arnold RM. Opening the black box: how do physicians communicate about advance directives? Ann Intern Med. 1998;129:441–9.
28. Tulsky JA, Chesnew MA, Lo B. How do medical residents discuss resuscitation with patients? JGIM. 1995;10:436–42.
29. Tulsky JA, Chesney MA, Lo B. See one, do one, teach one? House Staff experience discussing do-not-resuscitate orders. Arch Intern Med. 1996;156:1285–9.
30. Wilson IB, Green ML, Goldman L, Tsevat J, Cook EF, Phillips RS. Is experience a good teacher? How interns and attending physicians understand patients' choices for end-of-lie care. Med Decis Making. 1997;17:217–27.
31. Caring for the Dying: Identification and Promotion of Physician Competency-Educational Resource Document. American Board of Internal Medicine; 1996.
32. Blank L. Defining and evaluating physician competence in end-of-life care: a matter of awareness and emphasis. West J Med. 1995;163:297–301.
33. Barnard D, Quill T, Hafferty F, Arnold R, Plumb J, et al. Preparing the ground: contributions of the pre-clinical years to medical education for care near the end-of-life. Acad Med. 1999;74:499–505.
34. Weissman DE, Block SD, Blank L, Cain J, Cassem N, Danoff D, Egan K, Foley K, Meier D, Schyve P, Theige D, Wheeler B. Incorporating palliative care education into the acute care hospital setting. Acad Med. 1999;74:871–7.
35. Bowles T. USMLE and end-of-life care. J Palliat Med. 1999;2:3–4.
36. Schonwetter RS, Robinson BE. Educational objectives for medical training in the care of the terminally ill. Acad Med. 1994;69:688–90.
37. National consensus conference on medical education for care near the end-of-life. J Palliat Med. 2000;3:87–91.

38. Steel K, Ribbe M, Ahronheim J, et al. Incorporating education on palliative care into the long-term care setting. JAGA. 1999;47:904–7.
39. Danis M, Federman D, Fins JJ, et al. Incorporating palliative care into critical care education: principles, challenges, and opportunities. Crit Care Med. 1999;27:2005–13.
40. Nelson W, Angoff N, Binder E, Cooke M, et al. Goals and strategies for teaching death and dying in medical schools. J Palliat Med. 2000;3:7–16.
41. Simpson DE, Rehm J, Biernat K, Muchka S, Weissman DE. Advancing educational scholarship through the End of Life Physician Education Resource Center (EPERC). J Palliat Med. 1999;2:421–4.
42. Mullan P, Weissman DE, Ambuel PB, von Gunten CF. End-of-life care education in internal medicine residency programs: inter-institutional study. J Palliat Med. 2002;5:487–96.
43. Weissman DE, Mullan PB, Ambuel B, von Gunten CF. End-of-life curriculum reform: outcomes and impact in a follow-up study of internal medicine residency programs. J Palliat Med. 2002;5:497–506.
44. Mullan PB, Weissman D, von Gunten C, Ambuel B, Hallenbeck J. Coping with certainty: perceived competency vs. training and knowledge in end of life care. JGIM 2000;15(40 Suppl) (Abstract).
45. Weissman DE, Block SD. ACGME requirements for end-of-life training in selected residency and fellowship programs: a status report. Acad Med. 2002;77(4):299–304.
46. Sloan PA, Donnelly MB, Schwartz RS, Sloan DA. Cancer pain assessment and management by housestaff. Pain. 1996;67:475–81.
47. von Gunten CF, Ferris FD, Marquis D, DiPrima K, Ryan P, VanGeest J, Portenoy R, Emanuel L. The EPEC Project: education for physicians on end-of-life care. J Cancer Educ. 1999;14 Suppl 1:14.
48. von Gunten CF, Ferris FD, Robinson K, Sutton S, Meshenberg K, Martinez J, Molodyko N, Emanuel LL. The Education for Physicians on End-of-life Care (EPEC) project. J Cancer Educ. 2001;16(3 Suppl):14.
49. Ferrell B, Grant M, et al. End-of-Life Nursing Education Consortium (ELNEC). American Association of Colleges of Nursing. http://www.aacn.nche.edu/elnec.
50. White BC. The Macy report. Ann Emerg Med. 1995;26(2):239.
51. Allard P, Maunsell E, Labbe J, Dorval M. Educational interventions to improve cancer pain control: a systematic review. J Palliat Med. 2001;4(2):191–203.
52. Foley K. Advancing palliative care in the United States. Palliat Med. 2003;17:89–91.
53. von Gunten CF. Secondary and tertiary palliative care in US Hospitals. JAMA. 2002;287: 875–81.
54. US Supreme Court. No 95-1858, 96-110. Justice O'Connor, Justice Stevens concurring opinions.
55. Caring for the Dying: Identification and Promotion of Physician Competency-Educational Resource Document. American Board of Internal Medicine, Philadelphia; 1996.
56. Program Requirement for Residency Education in Internal Medicine. American Board of Internal Medicine, Philadelphia; 1998.
57. Morrison S, Meier D. America's care of serious illness: a state-by-state report card on access to palliative care in our Nation's Hospitals. Center to Advance Palliative Care: National Palliative Research Center; 2011.

Index

A
AACN. *See* American Association of Colleges of Nursing (AACN)
ABMS. *See* American Boards of Medical Specialties (ABMS)
ACA. *See* Affordable Care Act (ACA)
Accountable care organizations (ACOs)
   Michigan @HOMe Support Program, 65, 153–157
   Order of St. Francis (OSF) Health Care palliative care integration, 173–176
   PHS (*see* Partners health system (PHS))
   UnityPoint Health, 160–166
ACOs. *See* Accountable care organizations (ACOs)
ACOVE project. *See* Assessing care of vulnerable elders (ACOVE) project
ACSCAN. *See* American Cancer Society Cancer Action Network (ACSCAN)
ADs. *See* Advance directives (ADs)
Advance care planning (ACP)
   and ADs, 205–206
   community engagement, 181
   and NHs, 76
   quality improvement, 181
   systems redesign, 181
Advanced illness coordination services (AICS) project, 55
Advance directives (ADs)
   and ACP, 205–206
   end-of-life care, 6, 180
   policies, 85–86
Advance illness management (AIM) 49–57, 154–156
   Compassionate Care, 49
   and HOM, 154

Advance practice nurses (APNs), 25, 172, 232
Affordable Care Act (ACA), 53, 100, 131, 133–134
AICS project. *See* Advanced illness coordination services (AICS) project
AIM. *See* Advance illness management (AIM)
American Academy of Hospice and Palliative Medicine, 110
American Association of Colleges of Nursing (AACN), 228, 233
American Board of Internal Medicine (ABIM), 13, 229, 232
American Boards of Medical Specialties (ABMS), 115
American Cancer Society Cancer Action Network (ACSCAN), 195
   palliative care ad-dancer, 198, 199
   palliative care ad-mother, 198, 200
   quality of life, 196
American College of Surgeon's Commission on Cancer, 194–195
American Society for Clinical Oncology, 194
APNs. *See* Advance practice nurses (APNs)
Assessing care of vulnerable elders (ACOVE) project, 99
At Home Support™, 153–157

B
Beatitudes Campus, 77–78
Bluegrass palliative care consultation service, 76

C

Cancer
  ACSCAN, 196
  American Cancer Society and NPCRC, 194
  American College of Surgeon's Commission on Cancer, 194–195
  American Society for Clinical Oncology, 194
  CAPC, 194, 197
  Institute of Medicine reports, 193
  Joint Commission, 195
CAPC. *See* Center to advance palliative care (CAPC)
Care Planning Act, 55
CBPC. *See* Community-based palliative care (CBPC)
Centers for Medicare and Medicaid Innovation (CMMI), 82
Centers for Medicare & Medicaid services (CMS), 39, 85, 103–104, 130
  Dual eligibles, 128–131
  Hospice, 66–69
  Nursing Homes, 82–86
Center to advance palliative care (CAPC), 83, 116, 191–197
Choosing Wisely, 13–15
CMMI. *See* Centers for Medicare and Medicaid Innovation (CMMI)
CMS. *See* Centers for Medicare & Medicaid Services (CMS)
Comfort First model, care, 77–78
Community-based palliative care (CBPC), 47–57, 116–118
Cost, Palliative care impact on, 109–124

D

Disparities, health care, 19–26
Dual eligibles, 129–131, 137, 139

E

End-of-life care, 85, 120–122, 159, 180, 229
End-of-Life Nursing Education Consortium (ELNEC), 229, 233

F

Family and Medical Leave Act, 40
Family caregiving and palliative care
  AARP public policy institute, 32
  barriers, 37–38
  financial outcomes 34–35
  mental, physical and financial health, 33–35
  public policy, 40–42

H

Healthcare disparities. *See* Disparities, health care
Hospice
  clinical outcomes, 59
  disenrollment rate, 67–69
  education, 86
  expanded MHB eligibility, 63–64
  Medicare Hospice Benefit (MHB), 59, 79–82
  NHs, 75–76
  policy, 60–63, 66–67
  TEFRA, 61
Hospice and palliative nursing association (HPNA), 232

I

Institute of Medicine (IOM), 19, 23, 40, 43, 48, 93, 95, 193, 230
Interventions to reduce acute care transfers (INTERACT) tools, 82

K

Kaiser Permanente of Northern California (KPNC), 184–186

L

La Crosse Advance Directive Study (LADS), 180, 186
Liaison committee for accreditation of medical schools (LCME), 228, 233
Long-term services and supports (LTSS), 39–40, 127–130
  Medicare and Medicaid, dual eligibles, 127–131
  State Demonstrations to Integrate Care, 130
  family caregivers, 39

M

Maggie Allesee Center for Innovation (MAC), 154
Make-A-Wish Foundation, 208
Managed care organizations (MCOs)
  financing and delivery system, 138
  history, 1980–1990s, 139–142
  history, 2000-present, 142–144
  PACE programs, 139
Massachusetts general hospital (MGH), 158
MCOs. *See* Managed care organizations (MCOs)

Index 239

Medicaid
  dually eligible, 75, 83, 128–131
  managed care plans, 130, 131, 144
Medical and nursing education
  AACN, 233
  HPNA, 232
  IOM, 230
  LCME, 233
  palliative care education
    (*see* Palliative care education)
  palliative medicine, 227–234
  physician behavior, 225–226
  policy implications, 232–234
  RRCs, 233
Medicare advantage plans, 137
Medicare beneficiaries, 131–133
Medicare hospice benefit (MHB), 59–69
  Caregivers, 39
  expanded eligibility, 63–64
  fiscal intermediaries, 68–69
  home health coverage, 128–129
  NHs, 75–86
Medicare Modernization Act, 54–55
Medicare Prescription Drug, Improvement, and Modernization Act, 77
Medicare severity diagnosis related groups (MS-DRGs), 115
MGH. *See* Massachusetts general hospital (MGH)
MHB. *See* Medicare hospice benefit (MHB)
Michigan At HOME Support Program, 65, 153–157

N
National consensus project (NCP), 36, 95, 111, 112
National institute of nursing research (NINR), 192
National long-term care survey (NLTCS), 39
National palliative care research center (NPCRC), 191, 194–197
National Quality Forum (NQF), 36, 95–99
NHs. *See* Nursing homes (NHs)
NLTCS. *See* National long-term care survey (NLTCS)
NPCRC. *See* National palliative care research center (NPCRC)
NQF. *See* National quality forum (NQF)
Nursing homes (NHs), 73–87
  external palliative care consultation teams, 76–77
  hospice care, 75–76
  internal care teams and units, 77–79

Medicaid payment rates, 129
Medicare skilled nursing facility (SNF) benefit, 128–129

O
Older Americans Act, 39, 40
Omnibus Budget Reconciliation Act (OBRA), 61, 74, 75
Order of St. Francis (OSF) Health Care, 168–173
Overuse, medical services harms patients, 3–15
  ABIM foundation, 13
  Choosing Wisely, 13–15
  palliative care, 15
  PCORI, 13
  supply-sensitive care, 13

P
PACE. *See* Program of all-inclusive care for the elderly (PACE)
Pain, 216–218
Palliative Care and Hospice Education and Training Act (PCHETA), 198
Palliative care education, 225–234
Palliative care leadership center, 116
Partners Health System (PHS), 158–160
PAs. *See* Program announcements (PAs)
Patient-centered medical homes (PCMHs), 65–66, 139
Patient-Centered Outcomes Research Institute (PCORI), 13, 221, 222
Patient Centered Quality Care for Life Act, 24, 198
Patient Protection and Affordable Care Act (PPACA), 39, 40, 82, 139
PCHETA. *See* Palliative Care and Hospice Education and Training Act (PCHETA)
PCORI. *See* Patient-Centered Outcomes Research Institute (PCORI)
PHS. *See* Partners Health System (PHS)
PPACA. *See* Patient Protection and Affordable Care Act (PPACA)
Private sector innovation, 49–51, 55–56
Program announcements (PAs), 221

Q
Quality care, 100–104
Quality measurement, serious illness patients, 95–99
  ACOVE project, 99
  Agency for Healthcare Research and Quality (AHRQ) report, 96

Quality measurement, serious illness patients (*cont.*)
    NQF, 96
    PEACE project, 99
Quality of life
    medical interventions, 8
    national movement, 197–198
    oncology care, 193–194
    patient-and family-centered care, 37, 193–194
Quasi-experimental studies, 114

R
Randomized controlled trials (RCTs), 112–114
RCTs. *See* Randomized controlled trials (RCTs)
Requests for Applications (RFAs), 221
Research funding, 218–219
Research gaps
    design and methods, 220–221
    knowledge gaps, 219–220
Residency Review Committees (RRCs), 233, 234
Respecting Choices® (RC)
    ACP implementation, 181
    Australia, 182
    community engagement, 181, 186
    healthcare professionals, 180
    Honoring Choices® Minnesota, 182–183
    Honoring Choices Wisconsin, 184
    KPNC, 184–185
    LADS I, 180
    plans and quality, 185
    policy approach, 186
    populations, ACP approach, 186
    primary palliative care, 187
    progressive illness, coordinated care, 187
    quality improvement, 181
    systems redesign, 181
    training, 181
Respecting Patient Choices (RPC), 182
RFAs. *See* Requests for Applications (RFAs)
RRCs. *See* Residency Review Committees (RRCs)

S
Senate Finance Committee, 56
Senior Navigation and Planning Act, 55

Skilled nursing facility (SNF)
    and APNs, 172
    Medicare SNF benefit, 77, 81–82, 128–129
    quality of care, 82
SPARK©, 145–147
Specialist palliative care measurement model, 110–112

T
Tax Equity and Fiscal Responsibility Act (TEFRA), 61
Twin Cities Medical Society (TCMS), 182–184

U
UHC. *See* University Health System Consortium (UHC)
UnityPoint Health, 160–168
    Kaplan, Alan, 168
    Leaver, Bill, 166, 167
    metric evolution, 162–163
    palliative care integration, 160–161
    patient populations, 166–167
    physician certification and workforce, 161, 162
    Pioneer ACO, 161, 162
    program development, 163–165
    Reese, Monique, 168
    Vermeer, Kevin, 167–168
University Health System Consortium (UHC), 96, 140

V
Veterans health administration (VHA), 119–122
Visiting Nurse Service of New York (VNSNY)
    CHOICE Medicare, 145–146
    clinical team, 144–145
    cost saving, 146
    ESPRIT Medical Care, 144
    home health model, 144, 146
    patient stability and need, 147
    SPARK care management model, 145–147

CPSIA information can be obtained at www.ICGtesting.com
Printed in the USA
LVOW01s0833041014

407288LV00003B/8/P